ETHICS, LAW AND HEALTH CARE

ETHICS, LAW AND HEALTH CARE

A GUIDE FOR NURSES AND MIDWIVES

FIONA MCDONALD &

SHIH-NING THEN

BLOOMSBURY ACADEMIC

LONDON • NEW YORK • OXFORD • NEW DELHI • SYDNEY

BLOOMSBURY ACADEMIC
Bloomsbury Publishing Plc
50 Bedford Square, London, WC1B 3DP, UK
1385 Broadway, New York, NY 10018, USA
29 Earlsfort Terrace, Dublin 2, Ireland

BLOOMSBURY, BLOOMSBURY ACADEMIC and the Diana logo are trademarks of Bloomsbury Publishing Plc

First published in Great Britain 2019 by Red Globe Press
Reprinted by Bloomsbury Academic 2022

A catalogue record for this book is available from the British Library.

A catalog record for this book is available from the Library of Congress.

ISBN: PB: 978-1-352-00539-4

To find out more about our authors and books visit www.bloomsbury.com and sign up for our newsletters.

CONTENTS

LIST OF FIGURES

LIST OF TABLES

ABOUT THIS BOOK

The authors, who research and lecture in health law and ethics, believe that discussion of law and ethics for nursing and midwifery needs to be grounded in the realities of these professions, and be practically applicable to scenarios encountered on a daily basis by nurses and midwives. As such, we developed an approach – which is used in this text – to provide a practical framework within which nursing and midwifery students and professionals may apply their knowledge of law and practice to situations in their practice. We have used our experience in researching health law and ethics, and in teaching and refining a unit developed by us specifically for undergraduate nursing and midwifery students in Australia, to develop the content and approach outlined in this book.

Here we outline key features of this text and how it can be of most use to the reader.

Our approach to ethics

It is essential for nurses and midwives to have an understanding of ethical norms and how these apply to their day-to-day practice. As it is a requirement of their professions to know about and adhere to their codes of ethics and professional conduct, we have made these codes central to how ethics is explained in our text. In conjunction with this, we use the well-known principles approach (of autonomy, beneficence, non-maleficence and justice) to help clarify the main ethical issues that arise in any health care situation. In considering the codes and the four principles, nurses and midwives will gain an appreciation of the relevance of ethics and how they apply in practice.

In addition, throughout this book we have used examples of ethically contentious issues (see boxed text) to elaborate on matters of particular ethical complexity, such as abortion and euthanasia.

Our approach to law

Knowledge of relevant laws is a key professional requirement for practising nurses and midwives. In this text we have outlined and discussed what we believe to be the key laws relevant to nursing and midwifery practice. As the law often differs around Australia, we have made sure to highlight the differences between jurisdictions where necessary. In some chapters the law for each state and territory is explained separately, so students will generally only need to refer to the law in their own state or territory. We have used case law to highlight and illustrate legal principles that apply in Australia. Case law is also discussed in text boxes within each chapter.

Applying ethics and law

Given the importance we place on ensuring that nurses and midwives have knowledge not only of relevant ethical principles and the law but also of their application to real-life situations faced in practice, we also introduce an 'ethical decision-making framework' in Chapter 2. This provides students and practitioners with a structured approach to considering and applying the relevant ethical and legal principles to their practice. Crucially, at the end of the framework, conclusions should include what course(s) of action nurses or midwives ought to sensibly take if faced with such a situation. At the end of each chapter (except Chapter 3) we introduce a scenario that raises ethical and legal issues relevant to the chapter's contents. We suggest that the decision-making framework be used to work through the ethical and legal issues, and to make decisions as to what action ought to be taken.

Glossary

A glossary is provided at the end of the book containing brief definitions of key terms used throughout the text.

ABOUT THE AUTHORS

Fiona McDonald is an Associate Professor within the Faculty of Law at Queensland University of Technology and is Co-Director of the Australian Centre for Health Law Research. She is also an Adjunct Associate Professor in the Department of Bioethics at Dalhousie University, Canada. She teaches in the area of health law and ethics to law students and a range of health professionals. Fiona's research encompasses issues related to health governance and has four broad themes: the governance of health systems (including rural bioethics and disaster planning and response); the governance of health technologies; the governance of health professionals; and the governance of health organisations. Fiona's work has been published in a range of international and national journals, she has presented at a number of domestic and international conferences, and she has received grants and research fellowships to conduct research in this area. She is a co-editor of *Health Law in Australia*, 3rd edn (2018) and *Health Workforce Governance* (2012), and co-author of *Rethinking Rural Health Ethics* (2018).

Shih-Ning Then is a Senior Lecturer within the Faculty of Law at Queensland University of Technology and is a member of the Australian Centre for Health Law Research. She teaches in the area of health law and ethics to law students and a range of health professionals. Her research interests include issues relevant to groups that have not traditionally been given a voice in a health care context – with a focus on children and adults with decision-making difficulties. She engages with the broader health community through sitting on ethics committees, developing educational tools for health professionals and conducting empirical research in a health care setting. She maintains an active interest in law reform in the area.

ACKNOWLEDGEMENTS

In keeping with the spirit of reconciliation, we acknowledge the Turrbal and Jagera Peoples on whose lands we walk, work and live and we recognise that these lands have always been places of teaching and learning. We wish to pay respects to elders – past, present and emerging – and acknowledge the important role of Aboriginal and Torres Strait Islander peoples within Australia.

We would like to thank a number of persons and organisations who have supported the production of this book. We acknowledge the ongoing support provided by the Australian Centre for Health Law Research based at the Faculty of Law at Queensland University of Technology. We would like to thank the many nursing students who have influenced our teaching in this area, as well as our colleagues in the Law School and the School of Nursing for their continuing support. We would also like to thank Elizabeth Dallaston and Stephanie Jowett for research assistance.

We thank our editor Peter Hooper, who has been supportive of this edition of the book and the assistance provided by Red Globe Press.

We have endeavoured to state the law in this book as it stands at 1 November 2018.

Shih-Ning Then
Fiona McDonald
2018

LEGISLATION

INTERNATIONAL INSTRUMENTS

CASES

1

Ethics and law

Introduction

This book examines some important aspects of ethics and law that relate to the interactions nurses and midwives have with patients and families, colleagues, health organisations, the health system, the legal system, communities and society more generally. Ethics and law are crucial elements of nurses' and midwives' capacity to practise well. To be registered in Australia, nurses and midwives are required to have an understanding of ethics and law in relation to the provision of health care. The first chapter of this book therefore is an introduction to ethics and law, and discusses the interrelationship of ethics, law and health care.

What is ethics?

Ethics is a branch of philosophy. It has been described as 'the study of what we ought to do' (Kerridge et al. 2013, p. 3). It has a long history as people have been thinking, talking and writing about how we ought to act since we formed communities – indeed, ancient philosophies still inform our discussions. We still refer to the ideas of the ancient Greek philosopher Aristotle, which are thousands of years old. Other ethical traditions are even older. The fact that we are still talking about how we ought to act and what we ought to do points to the fact that these are complex and contentious ideas with a diversity of opinions and beliefs. Well-intentioned people can and do disagree about what is ethical and what is not. This raises a question about whether there is a right answer in respect of what is ethical or not or whether it is all relative. It might be argued that, despite a number of ways of talking about ethics, there is sufficient agreement on certain key principles that some answers will be more 'right' than others. However, there can be two (or more) responses to a question about whether certain types of conduct are ethical, and both responses can be justifiable on ethical grounds, although each answer is entirely different.

The specific field of ethics that focuses on health and health care is called bioethics. Bioethics concerns the moral, political and social issues raised by the clinical practice of medicine and health care in general, biomedical research and life sciences research (Viens and Singer 2008). Although the term 'bioethics' is fairly new, conversations about how health providers ought to behave in relation to patients, colleagues and communities also have an ancient pedigree. Hippocrates, another ancient Greek, remembered for the Hippocratic Oath, studied and theorised about how health providers, in his case physicians, should act.

A key aspect of philosophy, and its sub-branches ethics and bioethics, is that it requires argument, justification and reflection but also action. In engaging with ethics we need to critically engage with our values, the values of our professions and the values of our communities and/or societies, and be prepared to make arguments to justify our positions to ourselves and to others.

When we examine bioethics it is easy to suggest that the focus of ethical attention should be on the relationship between patients and health professionals. Historically, the relationship between patients and professionals was highly personal. However, the development of more complex societies and, over the past several centuries, complex systems to provide health care means that solely examining the relationships between patients and health professionals is insufficient for a robust examination of ethics in the health context. Ethical issues also affect organisations, communities, societies and nations. For example, a decision not to offer a maternity service in a rural community may have profound effects not only on women and their families but also on that community and its neighbours. Indeed, in an increasingly globalised world, bioethical questions have international scope – think for example of how we should manage a pandemic like avian flu, which is not restricted by national borders. The international scope of bioethics has been recognised through, for example, *the United Nations Education, Scientific and Cultural Organization's Universal Declaration on Bioethics and Human Rights* in 2005. Ethical analysis needs to cover the broader context.

Ethical schools of thought

There are several schools of ethical thought whose philosophical approaches can be used as tools to engage with ethical issues. This section of the chapter provides a brief introduction to some of the major ethical theories in the western tradition. First, a brief caveat: How we talk about and study ethics in western countries is influenced by the history of western civilisations with their focus on philosophies emerging from the ancient states of Greece, and (to a lesser extent) Rome, and from Europe and North America, and is often an essentially secular tradition. This history frames the way in which many of us discuss and use and teach philosophy, ethics and bioethics. However, it is not universal. Other cultures, for example, indigenous or religious cultures, may frame bioethical discussions in a different way, drawing on different values and ways of being (Garvey et al. 2004). These traditions may emphasise such values as obedience to God, and the importance of family, community and spirituality, as distinct from religion, to name but a few. Some of these perspectives are discussed in further detail in subsequent chapters, especially Chapter 5. We provide a list of further reading in this area at the end of the chapter.

Consequentialism

Consequentialism is a well-known and well-established ethical theory. Key theorists include Jeremy Bentham and John Stuart Mill. Consequentialism is complex, but in its most simple form theorists propose that the basis for determining if actions are right or wrong depends on whether those actions produce good consequences (general happiness and so on) for those affected. Actions that impact on a number of people will not make every affected person happy. The theory recognises this by suggesting that what is important is the 'greatest good for the greatest number'.

There are a number of critics of consequentialism and those critics focus on two questions:

➢ Do the ends always or ever justify the means? The classic, oft-cited example is torture. Can it ever be justifiable to torture a person if there is a perception that torture might compel the disclosure of critical information that could save lives? Does it make a difference in the acceptability of torture if there is an imminent threat to the life of an individual or the lives of a number of people? Can we distinguish between 'acceptable' torture, otherwise known as 'enhanced interrogation', and 'unacceptable' torture? Many would argue, and international law is clear, that torture of any sort is not acceptable and constitutes a crime against humanity.

➢ Could we, or should we, sacrifice the good of a few for the good of the many? Using a health-related example, consider organ donation.

Taken to its extreme, utilitarianism (a form of consequentialism) may suggest that it would be broadly beneficial, by increasing the general population's happiness, to kill, for example, homeless people, to use their organs for desperately needed organ transplants for 'socially worthwhile people'. As Illingworth and Parmet (2006) note, not only does it seem morally wrong to kill innocent people to benefit others, it involves a violation of the homeless people's right to be free from outside interference – to be left alone.

Deontology (Kantian ethics)

Deontology or Kantian ethics is another long-established theory. According to the German philosopher Immanuel Kant (1724–1804), when determining what is right or wrong what matters is the person's motives or intentions and the nature of the action itself. A good outcome can never justify a wrong action. Going back to the earlier torture example, if information was obtained as the result of torture and that information saved several lives or even thousands or millions of lives, a Kantian analysis would suggest that the outcome does not and cannot provide a justification for the fact that torture is inherently wrong. This approach also emphasises the universality of moral rules: that one must act only in ways one reasonably judges would be applicable to anyone in similar circumstances. Lastly, the approach emphasises respect for people. To paraphrase Kant: 'Act so that you treat people as an end and never as a means to an end.'

This approach too has its critics, who ask:

➢ What about rules that conflict?

➢ Could or should consequences make a difference? A strict deontological approach would suggest that if you opened the door and found a large man carrying a bloodstained axe on the doorstep who says 'Is Mary in? I want to kill her', you should not lie and say that 'Mary does not live here'. Instead, you must tell the would-be murderer the truth: 'Mary is in the bedroom changing the sheets on her bed.' There is a universal rule that people should not lie, as a lie is a morally wrong act and lying diminishes trust between people. According to this view a lie cannot be justified based on the consequences of that lie. However, many of us would think in these circumstances that a lie could be justified as the consequences of the lie are good (the man goes away and does not kill Mary) and therefore that there should be some exceptions to the universal rule about lying.

Virtue theory

Virtue theory is ancient, with its early proponent being the Greek philosopher Aristotle (384–322 BCE). This theory is concerned about an over-reliance on rules and focuses more on people's traits of character. At its core the theory suggests that a person who has certain moral values (justice, courage, temperance and so on) will naturally act in certain ways and will be unable to act in other ways. People should therefore try and develop the positive virtues and apply them to their lives, and in doing so will make 'good' decisions and be 'good'.

Critics raise a number of questions or concerns about this theory:

➢ How do we create virtuous people? Who determines what is virtuous or not?

➢ Does relying on traits of character provide sufficient guidance in tough situations?

➢ Even honourable and decent people sometimes do not know what to do. The case *Re A (children) (conjoined twins)* [2001] Fam 147 involved a question as to whether to separate conjoined twins. If the surgery was performed, one child would have no chance of survival and would definitely die. If the surgery was not performed, both children would die within months. The case reached the courts as two sets of honourable and decent people, the parents of the twins and the team providing treatment, could not agree on whether to undertake the surgery. The parents refused surgery based on their religious beliefs. The treating team thought the surgery was in the best interests of the child who would survive. The court agreed with the treating team.

The principles approach

The principles approach was developed by philosophers Tom Beauchamp and James Childress in 1979, specifically for the context of the health system. They developed several mid-level principles as a response to abstraction of higher level theories, such as consequentialism and deontology, which some found difficult to connect with the realities of their practice as health professionals. The principles were developed out of their experiences working as ethicists in the US health system. They claim that the principles play an important role in moral reasoning in the health context and are found in a number of ethical theories. In short, the principles form part of common morality. No one principle trumps the others – all are equally important. The four principles are:

> **Autonomy** – respect the capacity of individuals to make decisions about their own lives.

> **Beneficence** – foster the best interests of other persons and society at large.

> **Non-maleficence** – refrain from needlessly harming other persons.

> **Justice** – act fairly, distribute benefits and burdens in an equitable fashion and be accountable.

A key criticism of this approach is that without sufficient attention to the substance of these principles, they can become an 'empty checklist' and will be unable to give any guidance in difficult situations. Critics also raise the question of what happens if the principles conflict. How do we adjudicate between the principles? A further detailed discussion of the principles approach is contained in Chapter 2 and is used throughout this book.

Feminist theory

Feminist theory in relation to health care was developed in conjunction with the broader feminist movement. In general, feminist theory has focused on the ways in which ideas about gender affect perceptions of the world, what we notice and value, and how we conceptualise issues. It further examines how these perceptions are harmful to all, but are particularly constraining to women (Little 1996). For example, up until the 1990s women were often inappropriately excluded from health-related research on the basis of their gender. One justification was that women's hormonal cycles made it harder to study the effects of drugs (even more reason, one would think, for women to be participating in clinical trials as women would also be using the drugs). The exclusion of women from health research created risks when the results of research conducted only with male participants were generalised to women (Little 1996).

Feminist bioethics also challenges some concepts that might be inherently gendered. Many of the ethical theories discussed above are premised on an individual making a rational, unemotional choice about how to proceed. Traditional ethical theories may underplay 'the importance of the "emotional work" of life – of nurturing children, offering sympathetic support to colleagues, or displaying felt concern of patients' (Little 1996, p. 13). Gilligan (1982) developed the idea of an ethics of care in reaction to traditional theories that emphasised rationality and impartiality. In a paper examining women making decisions about abortion, she concluded that women made their decisions based on emotional responses connected to the idea of nurturing and the importance of human relationships, not in relation to the concept of justice which seemed to drive male decision-making. Crossthwaite (1994) has summarised the characteristics of an ethics of care as:

➢ a focus on relationships as opposed to individualistic ideas about rights.

➢ an awareness of the emotional needs of others.

➢ a concern about avoiding harm and nurturing people and relationships over concerns about justice and equality.

➢ a focus on the broader context within which a person is making a decision.

Some feminists, and others, have strongly critiqued the ethics of care suggesting that, as nursing and midwifery are female-dominated professions, by embracing the ethics of care nurses and midwives perpetuate stereotypes of female behaviour (Nelson 1992).

The feminist theory of relational autonomy also challenges the nature of individual decision-making noting that the majority of decision-makers make decisions relationally, that is, not just in pure self-interest but with regard to the interests of others as well. In other words, a decision is made considering the needs, expectations or demands of that individual and their family, friends, employers and the community. This is because we are constructed as persons through dependent relationships (children to parent and so on) and we maintain relationships as part of the social interactions that characterise the way in which we live our lives (Sherwin 1992).

Despite its not the traditional focus on gender, feminist theory is diverse and has developed beyond a strict gender orientation. At the base of feminist theory are three feminist-inspired presumptions:

1. The oppression of certain social groups exists (including women, gays, lesbians, bisexuals and queers, the disabled and ethnic or cultural minorities).

2. This oppression is a moral and political wrong.

3. Substantive efforts should be undertaken to mitigate/eliminate oppression.

Critics note that it is unclear whether feminist bioethics is meant to supplant or supplement other moral theories and approaches. Feminist bioethics can be rejected out of turn by negative stereotypes and a sense of threat perceived from its focus on examining issues from a non-mainstream perspective.

Rights-based approaches

Typically, rights-based theories are regarded as a form of deontology, but will be considered separately here. Advocates of a rights-based ethical approach suggest that rights are often central to moral judgement. What is a right? It could be said to be an entitlement to something or to take some action – an entitlement that no one should be allowed to prevent you from having or from doing. Rights help us protect the individual from the majority. So for rights theorists the focus is on whether an individual, group or community has a right and whether the conduct in question violates a right. Rights are held to be what Dworkin (1977) terms a 'trump' – the exercise of a right overrules any questions of utility (any broader benefit that might be argued to society).

Rights-based approaches to ethics have also attracted critique, suggesting that a focus on rights can be overly individualistic and antagonistic and may not be all that matters in some situations. Similar to the principles approach, critics also ask how conflicting claims to different rights are resolved.

In summary

Using these approaches there are clearly a number of ways in which one can frame an examination of ethical issues, and each approach has both its strengths and its shortcomings. Steinbock, Arras and London (2003, p. 9) note that 'moral reality is sufficiently complex that any one theory gives only partial insight ... view ... [ethical theories] as important but partial contributions to a comprehensive, although necessarily fragmented, moral vision'. In other words, it is often useful to use some or all of the ethical theories discussed in this chapter when considering a particular **ethical dilemma** in order to obtain a more comprehensive assessment of the implications of an issue. Having said this, this book focuses on employing the principles approach. It also focuses on the nursing and midwifery Codes of Ethics and Codes of Conduct (see Chapter 4), which provide profession-specific perspectives on how nurses and midwives ought to behave.

What is law?

If you ask a person on the street 'What is law' you will likely get some varied answers. In general, though, many of the people that you ask may emphasise some characteristics. For example, law may be described as a system of rules that regulate society, especially our behaviour as individuals, groups and organisations. They will likely go on to say that these rules are established by an authority with lawmaking power (Parliament or the courts) and are enforceable. If you just focus on the first part of the definition – a system of rules that regulate society, especially our behaviour as individuals, groups and organisations – you might ask, how do law and ethics differ if they are both about behaviour? You might note that law emphasises rules, but so do some ethical theories (deontology, for example). It is the second and third elements of the definition that partially distinguish law and ethics (the differences are further discussed in the next section of this chapter) as they focus on who makes the rules and the enforcement of those rules. Scholars who theorise about law would say that this definition comes from a school of thought called 'legal positivism'. Legal positivism essentially focuses on the legitimation of rules by an appropriate authority. In the Australian context this authority is the Crown, as represented by parliaments at the Commonwealth, state and territorial level, and the courts. It also focuses on the enforcement of these government-imposed rules by agents of the Crown (the courts, the police, government agencies – for example, the Australian Taxation Office or the Therapeutic Goods Administration – and so on).

Some people on the street might suggest that law arises from some divine or higher origin – in legal theory this is called 'natural law'. In the ancient Greek, and to a lesser extent Roman, traditions that divine origin was the gods. In more recent times the Christian tradition and the Islamic tradition, to name but two examples, claim that law comes ultimately from God or Allah. The pre-Revolution (1642) English tradition talked of the 'divine right of kings'. More secular approaches, many first developed in the twentieth century, claim a higher origin of law from some universal norm of what is right – human rights norms and laws come from this school of thought.

The postcolonial Australian legal system is a mix of positivism and natural law (generally, although not exclusively, in its secular form – focusing on human rights). The influence of natural law can be seen particularly in international law with a number of human rights-related conventions and declarations, some of which have been included in Australian law. It can also be seen in the influence certain religious perspectives have traditionally had in some morally contentious areas that are regulated by the law, such as abortion. Positivism is seen in the structure of the Australian legal system where what we know as law is created by democratically elected parliaments and/or by appointed judges in the law courts. Law is enforced by a variety of government actors. How the Australian legal system operates will be explained in detail in Chapter 3.

Legal systems are built on a number of presumptions. It is a central presumption in a democratic system that law should be publicly accessible by all.

Therefore in Australia legislation and legal cases are available online from a variety of sources and in hard copy in some libraries. Further to this, as law is accessible, the High Court of Australia has concluded that ignorance of the law is not an excuse that can be used to escape a criminal conviction (*Ostrowski v Palmer* (2003) 218 CLR 493). Nurses and midwives are deemed to have knowledge of the law in relation to nursing and midwifery practice and are expected to abide by its requirements.

There also needs to be some certainty in the law. In general, we should know what the law is, or might be, at a fixed point in time so we know what we need to do to comply with the law. The law can and does change, and it needs some flexibility to evolve, but some degree of certainty is also required. The more serious the consequences of breaching the law, the more certain it needs to be. In general, making a law with retrospective effect is considered to be bad as a person acted in a certain way at that time believing the law did not prohibit that type of conduct and it is not fair to change the law to make past actions illegal.

The way in which parliaments and the courts make law in Australia can be very slow. For example, the *Criminal Code* in Queensland dates from 1889. It has been updated on several occasions but some sections of the law remain as they were in 1889. While law can be slow to change, social and technological developments in the health field can occur very quickly. Reflecting on this, Justice Windyer wrote: 'Law is marching with medicine but in the rear and limping a little' (*Mount Isa Mines v Pusey* (1970) 125 CLR 383 at 395). In other words, law often struggles to keep up with changing developments, especially in relation to health services.

The law has long had a role to play in respect of regulating the delivery of health services. The oldest surviving written legal code – the Babylonian Code of Hammurabi (1795–1750 BCE) which can be viewed in the Louvre in Paris – has a section regulating health care delivery. In translation it reads: 'If a physician make a large incision with the operating knife and kill him, or open a tumour with the operating knife, and cut out the eye, his hands shall be cut off' (King 2008). Fortunately, over the many thousands of years since this law was passed, our views on the punishment of erring health professionals have changed. Yet law still plays a key role in regulating the health sector. The many laws that regulate health-related matters are collectively termed 'health law' and will be discussed in more detail in subsequent chapters.

The relationship between ethics and law

Law and ethics have a complicated relationship and in a health care context may be perceived as being somewhat interconnected. However, there are some important differences.

Lord Chief Justice Coleridge wrote: 'It would not be correct to say that every moral obligation involves a legal duty; but every legal duty is founded on a moral obligation' (*R v Instan* [1893] 1 QB 453). Law is often influenced by the values (the ethical or moral beliefs) of the individuals, group, communities and societies that are involved in creating the law in question – but this can be a positive or a negative. Sometimes laws will be passed by parliament that some, or many people, would regard as profoundly unethical, while being consistent with the moral beliefs of others. In a health context, think about laws passed in many parts of the world, in the 1930s particularly, that allowed the forcible sterilisation of women who were deemed unfit to breed because they may contaminate the 'purity' of the race – often due to their perceived intellectual or mental deficits. At the time, some regarded this action as unethical. There are many other examples. On some occasions people may make a difficult choice not to obey laws they firmly believe are unethical. This is often referred to as civil disobedience. Going back to the example about the forced sterilisation of women, today, forcible sterilisation seems to most, if not all, people to be profoundly unethical. This shows how ethical perspectives and the legal framework can change substantially as societal understandings of what is ethical and moral evolve. While the forced sterilisation of women as a consequence of government policy is now a historical fact in many nations, it may be a reality for women in some countries, especially women with disabilities, or HIV/Aids, or those from minority groups.

It has been suggested that the main difference between ethics and law is in the law's ability to end debate. As one author suggests:

> Unlike ethics, where reasonable people may continue to take opposing views and continually justify them using their own normative ethics, law requires that debates be finalised. Once parliament or the judges have created a binding legal norm there is no capacity for further legal debate. The legal norm therefore has been normatively closed in a way that ethical norms can never be. Legal systems are capable of providing final resolutions; ethical systems are not. (Kerridge et al. 2013, p. 8)

In practice, we cannot have rules for everything and we cannot have laws that cover every conceivable possibility. Not every problem in practice will have a legal solution. In situations in which law does not dictate an outcome, it is essential for nurses and midwives to be able to weigh up the ethical considerations involved in order to respond appropriately. Even when the law dictates action, ethics might influence how the action is taken. If the law says that blood must be provided to a teenager who has refused it because of religious belief, how would a nurse do this to maintain, as much as possible, the dignity of that individual and their family? This may be determined by reference to ethical norms.

This chapter has introduced you to the areas of ethics and law. How ethics and law might be relevant in the health care setting and how they influence the practice of nursing and midwifery are further developed in the following chapters in this book.

Further reading

Bowman, K. & Hui, E. 2000, 'Chinese bioethics', *Canadian Medical Association Journal*, 163, 1481–1485.

Coward, H. & Sidhu T. 2000, 'Hinduism and Sikhism', *Canadian Medical Association Journal*, 163, 1167–1170.

Daar, A. & Khitamy, A. 2001, 'Islamic bioethics', *Canadian Medical Association Journal*, 164, 60–63.

Garvey, G., Towney, P., McPhee, J., Little, M. & Kerridge, I. 2004, 'Is there an Aboriginal bioethic?', *Journal of Medical Ethics*, 30, 570–575.

Goldsand, G., Rosenburg-Yunger, Z. & Gordon, M. 2001, 'Jewish bioethics', *Canadian Medical Association Journal*, 164, 219–222.

Little, M. 1996, 'Why a feminist approach to bioethics?', *Kennedy Institute of Ethics Journal*, 6: 1, 1–18.

Markwell, H. & Brown, B. 2001, 'Catholic bioethics', *Canadian Medical Association Journal*, 165, 189–192.

Questions

Law does not always reflect ethical norms or what is 'morally right'. Provide an example, either from within Australia or internationally (past, present or proposed), where a law has not necessarily reflected an ethical norm.

Scenario

A nurse is driving along a main road before beginning his shift at a major tertiary hospital. About 10 minutes away from work he drives past the scene of an accident where a woman is lying beside her car. Other motorists have stopped to render assistance. No ambulance is yet on the scene. As he is already running late for work, he decides to keep driving.

➢ What ethical issues does this scenario raise?

➢ What legal issues need to be considered?

➢ Faced with these circumstances, what would you do and why?

2

Ethics and ethical and legal decision-making frameworks

Introduction

In Chapter 1 we provided a brief introduction to ethics. This chapter builds on that introduction. In the first part of the chapter we discuss ethical issues in practice, the relevant nursing and midwifery professions' Codes of Ethics and Codes of Conduct and examine ethical principlism (introduced in Chapter 1) in more detail. In the second part of the chapter we outline an ethical and legal decision-making framework that provides a structure to work through ethical or legal challenges that might arise during the practice of the professions of nursing or midwifery.

It is important to remind you at the outset that:

> Ethics is not a black-and-white subject, which you either know or don't know ... Ethics always involves thinking and feeling, study and practice, knowledge and intuition. As such, ethics involves the whole person of you the nurse [or midwife], and the whole person of the patient or client. This is a tall order; it is also a personal challenge. (Tschudin and Farr 1994, p. 55)

However, despite this, as Jiwani (2001) notes, 'the enterprise of ethics ... is based on the assumption that while there may not be one particular right answer ... some answers will be more right than others'.

The nursing and midwifery professions' Codes of Ethics and Conduct

In the nineteenth century nursing became a health profession under the guidance of Florence Nightingale. Midwifery was long established as a form of care (with references to it being found in the Bible) and began to form as an organised profession in the nineteenth century. Part of the process of establishing a health profession is that the professions in question enter into what has been termed a 'social contract' – an unwritten (implied) contract between the professions of nursing and midwifery and the public. In law a contract is entered into by at least two parties and each party provides what is termed 'consideration', or something of value to be offered to the other party, as part of their contract. The terms of the social contract between the professions of nursing and midwifery and the public are, simply put, that the public will go to the professions for nursing and midwifery care and treatment and, in return, the professions of nursing and midwifery make sure those professions provide satisfactory care and treatment. The consideration in each case is that the public will use or access services provided by nurses and/or midwives and allow some degree of self-governance by the nursing and midwifery professions and, in return, the professions promise to regulate the practice and conduct of nurses and midwives (discussed in more detail in Chapter 4).

One mechanism through which the professions do this is through establishing ethical and other standards for practice and conduct – Codes of Ethics and Codes of Conduct. These types of codes have a long history, with the medical profession's Hippocratic Oath being an early example of a code for ethical and professional practice. These documents are 'living' documents that evolve over time as the nursing and midwifery professions assess their role in our ever-changing societies and health care systems. A significant recent change has been the release of updated Australian Codes of Conduct for both nurses and midwives in 2017 and the adoption of international Codes of Ethics for both professions in 2018. All these documents seek to provide guidance to students, nurses and midwives working directly with patients in a clinical setting, or in any other nursing or midwifery setting (for example, research, management or education).

Codes of Ethics

Prior to 2018 nurses and midwives in Australia had national Codes of Ethics. However, in March 2018 these national codes were replaced with international Codes of Ethics. The Nursing and Midwifery Board of Australia, the Australian College of Midwives, the Australian College of Nursing and the Australian Nursing and Midwifery Federation jointly agreed to adopt the International Council of Nurses Code of Ethics for Nurses – referred to in this text as 'ICN Code of Ethics' (ICN 2012) – and the International Confederation of Midwives Code of Ethics for Mid-wives – referred to in this text as 'ICM Code of Ethics' (ICM 2014) – as the appropriate documents to guide ethical decision-making for nurses and midwives in Australia.

These high-level Codes of Ethics have been developed with consid-eration of broader international developments in human rights and the delivery of health services. In the preambles to both Codes of Ethics the importance of human rights to both professions is emphasised. As such, the Codes of Ethics for these professions draw not just on ethical theory but on human rights norms, indicating the nursing and midwifery profes-sions' commitment to respecting, promoting, protecting and upholding fundamental human rights (ICN 2012, pp. 1, 2; ICM 2014, p. 1).

Both Codes of Ethics have common purposes:

➤ To identify the fundamental ethical standards and values to which the nursing or midwifery professions are committed.

➤ To provide a reference point for self-reflection and reflecting on the conduct of others.

➤ To guide ethical decision-making and practice.

➤ To indicate to patients, families, colleagues and communities the profes-sions' commitment to upholding certain ethical values and human rights.

Both the ICN and the ICM Codes of Ethics acknowledge the reality that ethical analysis occurs at different levels and that ethical responsibilities are not just to patients. The Codes of Ethics recognise that ethical analy-sis occurs at an individual level with nurses and midwives needing to be self-reflective, needing to reflect on the needs of patients or women and infants (and families) and colleagues. It is also recognised that nurses and midwives should consider their responsibilities to communities.

Codes of Conduct

Unlike the Codes of Ethics, national Codes of Conduct exist for each profession that establish the minimum standards of conduct that a nurse or a midwife is expected to maintain while acting in a professional capacity in order to maintain the public's trust and confidence in the professions of nursing and midwifery in Australia (NMBA 2018a, see also Appendix A this; NMBA 2018b, see Appendix B this). Having national Codes of Conduct allows specific consideration of issues of importance in the Australian context – in particular to recognise the human rights of Aboriginal and Torres Strait Islander people. The Codes of Conduct are far more detailed than the Codes of Ethics, with both professions' Codes of Conduct dealing with the following:

➢ Legal compliance

➢ Person/woman-centred practice

➢ Cultural practice and respectful relationships

➢ Professional behaviour

➢ Teaching, supervising and assessing

➢ Research in health

➢ Health and wellbeing.

These Codes of Conduct are an important component of the social contract between nurses and midwives and the public. It is explicit in the codes that a breach of the Code of Conduct may provide grounds for disciplinary action (see Chapter 4 for further discussion).

Ethical theories

However, no Code of Ethics or Code of Conduct can possibly address all the ethical challenges a nurse or midwife may encounter in practice. This is where ethical theories can assist by further clarifying the ethical values that arise. As discussed in Chapter 1, there are a variety of ethical theories that can be used; however, in this book we focus on using the International Codes of Ethics and Australian Codes of Conduct supplemented by the use of the principles approach. A general introduction to the principles approach is set out in Chapter 1. The principles were developed in the late 1970s by philosophers Beauchamp and Childress (2013) to bridge the gaps between the abstract nature of much ethical theory, the realities of clinical practice, and common morality. They devised four principles that they suggest are at the heart of ethical analysis conducted in a health care context. These principles were derived from their observation of the key values that arose in the context of clinical practice but are also consistent with the values and perspectives of a number of religious and moral traditions.

The principles approach is not without its critics. Some suggest that, although there may be consistency between the principles and some religious and moral traditions, the principles are based in, and derived from, a western paradigm and are not universally applicable. Some suggest that use of the principles approach results in health professionals who are able to rattle off the four principles but who are unable to actually use the principles in a meaningful way in a clinical setting.

The intention is that these principles guide ethical reflection; they may not and, in fact, generally will not provide definitive answers, instead leaving some scope for judgement and flexibility in order to respond to specific contexts. There is no hierarchy between the principles – each is considered equally as important and critical. A challenge in using the principles is that sometimes the principles conflict and the model provides no guidance as to how to resolve such conflicts. Again this calls for a judgement to be made as to the relative importance of each principle and that judgement will be shaped by every person's individual and professional values and by the situation itself. Additionally, sometimes when a particular value is analysed it can result in two arguments: one supporting a proposed course of action and the other opposing it. For example, a best interests/harm argument could be made that an anxious patient or women should not be told of an adverse event as it might cause them psychological harm. But a best interests/harm argument could also be made that it is in the best interests of the patient to be told so that they can plan their care, do not feel as though they had been deceived, and can maintain trust in health professionals.

The four principles identified by Beauchamp and Childress are set out in Figure 2.1. These principles are discussed in more detail in the sections that follow.

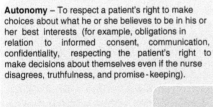

Autonomy – To respect a patient's right to make choices about what he or she believes to be in his or her best interests (for example, obligations in relation to informed consent, communication, confidentiality, respecting the patient's right to make decisions about themselves even if the nurse disagrees, truthfulness, and promise-keeping).

Beneficence – The duty to benefit others (for example, obligations to act in a patient's best interest and to undertake professional development and training).

Ethical Principles

Non-maleficence – The duty to do no harm and to protect others from harm (for example, obligations to provide care of an appropriate quality, to act in a manner that is consistent with the Code of Conduct, to not exploit patients, and to self-report and report others to appropriate authorities if there is a possibility that serious harm might result).

Justice – The threefold duty to: ensure the fair distribution of scarce resources (distributive justice); respect patient rights (rights-based justice); and respect morally acceptable laws and to be accountable for one's actions or inaction (legal justice).

Figure 2.1   Summary of Beauchamp and Childress's ethical principles

Autonomy

A key ethical norm in western liberal societies is autonomy – the right to choose for yourself what is in your best interest or how to live in accordance with your values – in other words, self-determination. A judge from the United States has described autonomy in the health context as 'Every human being of adult years and sound mind has a right to determine what should be done with his [or her] own body' (*Schloendorff v Society of New York Hospital* (1914) 211 NY 125 at 126). This is a limited expression of what autonomy means in a health context because the ethical principle of autonomy is more extensive than this and goes beyond bodily integrity.

If a competent adult has the right to make choices about what is in her or his best interest this creates an ethical obligation for nurses, midwives and other health professionals to respect individual autonomy. In practice, respecting an individual's decision-making capacity means that nurses and midwives must:

➤ Provide patients with the information that they need to make an informed decision.

➤ Support the making of informed decisions by patients, including through recognising some patients will need additional time and assistance in decision-making (supported decision-making) and advocacy.

➤ Effectively communicate with patients.

➤ Tell the truth.

➤ Keep information confidential (within limits).

➤ Respect a patient's privacy.

➤ Keep promises.

Above all, nurses and midwives must, in accordance with this principle, respect an individual's capacity to make decisions about what is best for them – even if that decision is to refuse treatment, to undertake a treatment option that the nurse or midwife does not believe is appropriate or to make a decision that does not accord with that nurse's or midwife's values. No matter how irrational, misguided or 'stupid' a nurse or midwife may think a decision is, if the patient is an adult and is judged competent, then their decision must be respected, even if it places their life at risk. Nurses and midwives can educate, inform and advise but, ultimately, in accordance with this ethical principle, they must respect the individual's right to make decisions and support the patient's exercise of their decision-making capacity, within the limitations described below. The position is a little more complicated in respect of infants, children, teenagers and adults with impaired decision-making capacity and these issues will be discussed in Chapters 5 and 6.

It is important to note that autonomy is a particularly important concept in western liberal democracies like Australia. These societies are built around the idea of rational individuals making decisions about how to live their lives. This does not accord with the societal values of all cultures or societies – even within Australia. Australia is increasingly diverse so in your professional practice you will encounter patients whose view of autonomy is different from yours. Some cultures and societies, such as Aboriginal and Torres Strait Islander societies, may have a more communitarian ethos where an individual's decision-making capacity is subsumed within that of the family or community (McGrath and Phillips 2008). For many traditional Aboriginal communities consent may be given by the individual in terms of signing off the paperwork but in reality is a function of the extended family and perhaps also key members of the community. This in turn may mean that different considerations apply in terms of confidentiality, privacy and the length of time required to obtain consent (McGrath and Phillips 2008) (see Chapter 7).

Feminist bioethicists also critique traditional notions of autonomy from within a western paradigm (Sherwin 1992). Even in traditional western societies feminist bioethicists suggest that the concept that we make decisions as individuals based on what is best for us as individuals is unpersuasive. They suggest that we exercise our autonomy relationally. Relational autonomy recognises that we generally do not make decisions only considering our personal interests but, in reality, we also consider the interests of others as part of our decision-making framework. For example, a person may delay a procedure because there is no one to look after their children.

All of this is to say that, although autonomy is a key concept in ethics and law, it may not be a concept that is understood the same way by all patients or accorded the same importance. Nurses and midwives need to be aware of this and consider what autonomy might mean for the patient and their family.

There are also limits on an individual's exercise of autonomy. The philosopher John Stuart Mill (1985) suggests that the only justifiable limitation on an individual's exercise of their autonomy is when the exercise of that autonomy may place others at risk of harm. In order to have peace, order and good governance we restrict an individual's choices when those choices have the potential to impact negatively or to harm others. For example, as a society we justify the compulsory hospitalisation of individuals with a mental illness who are posing a risk to others as necessary to protect the public. Some argue that further limits on an individual's autonomy may be imposed to protect that individual from self-harm. For example, as a society, in limited circumstances, we justify the compulsory hospitalisation of those individuals with a mental illness who are threatening self-harm, despite the fact that suicide is no longer illegal. We also make it illegal to possess and use a range of 'recreational' drugs. However, in some cases the desire to prevent an individual from self-harm was used to justify shielding patients from decision-making, concealing information or misleading or lying to patients, because it was presumed to be in their best interest – such as, not telling a patient she had a sexually transmitted disease in order to protect the patient's marriage. This approach has largely been rejected in western nations as being paternalistic as it undermines an individual's autonomy and is contrary to patient-centred care. However, in some circumstances, not providing a patient with information about their health status may still be considered appropriate in some cultural traditions. For example, in Japan and Korea it has traditionally not been considered appropriate to disclose cancer diagnoses to the patient (although attitudes towards this are changing) (Ells and Caniano 2002).

Justice

The ethical principle of justice has three faces: (1) distributive justice – ensuring the fair distribution of benefits and burdens; (2) rights-based justice – respect for patient rights; and (3) legal justice – respect for morally just laws and being accountable for one's actions or inaction.

The conversation about the distribution of benefits and burdens can occur at the societal level – for example, we ask questions such as: Who gets what from the health system? Are we providing enough resources to groups with poor health outcomes? However, these conversations can also occur at an individual level. An issue that was discussed in Western Australia was whether that state should provide funds to a young woman who was addicted to drugs to go overseas for her second organ transplant. That transplant would replace her first transplanted organ that had been damaged by her ongoing addiction. Should funding, even a loan, be provided to her when that money could be used in other areas of the health system to save another life or lives or to improve the quality of life of others? Should we make judgements about which individuals are 'worthy' of receiving services or should we be examining which individual is most likely to benefit from health care interventions? (ABC News 2010).

The second face of justice is rights-based justice – where one should respect patient rights. There are a number of sources of patient rights. In Australia, the Australian Charter of Healthcare Rights (the Charter) developed by the Australian Commission on Safety and Quality in Health Care (2008), is one source of moral rights for patients throughout Australia in all care settings. At an international level, the *United Nations Convention on Persons with Disabilities* and the *United Nations Convention on the Rights of the Child* recognise certain rights of people with disabilities and children.

The third face is legal justice – which is to act in a way that respects or complies with morally acceptable laws and to be accountable for one's actions or inaction. An example of a morally unacceptable law today would be a law that forcibly sterilises certain segments of the community. Accountability is also an important part of justice. Accountability can be in the prospective sense – of making a decision, acting on it or choosing not to act and assuming responsibility for any consequences that may follow. Or accountability can be in a retrospective sense – where your peers (formally or informally), a health complaints agency, a coroner, a court/ tribunal or you yourself hold you accountable for a past act or omission to act. Accountability is a critical part of the social contract between the professions of nursing and midwifery and the public as it is, in part, the basis on which the public's trust rests.

Beneficence

Beneficence is the duty to benefit and assist others, to care for their welfare and to always act in the best interests of the patient. This duty extends to the need for nurses and midwives to undertake professional development and training, to comply with the competencies expected of registered nurses or midwives, to collaborate effectively with others, to keep good records and to advocate for patients, or, in other words, to take positive steps to act in a patient's best interest. The necessity to act in the best interests of the patients is viewed as self-evident for nurses and midwives as caring lies at the heart of these professions. The principle of beneficence applies to individual patients but also to society as a whole. For example, the good health of a particular patient is an appropriate aim of nursing but so too is the prevention of disease through public health-related programs which benefit the population as a whole.

It is sometimes suggested that beneficence can only go so far. For example, nurses are duty-bound to seek to benefit their patients; however, what happens if two patients need treatment at the same moment? There has to be some criteria for deciding who receives treatment first (an issue discussed under the principle of justice), which means that, strictly speaking, the best interests duty to one of those patients has been breached. Another example of the difficulties comes when one considers the separation of conjoined twins when one twin will die as the result of the procedure but the other twin has a chance to live, but without separa-tion both will die. It is not in the best interests of both twins to die, but it is equally not in the best interests of one twin to die despite it being in the best interests of the other twin to live. Beneficence is not always as straightforward as it may seem and can raise complex ethical dilemmas.

Beneficence also may be problematic as, if carried too far, beneficence can become paternalism. This was discussed in respect of the principle of autonomy – you may remember the example where the health profes-sional's perception of what is best for the patient (preserving their mar-riage by not telling the patient of a diagnosis of a sexually transmitted disease) replaced the patient's determination of what is best for them (knowledge of the infection). When reflecting on your interaction with a patient or the interactions of colleagues with a patient, ask yourself whose agenda is being furthered? The patient's? Or are you or your colleagues, no doubt with the best of intentions, imposing your values or your inter-pretation of what is in that person's best interest onto that patient?

Non-maleficence

Non-maleficence is the duty to do no harm and to protect others from harm – this is a constant at the heart of all health care and at the heart of the nursing and midwifery professions. The principle of non-maleficence requires that nurses and midwives do not create a needless harm or injury to a patient, either through a nurse's or midwife's action or failure to act. The term 'needless harm' is used because the practice of providing health care often requires harm – for example, a needle-stick or a surgical incision. It is also important to note, to paraphrase Kenny and Giacomini (2005), when making ethical decisions it is often not a question of harming or not harming, but *how* to harm *and* benefit: Whom? How much? How cer-tainly? In what ways? It may not be possible to do no harm – the reality might rather be that a nurse or midwife should do the least possible harm.

Non-maleficence creates an ethical duty (reinforced by law) to provide a proper standard of care that avoids or minimises the risk of harm. Harm in this instance can be physical, emotional or psychological. This duty means that nurses and midwives are required, among other things, to:

➤ Provide care of an appropriate quality.

➤ Act in accordance with expected standards of professional conduct.

➤ Not exploit patients (financially, sexually or in any other way).

➤ Not kill patients, even out of mercy.

➤ Not commit criminal acts (for example, rape, indecent assault, torture, murder or selling drugs to patients).

➤ Self-report concerns about competence or conduct (that is, difficulties in performing certain functions, illnesses or addictions that inhibit performance, certain criminal convictions).

➤ Report others to appropriate authorities if their performance or conduct creates a possibility that serious harm to patients might result.

This principle affirms the need for professional competence.

Decision-making framework

The codes and ethical principles discussed above may not in isolation assist a nurse or midwife facing an ethical and/or legal problem in practice. A decision-making framework provides a process through which nurses and midwives can systematically consider the situation and its legal and ethical implications and come up with a conclusion or a course of action. There are a variety of decision-making frameworks available (see, for example, Swisher and Krueger-Brophy 1998; Purtilo 1999; NMBA 2007; Kerridge et al. 2013). However, in this book we are using the framework set out in Figure 2.2. The framework presented is one way to approach these issues but is not the only way. Ultimately, each nurse and midwife must reflect about ethics and ethical decision-making and take responsibility for integrating ethics (and legal knowledge) into their professional practice.

Step One: Identify issues and collect information

How do I identify or recognise an ethical issue?

The first question that many ask is 'how do I identify or recognise an ethical issue?' An ethical issue might be experienced in three ways:

1. As an **ethical violation** – incompetence or deliberate wrong-doing in the context of professional practice.

2. As an **ethical dilemma** – arising from a situation where there may be opposing but equally morally legitimate approaches to resolving a dilemma.

3. As **ethical distress** – moral distress (guilt, concern, distaste) arising from action or inaction – sometimes actions or inaction imposed on a person by another health professional, organisation or government.

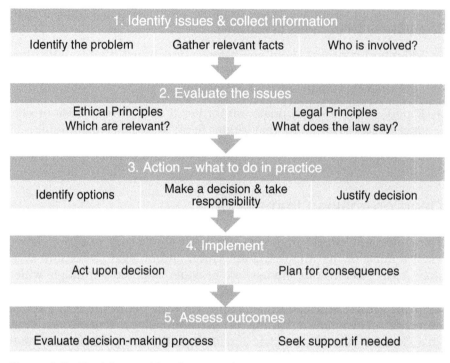

Figure 2.2 Decision-making framework

Ethical violations – incompetence or deliberate wrong-doing – place patients at risk and are unethical. Perhaps the most serious ethical violation one can imagine is when a health professional takes advantage of their position to murder their patients. In 1991 a nurse, Beverley Allitt, was convicted of murdering four children, attempting to murder three others and the grievous bodily harm of six other children in the paediatric unit at Grantham and Kesteven Hospital in the United Kingdom (UK Department of Health 1994). In Australia a nurse, Roger Dean, pled guilty to the murder of 11 nursing home patients and to eight counts of recklessly inflicting grievous bodily harm, as well as other charges, after he set fire to the nursing home where he worked (ABC News 2013). Reports have also been made of a Japanese nurse arrested for fatally poisoning patients in hospital (Sydney Morning Herald 2018). While such extreme deliberate wrong-doing is fortunately rare, other forms of serious violations, such as boundary violations involving sexual assault or misconduct, are less rare. Violations also include recklessness or incompetence; where, for example, a nurse or midwife deliberately chooses to ignore good infection control practices, such as handwashing, they may be considered reckless or they may not understand the importance of maintaining good infection control practices because they lack competence or are careless. In relation to violations, nurses and midwives have responsibilities to participate in professional development and to self-monitor their performance. Nurses and midwives also have an important role to play in exposing incompetence or deliberate wrong-doing to ensure that patients are safe. They may uphold this role by contributing to internal reporting and monitoring processes and, where institutional processes do not exist or are not responsive, by whistle-blowing (see Chapter 4). A recent Australian instance of whistle-blowing by a nurse was in 2004/2005 when Toni Hoffman, a nurse unit manager in the intensive care unit at Bundaberg Hospital, raised internally, and ultimately externally, concerns about the competence of Dr Jayent Patel. A Commission of Inquiry ultimately commended her for her actions and concluded that Dr Patel's conduct and practice were below the expected standard and that systems at Bundaberg Hospital were inadequate (Queensland Public Hospitals Commission of Inquiry 2005).

Ethical dilemmas – situations where there may be opposing but equally morally legitimate approaches to resolving a dilemma. An example of a significant ethical dilemma is illustrated by the legal case *Re A (children) (conjoined twins)* [2001] Fam 147. In that case the English Court of Appeal was asked to decide whether conjoined twins should undergo a surgical separation. Without the procedure both girls (referred to as Mary and Jodie for the purposes of the legal proceedings) would die within a relatively short period of time. However, the surgical separation would result in Mary's death – she would have no chance of survival. Jodie and Mary's parents refused the procedure based on their religious beliefs and, no doubt, the cruelty of the choice they were asked to make. The Hospital and the health care team were of the view that the surgery should proceed to save Jodie's life. In his judgement Lord Justice Ward of the Court of Appeal wrote: 'I cannot emphasise how much I sympathise with them [the parents] in the cruelty of the agonising choice they had to make. I know because I agonise over the dilemma too' (*Re A (children) (conjoined twins)* at 196). No doubt the health professionals involved in caring for the twins agonised over the dilemma as well. The Court of Appeal concluded in this case it was permissible that the surgery proceed, despite Mary's certain death, and that the refusal of the twin's parents could be overruled by the Court as it was in Jodie's best interests to live. The Court ordered that the surgery proceed. Mary died during the procedure. Jodie survived. This type of case is exceedingly rare, more commonly a patient or family may wish to refuse treatment when the health care team is convinced it is in the patient's best interest, at least from a clinical perspective.

Another example of an ethical dilemma that may confront nurses and midwives is that an individual's personal values may, at times, conflict with the values of the nursing and/or midwifery professions. An example of this may be in the midwifery setting where some nurses or midwives (and other health professionals) may feel conflicted between their personal values – that breastfeeding of newborn infants should always be attempted – and professional values that emphasise the right of a woman to make her own decision, including the decision not to attempt breastfeeding. This conflict may also cause ethical distress.

Ethical distress – moral distress arising from action or inaction – sometimes imposed on a person by another health professional, organisation or government. Moral distress might arise, for example, in the context of participating in the surgery to separate Mary and Jodie knowing that Mary would die as a direct consequence. Moral distress might also arise in the context of determining whether to report a colleague or to act as a whistle-blower (see Chapter 4). It might also arise when the policy of an institution conflicts with a nurse or midwife's professional values, for example when a decision is made by an institution to move a mental health outpatient service to a small block of shops at the edge of the city, with no effective public transport, further marginalising a vulnerable community.

Once you have identified the relevant issue (which may present as a violation, dilemma or through experiencing ethical distress or as a mixture of some or all of these) you should consider who is involved.

Who is involved?

This is an important part of Step One, as by identifying who is involved, or ought to be involved, it enables an evaluation to be made of each individual's or group's interests in the matter at hand. In some cases individuals or groups may have competing interests and it is critical to have an appreciation of these.

Gather information

It may be necessary to gather further information to assist in the decision-making. This could include medical information and contextual information (societal, organisational, familial and individual).

Step Two: Evaluate the issues

In this step you identify and apply relevant sections of the Codes of Ethics and the ethical principles to the issue(s) and identify any conflicts within or among them. Part of the process is to identify the perspectives and values of all those associated with the decision. Legal principles are also identified and applied in this step.

Step Three: Action – What to do in practice

In this step you identify and apply any relevant aspects of the Codes of Conduct to the issue(s). Considering and synthesising the results of your analysis of the relevant aspects of the Codes of Ethics and Conduct, the ethical principles and the law, you then identify the options for action or reach a conclusion and analyse the consequences/outcomes of each option or your conclusion. If there are options for action you should make a decision on how to proceed (at least in the short term) and clearly justify why that decision was reached, in particular how and why you balanced the ethical concerns. You must also, as part of this step, take responsibility for that decision.

Step Four: Implement

Act on the decision(s) reached in accordance with a plan to manage, as much as is possible, any foreseeable consequences of the action – for example, how do you discuss issues with the patient in such a way as to minimise anxiety? The decision should be documented and where relevant a care plan developed.

Step Five: Assess outcomes

In this step evaluate the decision-making process, your values and beliefs post-decision and the action taken, and seek support and assistance from your colleagues if you experience ethical distress. Depending on the situation, a nurse/midwife may recognise that it is desirable that she or he or the team seek additional training.

Decision-making framework: Example

Hilda is an elderly woman newly resident in a nursing home. She has moderate dementia. Her decision-making capacity varies from day to day – some days she is competent to make her own decisions and some days she is not. Hilda approaches the manager of the nursing home and asks to only be attended to by non-Asian nurses and caregivers.

Step One

Identify issues & collect information		
Identify problem	Who is involved?	Gather additional facts

Identify the problem:

> Hilda's request appears to amount to racial discrimination.

Identify who is involved:

> Hilda, Hilda's family (including who acts as her substitute decision-maker), staff at the nursing home, her General Practitioner (GP) and other residents of the nursing home.

Gather information:

> Hilda refuses to explain her request.

> Hilda's family confirm that in World War II Hilda was a prisoner of the Japanese and forced to act as a 'comfort woman' for troops. The Japanese Imperial Army in World War II forced captive women (from China, Korea, the Netherlands, Burma, Thailand, the Philippines, and Australia) into sexual slavery in military brothels ('comfort' stations). Survivors report being raped, beaten and otherwise tortured day and night, even by the (male) health professionals sent to check them for venereal disease. It is estimated that only 25 per cent survived and most were rendered sterile from rapes or disease.

> Hilda's GP confirms Hilda has post-traumatic stress disorder (PTSD) as a result of her experiences.

> Hilda's GP notes that Hilda has flashbacks due either to her PTSD or to her dementia.

> Hilda's GP notes that during her last hospital admission Hilda went into physical convulsions and fought violently when attended by a male Asian doctor.

Step Two

Evaluate the issues

Ethical principles
Which are relevant?

Legal principles
What does the law say?

ICN Code of Ethics for nurses

➢ Element 1: 'The nurse's primary professional responsibility is to people requiring nursing care ... In providing care, the nurse promotes an environment in which the human rights, values, customs and spiritual beliefs of the individual ... are respected.'

Hilda, as the patient, should be the primary focus. She could be physically or emotionally harmed if an Asian nurse provides care because of her PTSD/dementia. The history of her last hospital admission (convulsions) establishes that the risk is real.

➢ Element 3: 'The nurse, acting through the professional organisation, participates in creating a positive practice environment and maintaining safe, equitable social and economic working conditions in nursing.'

In this context, in order to maintain an equitable working environment it is important not to allow other nurses to be discriminated against by patients. However, in this case it appears that Hilda's desire to not have an Asian caregiver may be motivated by a desire to protect them and herself from harm, a harm she cannot control. In addition, an Asian nurse who attempts to provide care to Hilda may place herself/himself and/or colleagues at risk of physical, emotional or psychological harm. The risk of physical harm to staff is a real possibility, especially given Hilda's last hospital admission when she 'fought violently' when attended by a male Asian doctor. Emotional and/or psychological harm could result to nurses and to other staff from seeing a patient react so strongly to a nurse's presence. The safety and/or wellbeing of other residents may also be compromised through witnessing or being affected by Hilda's distress.

Ethical principles

Autonomy

As discussed earlier, in general the rights of patients to make decisions about what is in their best interests should be respected, but there are limits to autonomy if a person's decisions are likely to harm others. Hilda's request may harm members of staff by discriminating against them on the basis of race. This is a harm specifically recognised by the state as being of such concern that a specific law was created to prevent it.

Beneficence and non-maleficence

It seems in Hilda's best interest to agree to her request (beneficence) because of the extreme physical and emotional distress it would cause her if her request was not complied with. Equally, if you know that something will cause harm you have a responsibility to protect the patient from that harm (non-maleficence). More broadly, if Hilda is unable to control her physical, psychological and emotional reactions to Asian staff members (a possibility given her dementia and PTSD) she may inadvertently cause physical injury to staff or other patients or emotional distress to staff whose presence may trigger a reaction. Arguably there is also a duty to act in the best interests of others and to protect others, such as other patients and staff members from possible harm.

Justice

As discussed earlier there are three forms of justice – two seem particularly relevant here:

Legal justice – As a matter of legal justice to Asian members of staff the manager should respect the law and refuse to allow any form of discrimination against staff. However, are there any legal exceptions?

Distributive justice – Human resources are scarce and there is a question about whether it is fair to other patients to arrange staffing around the request of one patient.

What does the law say?

All the states and territories and the federal government have legislation that prohibits direct or indirect discrimination on the grounds of race (see Table 2.1). In this case Hilda's request is that staff be treated differently because of their ethnic backgrounds so her request, and any action taken to implement this request, would appear on its face to be discriminatory. The legislation all agrees that any motive for discrimination is irrelevant. So a beneficent motive, such as in this case to minimise harm to Hilda and others, is irrelevant. There also has to be some negative impact on an individual. In this case, nurses may agree that it is in everyone's best interest that any nurse(s) with an Asian

Table 2.1   Legislation relating to discrimination in Australia

Jurisdiction	Legislation
Commonwealth	*Disability Discrimination Act 1992*
	Racial Discrimination Act 1975
	Sex Discrimination Act 1984
	Age Discrimination Act 2004
	Australian Human Rights Commission Act 1986
Australian Capital Territory	*Discrimination Act 1991*
New South Wales	*Anti-Discrimination Act 1977*
Northern Territory	*Anti-Discrimination Act 1996*
Queensland	*Anti-Discrimination Act 1991*
South Australia	*Equal Opportunity Act 1984*
	Racial Vilification Act 1996
Tasmania	*Anti-Discrimination Act 1988*
Victoria	*Equal Opportunity Act 2010*
Western Australia	*Equal Opportunity Act 1984*

background not attend to Hilda and, assuming that staff allocation can be managed, there may be no negative impact and no perception of discrimination. Additionally, the legislation contains an exception for acts that are reasonably necessary to protect the health and safety of people at a place of work. Is this reasonably necessary to protect the health and safety of people at this place of work? Arguably, yes, based on Hilda's past history and her inability to control herself because of her dementia and PTSD.

Step Three

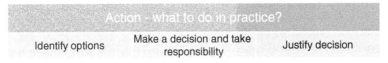

| Identify options | Make a decision and take responsibility | Justify decision |

Code of Conduct for Nurses

Principle 1.2(c) states that: 'Nurses must not participate in unlawful behaviour and understand that unlawful behaviour may be viewed as unprofessional conduct or professional misconduct.' Principle 3.2(d) also states that nurses must 'adopt practices that respect diversity [and] avoid bias, discrimination and racism'.

> Nurses should recognise the potential for discriminatory behaviour based on race and be familiar with anti-discrimination law to avoid engaging in unlawful behaviour.

Principle 2.2(a)/(c) states that nurses must 'take a person-centred approach to managing a person's care and concerns ... [and] advocate on behalf of the person where necessary'.

> Nurses should recognise that Hilda's concerns are legitimate ones and she is extremely vulnerable. Nurses should demonstrate understanding in relation to her position and advocate for steps to be taken to ensure she receives the best possible care and is not harmed.

Principle 2.3(c)/(d) states that nurses must 'act according to the person's capacity for decision-making and consent... [and] obtain valid authority before [providing] treatment'.

> One way of viewing Hilda's request is that she is refusing consent to care in specific circumstances (that is, if provided by an Asian health worker). However, as Hilda's capacity to make decisions varies from day to day, it will be necessary to involve her substitute decision-maker in any decision that is made.

Options

Ultimately, there seem to be two stark options:

Option 1 – refusing Hilda's request. This may cause serious physical, psychological and emotional harm to Hilda and to Asian staff. It may also contravene the principles of beneficence and non-maleficence, but comply with the law.

Option 2 – agreeing to Hilda's request. This seems to be in the best interests of Hilda, staff and residents. While on its face it may constitute direct discrimination against Asian staff, we need to investigate if it might fall within a permitted legal exception. It is important to note though that this would only become a *legal* issue if an affected individual chooses to make it an issue. If managed ethically for all involved, the law may not need to be invoked.

There is a conflict between ethical principles (autonomy and justice) and between some ethical principles and the law. Acting in Hilda's best interests by agreeing to Hilda's request may be harmful to any Asian members of staff because it looks like it may constitute discrimination. Balancing the risks here, if Asian staff care for Hilda, medical evidence suggests it is inevitable she will sustain at least psychological and emotional harm, if not physical harm, and the staff may sustain harm through experiencing moral distress. If there is no question that the Asian staff would lose their job and they would just not be rostered to attend to this one patient, the harm to them may fairly be considered limited or non-existent and perhaps, in the circumstances, arguably morally justifiable. A nurse concerned about the best interests of their patient might, in the circumstances, understand and be sympathetic to Hilda's request based on the fact that as her dementia progresses she is not able to control her reactions. The nurse may also not want to cause her to have a flashback to her traumatic past. In summary, it could be argued that a great harm is avoided through the imposition of a lesser harm. As mentioned earlier in the chapter, when making ethical decisions it is often not a question of harming or not harming, but *how* to harm *and* benefit: Whom? How much? How certainly? In what ways? (Kenny and Giacomini 2005).

However, the legislation is clear that it does not matter if the reason for the discrimination is beneficent as it will still amount to discrimination. So if the nursing home manager assents to Hilda's request and it negatively impacts on those staff it perhaps could be said that the nursing manager had discriminated against relevant staff members. But if this is so it may be that an exception could be made on occupational health and safety grounds – Does Hilda's condition pose an occupation health and safety risk? How might the nurse manager proceed?

Before a final decision is made additional information needs to be gathered so that the nursing manager and staff can decide how to proceed in the short term to gather the information so that a final decision can be made about how to manage Hilda's needs in the long term. Possible immediate options for action for nurses in this circumstance include seeking urgent expert advice from:

> Hilda's family (including her substitute decision-maker) about the best way to manage the situation based on their knowledge of her past.

> A geriatrician who specialises in dementia (with the patient's permission if she is to be identified). (As a practical matter the nurse manager needs to know how much physical, psychological and emotional distress will this cause Hilda. What are the risks to her and others? Is there any way in which Hilda's distress can be

managed other than potentially discriminating against staff? Are there any care requirements arising from the interaction between past trauma and dementia?)

➤ A lawyer about the relevant law and the impact of other laws – for example, are there occupational safety and health concerns for staff?

➤ Other nursing managers and aged care administrators (not disclosing identifiable details about the patient). How do other facilities deal with these types of situations? What do the regulators of nursing homes at the state and/or Commonwealth level suggest is good practice in these circumstances? What do Human Rights agencies say? The nursing manager should communicate with relevant staff, and probably their union representative, to discuss the problem.

Once additional information is received:

➤ A decision must be made.

➤ That decision must be justified – in other words, you need to be able to justify how and why you balanced the ethical principles and legal considerations.

➤ The nursing manager must take responsibility for the decision.

Step Four

Implementation	
Act on decision	Plan for consequences

A plan must be developed to implement the decision and that plan should include mechanisms to address any foreseeable consequences of the decision. For example, whether Option 1 or Option 2 is followed the decision should be documented. A care plan would need to be developed in conjunction with a geriatrician to manage Hilda's ongoing health needs and to plan for circumstances in which there is no other option than for an Asian nurse or other caregiver to provide care or treatment. The decision and its rationale must be communicated to Hilda and her family and to staff as the key stakeholders. Good practice would indicate having a staff training session on the effect of past trauma on dementia patients and mechanisms to manage the needs of such patients.

Step Five

Assess
Evaluate decision-making process   Seek support if required

The decision-making process should be evaluated. Did you consider everything? Was everyone who needed to be consulted, consulted? Have your values changed? How would you address a similar issue in the future? Was the action taken the best possible action that could have been taken? If not how could it be improved in the future?

Making ethical decisions is not easy – at times it may cause significant emotional distress. Do not hesitate to seek whatever support you need after a decision has been made. After dealing with a situation that raises some significant ethical issues, some facilities will undertake a formal debrief acknowledging the distress sustained by health professionals involved in the process.

Further reading

Veatch, R. 1995, 'Resolving conflicts among principles: Ranking, balancing, and specifying', *Kennedy Institute of Ethics Journal*, 5: 3, 199–218.

Questions

How would you balance conflicts between ethical principles?

What are the differences between ethical principles and the Codes of Ethics and Codes of Conduct in terms of their purposes, objectives and functions?

Scenario

(Adapted from Fry and Veatch, 2006, *Case Studies in Nursing Ethics,* 3rd edn.)

A 20-year-old patient, Blanche Smith, was admitted to a small regional hospital with signs of premature labour. The gestation of the foetus was uncertain. A midwife, Mary Jones, who had experience in neonatal care, and the obstetrician, Dr Angela Brown, were alerted. The obstetrician told

Blanche and her partner to prepare for the loss of the pregnancy. After a short labour Blanche delivered a small female infant who breathed spontaneously. Gestational age was estimated to be around 25 weeks. Mary anticipated that the infant would be given respiratory support and rushed to the nearest tertiary facility. However, Dr Brown stated that she was 'not sure we should be too aggressive with this patient' and decided that respiratory support should cease as Dr Brown thought the infant too small to survive. Mary disagreed, as she was experienced at treating infants in a similar condition. Mary asked whether the parents were aware of the child's condition and the small chance for survival if she was transferred to another facility. Dr Brown said she was going out to speak with the parents and 'they're too young to cope with the kind of problems the child will face. They'll have more babies.' Mary was told to keep the infant comfortable and to call Dr Brown when the child died. Dr Brown's first child had been born in similar circumstances and had significant disabilities as a result.

Apply the decision-making framework to this problem.

3

The Australian legal system

Introduction

The purpose of this chapter is to introduce the fundamentals of the Australian legal system to you. It is essential that nurses and midwives have a foundation understanding of what the law is and how it operates, as well as the specific laws that are discussed in later chapters. We cover the origins of Australian laws, what the difference is between different categories of law and introduce the court system that exists in Australia. We start by expanding on our discussion in Chapter 2 regarding what makes law and ethics different.

What is law? How does it differ from ethics?

In Chapter 1 we introduced the notion of law and how it differed from ethics. In that chapter we noted that law could be described as a system of rules that regulate society – especially our behaviour as individuals, groups and organisations – and that the rules are established by an authority with law-making power and are enforceable.

From earlier chapters we have seen that ethical principles or values can also be described as a system of rules that regulate society, however where they come from and whether such rules are universally acknowledged and enforced make them significantly different from legal rules. Unlike ethical principles and values, legal rules and principles are made by recognised authorities who are granted law-making power; in Australia these authorities are parliaments and the courts. Below we discuss how these law-making authorities create law (see 'Sources of law').

Another major difference between ethics and law is that there are recognised mechanisms of enforcing the law which do not exist for ethics. For example, if a person breaks the law it is generally understood that there will be detrimental consequences for that individual. Generally, the more serious the conduct resulting in breaking the law, the more serious the consequences will be for the individual and more severe the enforcement mechanism. For example, if you are driving above the speed limit and you are caught you may be fined, or perhaps have your driving licence taken away (if you have been caught multiple times). If the speed you were driving at was reckless and caused property damage or harm to others you may be charged with a criminal offence and possibly face jail time. All of these are recognised consequences of breaking the law and are used as a means of enforcing the law. While people may disapprove of your conduct if you act contrary to a particular ethical principle, no one has the ability to put you in prison for your action. Over time, however, ethical principles may influence the development of the law where sufficient consensus exists within the community regarding such conduct. So ethical principles may become law and as such become enforceable.

Law has the capacity to offer a degree of certainty on an issue. In most circumstances we can point to the legal rule, principle or piece of legislation that governs how we should act in accordance with the law. While people may disagree on whether the law on a particular issue is appropriate (and perhaps seek to have it changed in the future), people accept what the current law is and the consequences of not following that law. As Chapter 2 has highlighted, there is no such certainty in the application of ethical principles and values; people can hold legitimate and differing views about which ethical principle should guide a situation and, unlike the law, there is no written document or case which determines which ethical principle is 'right' in a given circumstance.

Laws on any particular topic do not, however, always stand still. As attitudes, opinions and common values in society develop over time, or differ from one society to the next, so law can also develop over time, or differ between States or Territories. The process of changing the law can be incremental and largely unintentional or can be led by government or lobby groups and lead to more substantial, immediate change (often called 'law reform') via laws created in parliament.

The law in Australia

While other forms of law predated colonisation in Australia – such as customary law exercised by Aboriginal and/or Torres Strait Islanders – what we recognise as our legal system today was brought here by the British. As such, the system of law we have today is largely inherited from, and similar to, the system that exists in England. It is sometimes referred to as a 'common law system' (as opposed to a 'civil law system' which exists in some European countries). Forms of customary law still coexist alongside our common law system but these laws are not officially recognised by governments and not widely practised. Here the focus of the chapter is on the common law system.

Sources of law

In a common law system, such as the one that exists in Australia, there are two main sources of law: law produced by governments (which we will call parliament-made law) and law made through cases being heard in the courts (which we will call case law or common law). In subsequent chapters we refer to both types of law. Here we explain how laws are created from these two sources.

Legislation (parliament-made law)

Each government in Australia, whether a State, Territory or the Commonwealth government, has power to make certain laws to dictate what should or should not occur. Each government has power over its 'jurisdiction' – the geographic area it controls and the people that are subject to that government. How governments create law is to pass legislation (also known as 'Acts' or statutes) on particular topics. Legislation are written documents which outline what the law is. They are created by the parliament of each government, this is why we call it 'parliament-made' law.

Parliament-made law starts life as a 'bill' introduced into parliament – a 'bill' is a written draft document of the proposed laws. This bill is then debated by those within parliament who may agree to changes to the bill. When sufficient consensus is achieved in parliament, the bill is enacted as a piece of legislation and becomes binding law in that jurisdiction.

Case law (common law)

Another source of law in Australia is law that develops through cases decided by judges in our court system. The Australian court system and the doctrine of precedent is explained below (see 'The court system in Australia'). Although governments in Australia have the power to enact legislation, sometimes no legislation exists on a particular issue. If there is no legislation, it will often be left up to judges in the court to decide cases in accordance with previous cases (see the explanation of the doctrine of precedent below). Principles of law have developed over time that are applied in cases by judges. These principles are recognised in case law.

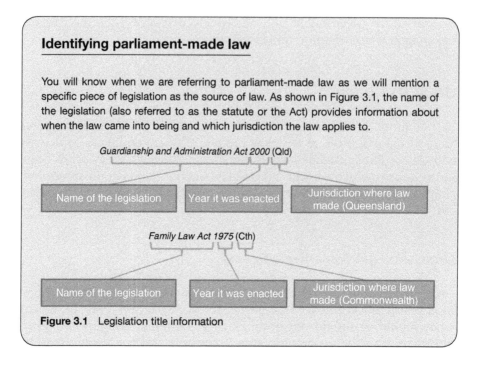

Identifying parliament-made law

You will know when we are referring to parliament-made law as we will mention a specific piece of legislation as the source of law. As shown in Figure 3.1, the name of the legislation (also referred to as the statute or the Act) provides information about when the law came into being and which jurisdiction the law applies to.

Guardianship and Administration Act 2000 (Qld)

| Name of the legislation | Year it was enacted | Jurisdiction where law made (Queensland) |

Family Law Act 1975 (Cth)

| Name of the legislation | Year it was enacted | Jurisdiction where law made (Commonwealth) |

Figure 3.1　Legislation title information

Case law is also often referred to as 'common law'. Unlike parliament-made law where a written document – the legislation – is produced which contains the relevant laws, the principles of case law are contained within the judges' reasons in decided cases.

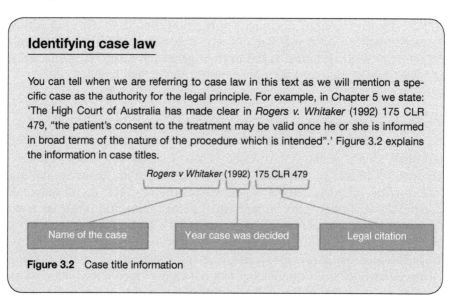

Identifying case law

You can tell when we are referring to case law in this text as we will mention a specific case as the authority for the legal principle. For example, in Chapter 5 we state: 'The High Court of Australia has made clear in *Rogers v. Whitaker* (1992) 175 CLR 479, "the patient's consent to the treatment may be valid once he or she is informed in broad terms of the nature of the procedure which is intended".' Figure 3.2 explains the information in case titles.

Rogers v Whitaker (1992) 175 CLR 479

| Name of the case | Year case was decided | Legal citation |

Figure 3.2　Case title information

Case law influences parliament-made law, as often judges in the courts are asked to decide how legislation should be interpreted. For example, cases may be brought to court that debate what a section in legislation means. Or the court may be asked whether this section applies in this particular circumstance. In this way both types of law coexist and complement one another.

Inconsistencies between legislation and case law

However, sometimes there may be an inconsistency between case law and legislation. If this occurs, to the extent that a piece of legislation is inconsistent with existing case law, the legislation prevails.

Example

There is a common law principle that states that health professionals, including nurses and midwives, owe a duty of care to their patients. This duty of care usually commences from when the nurse or midwife takes on the care of the patient – for example, at the start of their shift. The common law does not extend a health professional's duty of care to strangers whom they have never seen or cared for.

Let us assume that in Western Australia a new piece of legislation (the *Fictional Duty of Care Act 2018* (WA)) is enacted which requires all nurses and midwives to owe a duty of care to persons within a 1 km radius of their place of residence.

This piece of legislation is inconsistent with the common law principles regarding when a duty of care is owed and, as such, the legal principles in the legislation prevail, requiring nurses and midwives to owe a duty of care to a much wider range of people.

Australia as a federation

While Australia derives its legal system from the United Kingdom, unlike that country Australia as a nation is a federation. This means that the country is made up of different States (New South Wales, Queensland, South Australia, Tasmania, Victoria and Western Australia) and Territories (the Australian Capital Territory and the Northern Territory) that each have its own government. In conjunction, there exists the Commonwealth government (also known as the federal government). Every person in Australia is subject to the laws within their own State or Territory (either legislation or case law) and also relevant laws of the Commonwealth.

Despite the overlap of government power between State/Territory and the Commonwealth governments, this is usually not a problem. This is because Australia as a nation was created by a legal document known as the *Commonwealth of Australia Constitution Act* (the *Constitution*). In the *Constitution* the Commonwealth has defined powers in which it can legislate. Any powers which are not allocated to the Commonwealth can be determined by the States. For example, the administration of the pharmaceutical benefits scheme is a matter for the Commonwealth government to legislate on under Section 51 (xxiiiA) of the *Constitution* which provides, among other things, that the Commonwealth parliament has power to make laws regarding 'pharmaceutical, sickness and hospital benefits'. In contrast, issues regarding transplantation of human tissue is an issue left for the States and Territories to legislate on. This means laws regarding the pharmaceutical benefits scheme are Commonwealth laws, whereas laws governing the transplantation of human tissue are made by each State and Territory.

Conflicts between Commonwealth and State laws

Occasionally there is an overlap between laws of the Commonwealth government and those of a State or Territory. In such cases it is possible for the two laws to require different things and results in an inconsistency between the Commonwealth law and the State/Territory law.

The *Constitution* provides a way to resolve these inconsistencies between Commonwealth and State/Territory parliament-made law. Section 109 of the *Constitution* states that where an inconsistency exists between a Commonwealth and State/Territory law, the Commonwealth law should be followed.

Commonwealth law or State law?

Let us assume that Queensland has legislation (the *Fictional Biological Materials Act 2016* (Qld)) that requires biological materials (such as used syringes, swabs, bandages, etc.) to be disposed of in a certain manner. However, in 2017 the Commonwealth government introduced legislation (the *Fictional Procedures in Hospitals Act 2017* (Cth)) which standardised the way certain procedures had to be carried out in hospitals which receive Commonwealth funding. This included procedures for disposal of biological materials which were required to be disposed of in a different way from that outlined in the *Fictional Biological Materials Act 2016* (Qld).

▶

◀

Which procedures for disposal of biological material should a nurse or midwife follow in Queensland and why? Section 109 of the *Constitution* provides that, in the event of an inconsistency, the Commonwealth law should prevail. Therefore the *Fictional Procedures in Hospitals Act 2017* (Cth) should be followed.

The court system in Australia

In this part of the chapter we specifically consider how case law is created through the doctrine of precedent and examine the system of courts that exists in Australia.

The doctrine of precedent

One of the sources of law in Australia is case law which is generated through decisions of judges in the courts. Case law comes about through what is known as the 'doctrine of precedent'. Applying this doctrine means that the legal principles applied in past decisions should be followed in future cases where the facts are similar. Therefore, principles which applied in past cases are reapplied to a new but similar set of facts in a later case. In this way legal principles in cases are applied in a predictable manner in accordance with similar past cases. While the application of the doctrine of precedent attempts to minimise arbitrary decision-making and is easily stated, it is not always easily applied. The application of legal principles to a given set of facts is always open to interpretation and this is why, in many cases, the two parties coming before the court will disagree as to whether a previous case applies and, if it does apply, how it should be applied in the given case.

The doctrine of precedent applies so that lower courts must decide cases in accordance with higher court decisions. Judges are not bound to follow the decisions of cases decided in courts lower in their jurisdiction's court hierarchy or from a different court hierarchy (see Figure 3.4).

Sometimes a court from a different Australian State or Territory or a different country may make decisions relevant to a case. While the decision of a court from a different Australian state or even a different country is not binding on a court – that is, the doctrine of precedent does not apply – the court may find such cases from other jurisdictions to be helpful in deciding the current case. In this way, although the court is not 'bound' to follow the other courts' decisions, it may find such cases 'persuasive'. For example, the Supreme Court of Western Australia is not bound to follow decisions of the Supreme Court of Queensland but, where a case with similar facts and similar legislation exists, it may find the previous decision of the Supreme Court of Queensland on an issue to be 'persuasive'. Similarly, the High Court of Australia is not bound by the doctrine of precedent to follow any other court decisions but it may look at how similar cases have been decided in the highest courts in other countries, such as the United Kingdom's House of Lords or the Supreme Court of New Zealand, and find their reasoning to be persuasive in Australia.

Australian courts

The court system in Australia is relatively complex, as it reflects our federated national structure. Within each State and Territory there is a hierarchy of courts, and concurrent with these State and Territory court hierarchies exists the Commonwealth courts (also known as the federal courts). Figure 3.3 provides an overview of the court system in Australia.

State and Territory courts

Within each State and Territory exists a hierarchy of courts. Typically the courts at the bottom of the hierarchy deal with minor breaches of the law (traffic offences, monetary disputes of a low value, etc.), while the courts at the upper end of the hierarchy deal with the more serious breaches of

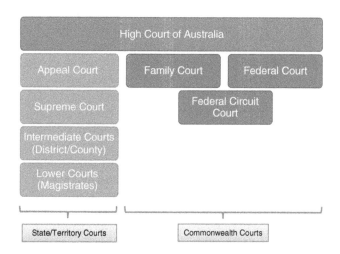

Figure 3.3 The court system in Australia

Tribunals and courts

In addition to these courts, a system of tribunals also exists next to the courts. It is important to understand that tribunals are not the same as courts, although they may exercise similar functions. Instead they have a limited quasi-judicial role – partly administrative, partly judicial.

The scope of matters that tribunals can hear is always defined by legislation. They are usually established to deal with specific types of matters. When matters from tribunals are appealed, those matters may end up being heard by a court in the court system.

In later chapters we refer to various tribunals that have a role in resolving health care issues alongside the courts.

---

the law (murder, manslaughter, monetary disputes of a high value, etc). While additional courts exist in each jurisdiction – such as the Coroner's Court (discussed in the section 'Coronial investigations') – here we focus on the principal courts in Australia which are most relevant.

Each State and Territory has an Appeal Court which sits at the top of their hierarchy. This is the highest court in that State or Territory and only the Australian High Court sits above it. Cases may be heard in lower courts and proceed to the Appeal Court where one party in a case wishes to dispute the finding in the lower court. Usually they will allege that the lower court did not apply the legal principles correctly. When a party appeals the lower court decision it will often end up being heard by the Appeal Court in that State or Territory.

The doctrine of precedent in State/Territory courts

Example: The Court of Appeal of Western Australia makes a decision that the definition of 'health professional' in the *Fictitious Health Care Act 2003* (WA) includes midwives working independently of hospitals. In a later case the Supreme Court of Western Australia hears a case that requires them to determine whether a midwife working privately and independently of any health care facility falls within the definition of 'health professional' in the *Fictitious Health Care Act 2003* (WA). The doctrine of precedent requires the Supreme Court of Western Australia to follow the legal interpretation of the definition in the *Fictitious Health Care Act 2003* (WA) determined by the Court of Appeal of Western Australia (see Figure 3.4).

▶

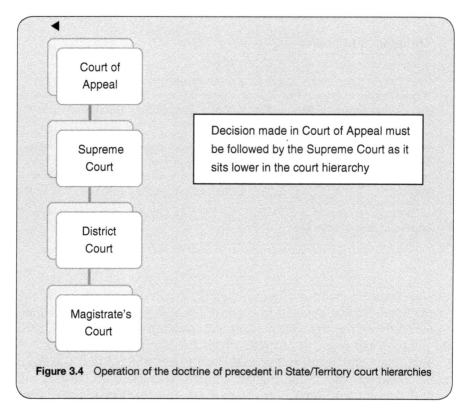

Figure 3.4   Operation of the doctrine of precedent in State/Territory court hierarchies

As shown in Figure 3.3, the High Court of Australia sits at the top of the State/Territory hierarchies.

Commonwealth courts

In conjunction with the State/Territories court hierarchies, there exists a system of Commonwealth courts. These courts will also sometimes be called on to resolve health care matters. In the Commonwealth system there exist the Federal Courts, the Family Court and the Federal Circuit Court. As discussed in Chapter 6, the Family Court in particular is relevant to issues involving child patients as it may be called on to resolve issues relevant to a child's health care.

As shown in Figure 3.3, the High Court of Australia also sits at the top of the Commonwealth court system.

The High Court of Australia

The High Court of Australia is the highest court in our country (see Figure 3.3). It sits at the top of each State/Territory court hierarchy and at the top of the Commonwealth court system.

The doctrine of precedent applies so that, where the High Court makes a decision, all the courts in the States/Territories and the Commonwealth court system are bound to follow the legal principles stated by the High Court when a similar case appears in those courts.

As noted above, the High Court is not bound to follow the decisions of any of the State, Territory or Commonwealth courts below it. It is also not bound to follow the decisions of any courts of other countries. However, it may find such cases to be helpful or 'persuasive' in deciding cases that come before it.

Categories of law

Having outlined the system of courts that exists in Australia, we now consider some categories of laws. Here the distinctions between two categories of law – civil and criminal – will be explained.

Criminal law

Criminal law imposes a set of rules on society to generally dictate what is acceptable behaviour and what is not. However, it should be noted that what is considered acceptable in a society may differ over time and between different countries (see, for example, Chapter 11 regarding the euthanasia and assisted suicide debate and consider community attitudes to issues such as abortion in Chapter 12). If a citizen does not abide by these rules they will be in breach of the law and commit an offence or a crime. As a consequence they may be subject to sanctions such as fines or imprisonment. The purpose of the criminal law is punishment for the wrongs committed.

The scope of criminal law is broad; it covers relatively minor offences, such as minor traffic infringements, through to the most serious crimes, such as assault, drug offences and murder. Criminal law can take the form of legislation (particularly in Queensland and Western Australia where most crimes are contained within legislation known as a criminal code) or case law. In a health care setting nurses and midwives need a working knowledge of offences concerning the person – such as assault and battery, manslaughter and murder (we discuss each of these offences in Chapters 5 and 11). Although it would be rare that a nurse or midwife would be alleged to have committed such crimes, unfortunately, it is not unheard of (see, for example, 'Ethics violations' in Chapter 2).

For breaches of the criminal law – where offences are alleged to have been committed – the usual process for allocating blame and punishment is a matter for the courts. Where it is alleged that a crime or offence has been committed, the police will usually be called on to investigate and decide whether or not to charge the person and refer the matter to the relevant State/Territory or Commonwealth director of public prosecutions. The prosecutor decides whether that evidence is sufficient to prosecute the matter in the courts. As such, it is the relevant government – in the guise of the government prosecutor – who decides whether to proceed with a criminal matter (unlike civil matters which can be pursued by individuals). The person charged with the offence is called the accused. When a criminal matter comes before the courts, it is up to the prosecution to show that all the elements of the offence have been satisfied. This is known as the prosecution having the burden of proof.

A person charged with a criminal offence is presumed innocent until proven guilty. The prosecution has the task of proving beyond reasonable doubt that the person charged committed the offence. This threshold level of beyond reasonable doubt is known as the standard of proof. Depending on the alleged offence, whether it has been shown beyond reasonable doubt that the accused committed the crime may be decided by a judge or by a judge and jury.

Punishment may take the form of imprisonment, fines, community service orders or other types of sanctions.

Civil law

Civil law differs from the criminal law in that it allows individuals to take action against others for perceived wrongs that have been inflicted on them. It does not involve the police or the government prosecutor. Its purpose also differs from the criminal law; while criminal law is concerned with justice and punishment, the civil law is concerned with compensation – normally in the form of money – to individuals who have suffered a wrong.

Civil law encompasses many areas of law, including negligence, contract and family law. We deal with many of these areas of civil law in later chapters (see, for example, Chapters 6 and 8). The person who brings a civil action is the person who has suffered a wrong – usually in the form of receiving an injury or having suffered property damage due to the actions of another. The person who brings the action is known as the plaintiff and the person brought to court to defend the action is known as the defendant. Unlike in the criminal setting, where the standard of proof is beyond reasonable doubt, in the civil action the plaintiff must satisfy a lower standard of proof. The plaintiff must show that on the balance of probabilities the defendant caused the plaintiff's harm (i.e. it is more likely than not that the defendant caused the plaintiff's harm).

For example, in a health care setting a patient may bring an action against a nurse for negligent care which resulted in the patient sustaining a physical injury. The patient is the plaintiff, the nurse is the defendant, the civil action is negligence and the patient would be seeking money in the form of damages as compensation for the injury they received.

Table 3.1 outlines the key differences between the areas of criminal and civil law.

Table 3.1 Key differences between criminal law and civil law

	Civil law	Criminal law
Purpose of the action	Compensation	Justice/punishment
Who can bring an action	An individual	The state
What is the person bringing the action called	Plaintiff	Prosecutor
What is the person subject to the action called	Defendant	Accused
What is the standard of proof	On the balance of probabilities	Beyond reasonable doubt
What is the outcome of a successful action	Damages (usually in the form of monetary compensation)	Punishment (usually in the form of imprisonment, fines or other sanctions)

Other relevant areas of law in health care

Two further areas of law of importance in the health care context are that of disciplinary action and coronial investigations. As nurse and midwives are subject to regulation from their professional body, an understanding of what disciplinary action is and how it differs from other types of law (such as criminal law) is necessary. In addition, in a clinical setting it is not unusual for the coroner to be involved when some patients die. As such, it is helpful for nurses and midwives to know what the coroner's role is and what it means to be involved in a coronial investigation or inquest.

Disciplinary action

Like many other health professionals, midwives and nurses are subject to professional regulation. The Nursing and Midwifery Board of Australia, under the auspices of the Australian Health Practitioner Regulation Agency, is the relevant professional body for nurses and midwives (although the situation differs in New South Wales). We discuss the role of these agencies in greater detail in Chapter 4.

For the purpose of this chapter it is necessary to understand that professional bodies have certain powers to discipline members of their profession. Information about conduct that may require disciplinary action can come from a number of sources, including where a patient makes a complaint to the relevant State or Territory Healthcare Complaint Agency. These agencies are established by legislation and are given specific powers to manage patient complaints (see *Human Rights Commission Act 2005* (ACT); *Health Care Complaints Act 1993* (NSW); *Health and Community Services Complaints Act* (NT); *Health Ombudsman Act 2013* (Qld); *Health and Community Services Complaints Act 2004* (SA); *Health Complaints Act 1995* (Tas); *Health Complaints Act 2016* (Vic); *Mental Health Act 2014* (Vic); *Health and Disability Services (Complaints) Act 1995* (WA)).

The action taken by professional bodies, such as the Nursing and Midwifery Board of Australia, is separate from the criminal law and civil law actions described above. The power of professional bodies to discipline members is usually limited to excluding them from practising, or imposing limitations on their ability to practise, as a professional. For example, the outcome of disciplinary action against a nurse may be to impose conditions on the nurse's scopes of practice, to suspend their registration for a period of time or to de-register them.

Disciplinary action may, however, be taken in conjunction with a civil or criminal action against a nurse or midwife. For example, a midwife who has been charged with the criminal offence of stealing pharmaceuticals from a hospital in which they are employed may also be subject to disciplinary action by the Nursing and Midwifery Board of Australia. The purposes of these actions are, however, different. As shown in Chapter 4, the purpose of disciplinary action is protection of the public, whereas we know that the purpose of the criminal law is punishment. Similarly, the purpose of the civil law is different again – it being concerned with compensation.

Coronial investigations

Coronial investigations focus on discovering the circumstances of a death so that the coroner can inform the family and the public as to how the death occurred. The purpose of such investigations is not to attribute blame to any particular person or entity. The coroner acts within the jurisdiction of the Coroner's Court, one of which exists in each jurisdiction. While it is a court, it differs from other courts in that the coroner is able to independently investigate a death and does not rely on two parties presenting two sides of an argument (as occurs in other courts).

In each State and Territory in Australia legislation exists which creates the role of the coroner. Typically, the role of the coroner across Australia is to investigate the circumstances of certain deaths (generally known as 'reportable deaths') and to report their findings. Their powers of investigation extend to holding inquests and ordering autopsies to determine the cause of death. An inquest is an inquiry led by a coroner to determine why a death occurred and these hearings are generally open to the public. Witnesses may be called during an inquest. Not all deaths that the coroner investigates require a public inquest; in fact the majority will not have an inquest held.

Understanding the role and the consequences of coronial investigations is relevant to nurses and midwives as they may be called on to provide information or evidence to the coroner when a patient they have been caring for dies in certain circumstances. You may be asked by your employer, a hospital lawyer (who acts for your employer) or the police for a statement. If asked to provide a statement, you are entitled to legal representation which is often provided by your insurer or your union (if you are a member).

In addition, some coronial findings may impact directly on nurses and midwives where adverse findings are made about their conduct. Where this is the case, the outcome of a coronial investigation may, indirectly, lead to disciplinary, civil or even criminal action against a nurse or midwife (see the section 'Interaction between coronial inquests and other proceedings (disciplinary, criminal)'). Some nurses and midwives find their involvement in coronial inquests – even when there is no likelihood of adverse findings being made against them – to be a stressful experience due to their misunderstanding of what a coronial investigation involves.

In investigating deaths the coroner is generally required to establish:

➢ the identity of the deceased;

➢ the circumstances surrounding the death; and

➢ the cause of death.

Typically the legislation in the States and Territories require unexpected, unnatural or violent deaths and deaths resulting from an accident or injury to be reported to the Coroner. In addition, there exist specific provisions regarding deaths relevant to the health care context which must be reported and which are most relevant to midwives and nurses. The situations in which these deaths must be reported are outlined in Table 3.2.

Outcomes from coronial investigations

As already noted, the principal outcome from all coronial investigations is to determine the identity and cause of death. However, in addition, the

Table 3.2 Situations in which deaths must be reported

State/Territory	Deaths which must be reported that are most relevant to the health care context.	Legislation
Australian Capital Territory	A death that appears to be completely or partly attributable to an operation or procedure or where the Chief Coroner considers circumstances should be better ascertained.	*Coroners Act 1997* (ACT)
New South Wales	A death that occurred that was not the reasonably expected outcome of a medical, surgical, dental or other health-related procedure.	*Coroners Act 2009* (NSW)
Northern Territory	A death that occurred during an anaesthetic or as a result of an anaesthetic and is not due to natural causes.	*Coroners Act* (NT)
Queensland	A death that occurred after receiving or failing to receive health care where it is likely to have caused or contributed to the death and an independent person would not have reasonably expected it to have caused or contributed to the death.	*Coroners Act 2003* (Qld)
South Australia	A death that occurred during, as a result or within 24 hours of a surgical procedure or invasive medical or diagnostic procedure or the administration of an anaesthetic, or that occurs within 24 hours of a person being discharged from hospital or having sought emergency treatment at a hospital.	*Coroners Act 2003* (SA)
Tasmania	A death that occurred during a medical procedure, or after a medical procedure where the death may be causally related to that procedure, and a doctor would not immediately before the procedure have reasonably expected the death.	*Coroners Act 1995* (Tas)
Victoria	A death that occurred during a medical procedure or following a medical procedure where the death is or may be causally related to the procedure, and a doctor would not immediately before the procedure have reasonably expected death.	*Coroners Act 2008* (Vic)
Western Australia	A death that occurred during an anaesthetic or as a result of an anaesthetic and is not due to natural causes.	*Coroners Act 1996* (WA)

legislation in every State and Territory in Australia provides that the coroner can also 'comment' and make recommendations regarding 'public health or safety'. In cases where the death was considered preventable, the coroner may recommend steps be taken to prevent a death in similar circumstances in the future.

The example below demonstrates how such recommendations may affect nursing and midwifery practice.

The case of Bela Heidrich (Inquest into the death of Bela Heidrich, Queensland Coroner's Court, 2008/562, 29 June 2011)

The Queensland case of Bela Heidrich involved the coroner investigating the death of newborn Bela while her mother was in hospital. The coroner made findings that Bela died through suffocation while being breastfed in bed with her mother shortly after birth. Her mother had fallen asleep while breastfeeding. As well as making these findings, the coroner also made a series of recommendations to Queensland Health, which suggests how the conduct of nurses and midwives who care for mothers and newborns following birth could be improved.

Recommendations, which would be relevant for nurses and midwives, included:

- That Queensland Health consider whether it should have a policy which specifically requires the following steps to be taken before breastfeeding lying down by a new mother occurs:

  a) That a risk assessment be conducted to consider the condition of the mother, in particular that she is lucid and awake and that this is noted in the patient's medical records;

  b) That the mother be given some information about the dangers of falling asleep and be provided with a buzzer to be able to contact staff in the event she becomes tired, the baby has stopped feeding or is unsettled; and

  c) That a determination be made about the level of supervision required and this be noted in the patient's medical records.

This case demonstrates how relevant recommendations may be made by a coroner to reduce the risk of death occurring in similar circumstances.

Where the coroner makes recommendations to State or Territory government departments, there is an obligation for those departments to act and consider implementing the relevant changes recommended.

Interaction between coronial inquests and other proceedings (disciplinary, criminal)

Sometimes the coroner will make a finding adverse to a health care institution or health professional despite the fact that the purpose of such investigations is not to allocate blame. However, the coroner does not have powers to start criminal, civil or disciplinary action against an institution or professional and, indeed, is prevented from commenting on the criminal liability of persons (*Coroners Act 2003* (SA), s 25(3); *Coroners Act 2008* (Vic), s 69(1); *Coroners Act 1995* (Tas), s 28(4); *Coroners Act 2009* (NSW), s 82(3); Coroners Act (NT), s 34(3)).

In the majority of States and Territories the legislation specifically states that the coroner can refer a matter to the State/Territory prosecution for their consideration about whether to pursue a matter and charge a person with a criminal offence (*Coroners Act 1997* (ACT), s 58; *Coroners Act 2003* (Qld), s 48(2); *Coroners Act* (NT), s 35(3); *Coroners Act 2008* (Vic), s 49(1); *Coroners Act 1995* (Tas), s 30(3); *Coroners Act 2009* (NSW), s 82(2)(b); *Coroners Act 1996* (WA), s 27(5)).

In Queensland and Western Australia the legislation specifically states that the coroner can refer potential misconduct to professional bodies for consideration of disciplinary action. This would include referrals to the Australian Nursing and Midwifery Board (*Coroners Act 2003* (Qld), s 48(4); *Coroners Act 1996* (WA), s 50). In other States and Territories, the legislation, although worded more generally, would also allow the coroner to refer matters to professional bodies (Staunton and Chiarella 2012, p. 294).

Overview

This chapter has introduced the basics of what the law is and how it operates within the context of the Australian legal system. An appreciation of the legal background and principles discussed in this chapter is a necessary precursor to understanding the law in the chapters that follow.

Further reading

➢ Forrester, K. & Griffiths, D. 2014, *Essentials of Law for Health Professionals*, 4th edn, Elsevier: Sydney, chaps. 1–2, 10.

Questions

What effect do the following hypothetical laws have on a nurse's legal obligations in your State or Territory?

1. A case has just been decided in the New South Wales Supreme Court in relation to health care. This case has received a lot of media attention as it changes the previous law.

2. A recently amended section of Commonwealth legislation sets out what nurses must do in relation to the disposal of dangerous drugs but this is different from the procedure set out in the legislation in your State or Territory.

3. A recent decision of the United States' Supreme Court (the highest court in the United States) sets a new precedent making it mandatory for nurses to disclose patient information if the nurse has information that a patient intends to harm a third person.

Scenario

Paul is a nurse at a public hospital. He administers the wrong dose of medication to a patient and the patient subsequently dies. The patient's family wants legal action taken against Paul. Based on these limited facts, is Paul's case likely to be a civil or a criminal matter? What other avenues might be open to the family? What factors have you considered to reach your conclusion?

4

Ethics, law and nursing and midwifery practice

Introduction

In Chapter 2 we discussed the 'social contract' – the unwritten implied contract between the professions of nursing and midwifery and the public. The terms of this social contract are that the public will go to those professions for nursing and midwifery care and treatment. In return, the professions of nursing and midwifery make sure those professions provide satisfactory care and treatment by regulating the practice and conduct of nurses and midwives. So how do the professions do this? What are the implications for nursing and midwifery practice? Do any other responsibilities arise from the social contract? Nurses and midwives are responsible and accountable to their patients, their colleagues, their profession, the public, regulatory bodies and their employers for maintaining their professional competence, practising in accordance with accepted standards and in compliance with the law.

Ethics and nursing and midwifery practice

The principles approach

Justice

The most immediately relevant face of justice, when talking about nursing and midwifery practice, is legal justice – which in Chapter 2 was defined as 'respect for morally just laws and being accountable for one's actions or inaction'. What implications does this have for nursing and midwifery practice?

Respect for morally just laws

It is hard to imagine that anyone could suggest that the legal framework put in place to regulate the professions of nursing and midwifery is not morally just when its primary purpose is to protect the public. The mandatory reporting provisions contained within the legal framework, where one registered health professional is required to report another registered health professional in some circumstances, have been more contentious. Although generally supported by the professions of nursing and midwifery, there have been concerns raised about the potential impact on overseas-trained nurses (Kochardy 2010), impaired health professionals (Australian Health Ministers Advisory Council 2017) and professional self-regulation (Jackson and Parker 2009). Some of these concerns are arguably, at the very least, balanced, if not overruled, by the potential harms resulting to patients and to the public's trust in the health professions if a health professional continues to practise in an unsafe manner.

Accountability

Accountability is an important facet of justice (Sharpe 2004). It is also an equally important part of the social contract. The understanding that a health profession will hold its members to account for any actions or omissions in a professional (and, rarely, in a personal) context is key to the social contract and to the understanding of the principle of justice. However, upholding the principle of justice is not just an institutional obligation but also a personal one. This would involve a nurse or midwife being honest about events that have occurred. This honesty may be in terms of keeping accurate records, participating in disclosure processes and not seeking to avoid accountability, for example by concealing events, falsifying records or lying. There is also arguably a positive ethical obligation: that nurses and midwives may have an obligation to their profession and to the general public to take action, generally through reporting the activities of other individuals, organisations or systems that are not acting in the interests of patients or the public. This is also a form of being accountable to the public for one's knowledge.

Distributive justice

Distributive justice refers to the fair distribution of resources, which recognises that nurses and midwives are themselves valuable resources, integral to the operation of the health system. As such, the fair distribution of human resources matters in ensuring healthy outcomes for all Australians. Nurses and midwives under this principle need to consider resource implications and advocate for patients and populations.

Rights-based justice

Rights-based justice (respecting patient rights) is another aspect of justice which indicates that nurses and midwives should practise in a manner that enables patient rights and human rights more generally.

Beneficence and non-maleficence

The principle of beneficence suggests that nurses and midwives must practise safely, competently and ethically to act in the best interests of their patients. The principle of non-maleficence suggests nurses and midwives have a duty to do no harm and to protect patients from harm. These principles are connected in the context of nursing and midwifery practice.

The principles of beneficence and non-maleficence jointly suggest that nurses and midwives should not exploit patients. Both principles recognise the relative power imbalances between health professionals and patients due to the training, the professional and social status of the health professional, the particular vulnerability of some patients due to their illness, and the general vulnerability of patients who may have a lesser knowledge of health care or of the health system. Even patients who are trained health professionals may admit that the experience of being a patient can be disorientating and disempowering, despite their knowledge and expertise. Given this, these principles speak to the importance of nurses and midwives maintaining professional boundaries. Professional boundaries are the boundaries between a professional and therapeutic relationship and a personal relationship between nurses and/or midwives and patients, also their spouses and partners and family.

It is not in a patient's best interest if a nurse or a midwife practises outside their scope of practice (except in an emergency), lacks competence or seeks to exploit patients and indeed these types of practice might cause harm to patients, the public and/or colleagues. It is also arguably not in patients' best interests if a nurse or midwife knows another health professional lacks competence and yet does nothing to safeguard patients. These principles would seem to create a corresponding obligation to take positive action to report potential risks before and after they eventuate. The principle of beneficence also creates an obligation to undertake professional development and training.

Autonomy

The principle of autonomy in a health care context is premised on a patient's right to make choices about their best interests. This could suggest that patients should be told if there are any concerns about the nurse's or midwife's health, competence or conduct, if those concerns may pose a risk to that patient. However, the principle of autonomy is also relevant to a nurse or midwife as they must make choices (exercise their autonomy) about how they are going to practise their profession and interact with their patients and co-workers. Having said this, the professions of nursing and midwifery emphasise caring for others and patient-centred care. This implies that, although a nurse or midwife is an autonomous actor, his or her exercise of autonomy in a professional context is constrained by a need to put the interests of others before self-interest.

The nursing and midwifery codes

As discussed in Chapter 2, one mechanism through which the professions uphold their part of the social contract is through establishing ethical and other standards for practice and conduct. In Australia, this has been done through the use of Codes of Ethics from the ICN and the ICM and the creation of Codes of Conduct by the Nursing and Midwifery Board of Australia for each profession. In that context the Codes as a whole are relevant to ensuring the integrity and professionalism of nursing and midwifery practice. Having said that, there are specific principles that are particularly relevant to the practice of nursing and midwifery.

Competence

Competence is a key aspect of discussions around the ethical principles of beneficence and non-maleficence and is central to the Codes of Ethics and Conduct for both professions. Principle 2 of the ICN Code of Ethics relevantly notes: 'The nurse carries personal responsibility and accountability for nursing practice, and for maintaining competence by continual learning.' The ICM Code of Ethics (II c) states: 'midwives use up-to-date, evidence-based professional knowledge to maintain competence in safe midwifery practices.' The Code of Conduct for Nurses also notes in Principle 2.1 that 'nurses apply person-centred and evidence-based decision-making, and have a responsibility to ensure the delivery of safe and quality care. Nurses must a. practice in accordance with the standards of the profession and broader health system ...' Similarly, the Code of Conduct for Midwives at Principle 2.1 uses identical wording, although 'person-centred' is replaced by 'woman-centred'.

As noted above, there seems an ethical imperative for nurses and midwives to further beneficence and non-maleficence by participating in professional development. This is clear in the ICM Code of Ethics which notes at II f that 'midwives actively seek personal, intellectual and professional growth throughout their midwifery career, integrating this growth into their practice'. This obligation is implicit in the ICN Code of Ethics Principle 2: 'The nurse carries personal responsibility and accountability for nursing practice, and for maintaining competence by continual learning.' Both Codes of Conduct (1.1.c) note that completing professional development is a legal requirement.

Questioning and reporting

The statements outlined above speak to the necessity of retaining professional competence, but what should a midwife or nurse do if there is concern that a health professional's competence or conduct is in question? Some health professionals, particularly doctors, have expressed concerns about questioning and reporting concerns about competence or conduct in terms of the consequences for themselves and for other health professionals, although others see reporting as a protective mechanism (Kingston et al. 2004). Others note that if health professionals are not seen to be acting to protect patients by raising legitimate concerns, no matter the consequences to themselves, it may damage public trust in the health professions (Jackson and Parker 2009). The ICN Codes of Ethics emphasise the importance of questioning and reporting issues in respect of competence and conduct. For example, Principle 4 in the ICN notes: 'The nurse takes appropriate action to safeguard individuals, families and communities when their health is endangered by a co-worker or any other person.' The Codes of Conduct also note that nurses and midwives should abide by any reporting requirements (1.1.a and 7.1.e).

Reporting does not just relate to the actions of other health professionals. The Codes of Conduct are clear that nurses or midwives should self-report to an appropriate authority personal health limitations that may compromise their ability to practise safely (7.1.e). Principle 7 of the Codes of Conduct also emphasises the importance of nurses and midwives having a 'responsibility to maintain their physical and mental health to practise safely and effectively'.

Conscientious objection

The ICM Code of Ethics (III c, d) recognises that at times there may be a conflict between a midwife's personal or religious values and the provision of some types of health services. Accordingly, it recognises that midwives are entitled to conscientiously object or refuse to participate in the provision of certain types of health services. This is also stated in the Codes of Conduct (4.4.b) but it is noted that they must inform the patient of their objection and make sure that the person has alternative care options. Commonly used examples of conscientious objection are that some people have a religious or moral objection to abortion on the basis that to terminate a foetus is to terminate a potential or actual life and some object to providing assistance in dying (assisted suicide or voluntary euthanasia).

Professional boundaries

The maintenance of professional boundaries is a key part of nursing and midwifery practice. Professional boundaries are the limits on relationships between a nurse/midwife and a patient(s) and the patient's significant others, which includes under- or overinvolvement in the provision of care. The Codes of Conduct for both professions contain Principle 4.1 Professional boundaries. Both Codes are clear: nurses and midwives have a responsibility to maintain professional boundaries between themselves and patients and others involved in that person's care (i.e. partners, family).

Sexual relationships with a current or past patient may also be held to be inappropriate in most circumstances, even when the patient has consented (Codes of Conduct 4.1.d). Both Codes of Conduct also address gifts and state that only token gifts of minimal value should be accepted (4.5.b) and that nurses and midwives should not 'accept, encourage or manipulate people to give, lend or bequeath money or gifts that will benefit a [nurse or midwife] directly or indirectly' and 'not become financially involved with a person who has or will be in receipt of their care, for example through bequests, powers of attorney, loans and investment schemes …' (4.5.c, d).

It is not just with patients that professional boundaries need to be maintained but also with family, friends and those with whom one has a non-professional relationship. Nurses and midwives need to exercise caution when providing advice and should not be required to provide nursing or midwifery care to those with whom they have close personal relationships (Codes of Conduct 4.1.c).

Law and nursing and midwifery practice

Professional regulation

The social contract sees partial expression in the legal framework that regulates health professionals. This framework enables the professions to provide assurances that persons are qualified to practise as a nurse or midwife (for example, that someone who claims to be a nurse actually has the right training and skills and retains them) and provides mechanisms to protect the public from professionals whose competence or conduct places the public at risk.

As discussed in Chapter 3, the Australian Constitution allocates specified responsibilities to the Commonwealth government. The responsibility for regulating health professionals was not allocated to the Commonwealth in the Constitution, leaving such regulation to be the responsibility of the states and territories. As a consequence, until 2010, Australia had eight different systems to regulate health professionals. This was considered to be problematic as it meant that a midwife in one state, for example, might be dealt with in the legal framework in a different way than they would be dealt with in another state or a nurse would be dealt with in a different way than would a dentist (Productivity Commission 2005). In addition, the different legal frameworks made it difficult for a nurse or midwife to move from state to state as they would have to re-register each time, negatively affecting workforce mobility (Productivity Commission 2005). After several years of negotiation the Commonwealth, states and territories reached an agreement for a national framework to consistently regulate a number of health professions across all Australian states and territories (Council of Australian Governments 2008). Although there was a national agreement, because the states and territories have the power to regulate in this area, each state and territory had to pass legislation to enable the national agreement to be put in place. It was agreed that Queensland would pass the legislation and the other states and territories would pass legislation that essentially said that the law in Queensland would be the law in that state or territory (with the partial exception of New South Wales and, more recently, Queensland). Accordingly, the relevant law is the schedule to the *Health Practitioner Regulation National Law Act 2009* (Qld) (all references to 'the Act' in this chapter are references to the schedule in this Act) which came into effect on 1 July 2010.

Regulated Health Professions – July 2018

Aboriginal and Torres Strait Islander Health practice

Chinese medicine

Chiropractors

Dental (dentists, dental hygienists, dental prosthetists, dental therapists)

Medical

Medical radiation practice

Nurses and midwifery

Occupational therapy

Optometry

Osteopathy

Paramedicine

Pharmacy

Physiotherapy

Podiatry

Psychology

The purpose of the Act and the legislative scheme for the regulation of health professionals is explicitly set out in section 3(2)(a) of the Act, including to: 'Provide for the *protection* of the public by ensuring that only health practitioners who are suitably trained and qualified to practise in a competent and ethical manner are registered' (emphasis added).

The Act also established the Australian Health Practitioners Regulatory Authority (AHPRA) which provides support to the National Boards for each profession (for nursing and midwifery the Nursing and Midwifery Board of Australia) through establishing a national process for applications for registration, national registers for each health profession, and a process for receiving and addressing mandatory and voluntary reports and self-reports. National registers are publicly accessible and enable a person to confirm that a professional is registered and the status of that registration. There are separate registers for nurses (including registration as an enrolled nurse and endorsement as a nurse practitioner) and midwives (including endorsement as a midwife practitioner or as an eligible midwife), although there can be dual registration as both a nurse and a midwife. Nurses and midwives can also be endorsed in respect of prescribing or administering scheduled (restricted) medicines. A nurse or midwife can also choose to be on the practising or non-practising register. There are also registers for student midwives and nurses.

Registration

The first element of the social contract requires that the public knows that, when it seeks health care services from a nurse or midwife, the person claiming to be a nurse or midwife has the requisite training and qualifications required by the professions of nursing and midwifery. A person must be registered to use the titles nurse, midwife or registered health professional (ss 113, 116). If a professional is registered in one state or territory they can now practise in any other state or territory without re-registering. A person may be registered if they:

➤ are qualified;

➤ have completed any required period of supervised practice;

➤ have completed required exams or assessment;

➤ are suitable; and

➤ are not disqualified (ss 42, 57, 62).

A national board may decide not to register a person if:

➤ the person is impaired (has a health condition that might affect their ability to practise safely);

➤ the person has a criminal history;

➤ proceedings are underway against the person;

➤ the person lacks English competency; or

➤ the person's registration was suspended or cancelled elsewhere (s 52).

However, if the registration body has a concern about a person's capacity or suitability to practise it may impose conditions on the person's registration (s 52) – allowing them to practise but imposing limitations on what they can do in order to protect the public.

A key issue is whether the person is considered unsuitable to practice and therefore not fit to be registered – this goes back to the element of the social contract which emphasises that the public must be able to trust the professions of nursing and midwifery to maintain the integrity of the profession. The cases set out below discuss these issues.

***Chan v The Nurses Board of Western Australia* [2005] WASAT 115**

Chan had previously been registered as a nurse but her registration had lapsed after she had been convicted of theft and fraud and sentenced to nine years in prison. Chan was on parole when she applied for registration and did not advise the Board of her status. Her application for registration was refused on the grounds that the offence she had been convicted of made her unsuitable to practise as a nurse. It was held that the criminal convictions fundamentally undermined her claim to be trustworthy and of an honest character. The Court considered that the time that had elapsed since Chan's conviction was too short for her to suggest her integrity had been restored.

***HCCC v Martin* [2009] NSWNMT 3**

Martin was an enrolled nurse who had been convicted of two counts of indecent assault of a person below 16 years of age and one of having intercourse with a person under 16 years of age by a person in authority; there were two similar charges relating to sexual intercourse that were also taken into account. The victim was his daughter. She was 8 years old when the indecent assaults began and 12–13 when her father first had intercourse with her. He was sentenced to a non-parole period of four years and one month. On his release he applied for re-registration. The Tribunal was particularly concerned about Martin's lack of insight into the harm he had caused his daughter. The Tribunal held he was unfit to practise nursing as he was not of good character and should not be re-registered. To protect the public the Tribunal ordered that Martin could not re-apply for registration for another four years and recommended extensive counselling in the interim.

It is a fundamental principle of our criminal justice system that after a criminal conviction a person can rehabilitate themselves in the eyes of society. The cases discussed above are consistent with that principle. In both cases the Court and/or Tribunal made it clear that the applicants could reapply for registration at some point, if they could establish, to the satisfaction of the registration body, that they had been rehabilitated.

Endorsements to registration

A Board can also place an endorsement on a nurse's or midwife's registration, indicating they have some special qualification or privilege.

Endorsement for scheduled medicines

Section 94(1) of the Act allows the Board to endorse the registration of a nurse or midwife as being qualified to 'administer, obtain, possess, prescribe, sell, supply or use a scheduled medicine or class of scheduled medicines' in certain circumstances. Authorisation for the nurse or midwife to actually do this must first be obtained from the jurisdiction in which the nurse or midwife is practising pursuant to other legislation (usually drugs and poisons legislation). The endorsement must specify the scheduled medicine or class of medicines, what use is permitted and the date the endorsement expires (s 94(2)). Nurses and midwives can currently be endorsed as practising in rural and remote areas, or as an eligible midwife (they can prescribe scheduled medicines).

Specialist endorsement – nurses

Section 95 permits registered nurses to be given endorsement as a nurse practitioner, assuming they have the relevant qualifications and meet relevant registration standards. It authorises a nurse to use the title 'nurse practitioner' and sets out any conditions for practice as a nurse practitioner (in other words it establishes the nurse practitioner's scope of practice including their qualifications in respect of medications). Nurse practitioners will still have to be authorised by the relevant state or territorial authorities in respect of medications.

Nurse practitioners are permitted to apply for a provider and/or prescriber number from the Medicare Benefits Schedule (MBS) and the Pharmaceutical Benefits Scheme (PBS) under the *Health Legislation Amendment (Midwives and Nurse Practitioners) Act 2010* (Cth). This will enable their patients to access some MBS rebates and PBS prescriptions. There are specific requirements for collaboration under the *National Health (Collaborative Arrangements for Nurse Practitioners) Determination 2010* (Cth) sections 5–7.

Notation – midwives

The Maternity Services Review recommended MBS/PBS benefits for some services provided by what they termed 'eligible midwives' (a specific class of midwives). A notation needs to be placed on the registration of members of this class of midwives indicating they have the qualifications to access MBS (s 38(2)).

Renewal of registration

It is not sufficient that a professional has the requisite qualifications and training and is suitable to practise when he or she enters the profession. The social contract requires the maintenance of competence and conduct to sustain the public trust. Accordingly, each year the Act requires that a nurse or midwife must renew their registration to provide the professions and the registration body with data on which they can determine whether a professional should stay registered. As part of this process nurses and midwives must provide a statement that they:

➤ Do not have an impairment impacting on the safety of their practice;

➤ Meet recency of practice requirements (i.e. it is recognised that if a person is not practising, for example as a midwife, for several years the professional is likely to lose their skills and so if admitted back to practise may place patients at risk);

➤ Have completed continuing professional development (CPD);

➤ Hold professional indemnity insurance;

➤ Maintain the right to practise; and

➤ Do not have a complaint made against them (s 109).

The Health Ombudsman v Jamieson [2017] QCAT 172

A registered nurse stole three boxes of antibiotics from her employer. She pled guilty before the court and was sentenced without the court recording a conviction. She did not notify the National Board under section 130 of the Act (see below). She also made a false declaration when she applied to renew her registration when she ticked 'no' to the question 'since your last declaration to AHPRA, has there been any change to your criminal history in Australia that you have not declared to AHPRA?' knowing that she had been charged and convicted for theft. The Tribunal found she has committed professional misconduct. She was reprimanded. She had earlier voluntarily de-registered herself.

The Health Ombudsman v Chambers [2017] QCAT 362

The registered nurse scrubbed up and entered the operating theatre to work as part of the anaesthetics team. She had a conversation with the Anaesthetist, who reported

▶

◄

to the scrub nurse that the nurse appeared drunk. The scrub nurse confronted her. The registered nurse left theatre and was found asleep in recovery 20 minutes later: her pupils were dilated, left the theatre she was loud, abusive, agitated and aggressive. Police were called and reported she was glassy eyed, erratic and smelt of alcohol. Her employment was terminated. She was charged with resisting arrest and driving under the influence of alcohol and convicted on both counts. She did not inform the Board of her convictions. The Tribunal reprimanded and fined her.

Self-reporting

Significant issues may arise during the registration period that the registration authority also needs to know about to protect the public. Section 130 of the Act requires that a nurse or midwife must advise the registration body if:

➤ They are charged with a criminal offence (that would, if the person is convicted, be punishable by more than 12 months' imprisonment);

➤ They are convicted of an offence punishable by imprisonment;

➤ They no longer carry indemnity insurance;

➤ Their right to practise at a hospital is withdrawn, suspended or restricted;

➤ Their authority to prescribe drugs is withdrawn;

➤ A complaint is made against them; or

➤ Their overseas registration is cancelled, suspended or conditions are imposed on it.

Obligations

The Act also imposes some obligations on nurses and midwives, again as part of the maintenance of the social contract. CPD is required to ensure nurses and midwives remain up to date with developments in their professions and to maintain the public's trust. Accordingly, the Act requires that all registered health professionals complete CPD (s 128). As of 2018 this requires that nurses and midwives participate in 20 hours of relevant CPD per year. If the nurse or midwife has any endorsements on their registration an additional 10 hours of CPD per annum is required. The nurse or midwife must keep evidence of participation.

In addition, all registered health professionals must hold professional indemnity insurance (s 129). There are two reasons for this. First, insurance is necessary to ensure that if a patient sustains an injury as the result of the negligent provision of a health service some compensation will be forthcoming. Second, insurance enables a health professional to be represented by a lawyer. Indemnity insurance may be provided by an employer as part of the contract of employment or it may be purchased by the individual nurse or midwife. Students are not required to have insurance nor are non-practising nurses or midwives.

Mandatory reporting

Mandatory reporting requirements were introduced into law in Australia because there had been a string of cases (in Australia and outside it) where there was a perception that widely shared concerns by health professionals about a particular health professional may not have been reported, particularly to the registration body for that profession (McDonald 2018). The lack of reporting was perceived, in some instances, to have led to patient harm and caused public disquiet. While the necessity to report a fellow health professional who may be causing harm is an ethical obligation – connected with beneficence and non-maleficence (see the discussion above) – the passing of the mandatory reporting provisions in the Act may be seen as an element of the social contract as it now requires health professionals to report to serve what governments consider to be the public interest. The Act now makes it mandatory for health professionals to report other health professionals in certain circumstances. Section 140 of the Act states that a registered health professional must notify the AHPRA if he or she has a reasonable belief (a belief supported by good reasons) that another registered health professional has:

➢ Practised while intoxicated (alcohol or drugs);

➢ Engaged in sexual misconduct during the course of professional practice;

➢ Placed the public at risk of substantial harm because of an impairment; or

➢ Placed the public at risk of harm because he or she practised in a way that constitutes a significant departure from accepted professional standards.

Reporting may be done electronically, by mail, by phone or in person.

Two jurisdictions have placed limitations on mandatory reporting on health-related matters. In Queensland under the *Health Ombudsman Act 2013* (Qld) s 325(25) the obligation does not apply to a health professional providing treatment to another health professional if the treating professional does not believe that the impairment will place the public at substantial risk of harm. In Western Australia section 4(7) of the *Health Practitioner Regulation National Law (WA) Act 2010* (WA) states mandatory reporting is not required if the health professional is providing health services to the second health professional or student.

This aspect of the mandatory reporting framework is currently under review nationally (Australian Health Ministers Advisory Council 2017).

Intoxication

The requirement to report intoxication only arises in a professional context – did the nurse or midwife see a registered health practitioner who was intoxicated by alcohol or drugs while practising as a registered health professional? Refer to *The Health Ombudsman v Chambers* [2017] QCAT 362 at p. 67–68.

Sexual misconduct

The Codes of Conduct state that nurses and midwives should avoid sexual relationships with a person with 'whom they [the nurse or midwife] have currently or had previously entered into a professional relationship. These relationships are inappropriate in most circumstances' (4.1.d). The Guidelines for Mandatory Notifications (APHRA 2014b, p. 8) state that:

> sexual misconduct also includes making sexual remarks, touching patients or clients in a sexual way, or engaging in sexual behaviour in front of a patient or client. Engaging in sexual activity with a person who is closely related to a patient or client under the practitioner's care may also constitute misconduct … Engaging in sexual activity with a person formerly under a practitioner's care (i.e. after the termination of the practitioner–patient/client relationship) may also constitute sexual misconduct. Relevant factors will include the cultural context, the vulnerability of the patient or client due to issues such as age, capacity and/or health conditions; the extent of the professional relationship; for example, a one-off treatment in an emergency department compared to a long-term programme of treatment; and the length of time since the practitioner–patient/client relationship ceased.

Jacobsen v Nurses Tribunal & Anor (Unreported, Supreme Court of New South Wales, 3 October 1997)

Jacobsen was a registered mental health nurse and a member of a rehabilitation scheme run by a health authority. He was the case manager for a female patient variously diagnosed with schizophrenia and manic depression. The patient's marriage had broken down, her ex-husband had the children, and she wanted to have her children move back in with her. It was decided that the patient and two of her children should move into the nurse's house as paid boarders. He would cease to be her case manager. She moved in three weeks after he had ceased being her case manager. He did not advise his employer of the arrangement. When the employer discovered it they suggested it was inappropriate that she remain living in his house.

Three months after she moved out they established a seven-month sexual relationship. The NSW Tribunal found him guilty of unsatisfactory professional conduct because he:

- Invited her to live in his house and entered into a sexual relationship without properly terminating the professional relationship.

- Ended a professional relationship with a patient when about to commence a personal one.

Because the matter as a whole was so serious, it amounted to professional misconduct (the most serious charge).

Jacobsen appealed. The Court held that he was aware that the woman's mental disorders made her vulnerable to exploitation. Despite this Jacobsen fostered the non-professional relationship between them. Although care was transferred, it did not terminate Jacobsen's power and influence over her. He still had all the confidential information he had gained about her and it was implicit that he would still assist her and be partly involved in her care. The Court agreed that his conduct amounted to professional misconduct because of the seriousness of his breach of standards and de-registered him for six months.

Nursing and Midwifery Board of Australia v Stephenson [2016] SAHPT 6

A registered nurse engaged in a sexual relationship with the spouse of a patient when providing palliative care to the patient. The nurse also engaged in sexual contact while the nurse's 15-year-old female relative. The nurse was de-registered and he was disqualified from applying for registration for a period of four years.

Sexual misconduct, as is evident in the Jacobsen case described above, may occur with a former patient, although relevant factors will include vulnerability, the extent of the previous professional relationship and the length of time since the professional relationship was terminated. Sexual misconduct will also apply when a nurse or midwife has a sexual relationship with the partner of a patient.

Impairment

Another ground to report a registered health professional is impairment. 'Impairment' is defined in section 5 of the Act as:

> a physical or mental impairment, disability, condition or disorder (including substance abuse or dependence) that detrimentally affects or is likely to detrimentally affect a registered health professional or applicant for registration's capacity to practise the profession or the student's capacity to undertake clinical training.

Many, if not all, nurses and midwives will have an impairment at some point in their professional life. The mere existence of an impairment is not sufficient to trigger a report. The impairment must detrimentally affect the professional's, applicant's or student's capacity to practise and must place the public at risk of substantial harm. An example of an impairment that affects capacity to practise and that was considered substantial enough to place the public at risk of substantial harm is set out below.

HCCC v Marr [2008] NSWNMT 3

Marr was an enrolled nurse. There were multiple serious concerns raised about her competence, including that she attempted to give juice and food to patients who were nil by mouth and insulin to a patient who had a blood sugar level of below six, she did not follow aseptic technique or basic infection control procedures, she had attempted to commence an infusion before the placement of a PICC line had been confirmed by x-ray and so on. After concerns had been raised by her colleagues her employer had provided her with opportunities for training and mentoring and had assigned a registered nurse to shadow her; as a result of this there had been no harm to patients. Ultimately, the Health Authority reported its concerns to the registration body. On examination Marr was found to have severe depression and a paranoid personality disorder. Her employer was concerned that she posed a substantial risk to patients and to herself, a concern shared by the examining psychiatrists. Because the nature of her impairment posed a substantial risk of harm to patients the Tribunal removed her name from the register. The Tribunal ordered that she could not apply for re-registration for a period of two years. Owing to the seriousness of her condition and the level of risk she posed, the Tribunal thought it possible she would never be re-registered.

Professional standards

The final ground to report is a reasonable belief that a registered health professional has significantly departed from accepted professional standards placing the public at risk. This is a high threshold and a judgement needs to be made about what is a significant departure from professional standards. Conversely, there needs to be only some level of risk posed to the public.

It is especially difficult when a nurse or midwife has concerns about a person from another health profession, as it is not always easy to assess the standards of another profession. It might be easier for a member of one health profession (e.g. nursing) to assess a health professional from a different health profession (e.g. medicine) if the professions work closely together and have a good understanding of what constitutes accepted professional standards for the other profession. In general the threshold to decide whether or not to report is high (significant/substantial) and the focus is on behaviour that puts the public at risk of harm – not that the nurse or midwife does not like the way a person does their job, feels they could do it better or there is another accepted way of doing it that the health professional prefers.

Section 141 of the Act states that a nurse or midwife does not need to report to APHRA if he or she formed a belief that another registered health professional should be reported while:

➢ Acting for a professional indemnity insurer

➢ Providing legal advice

➢ Sitting on a quality assurance committee.

Nor do they need to advise APHRA if the nurse or midwife reasonably believes it has already been informed (s 141).

What if you do not report when you should? Failure to make a mandatory report or failure to comply with a self-reporting obligation is grounds for disciplinary action (ss 128, 129, 130, 141). In *Medical Board of Australia v Al-Naser* [2015] ACAT 15 disciplinary proceedings were brought against Dr Al-Naser for a number of matters, including a failure to make a mandatory notification against another doctor, Dr Khalil, who was a colleague and employee. A patient told Dr Al-Naser on six occasions that she was having a sexual relationship with Dr Khalil but he did not report this. The Tribunal reprimanded him and conditions were imposed on his practice. He was required to undertake an ethics and communication course, meet with a mentor regularly and pay costs.

Voluntary reporting

The Act also makes provision for health professionals to voluntarily report other health professionals when they have concerns about that person but where those concerns are not sufficient to require a mandatory report. Under the Act a health professional may voluntarily report to APHRA concerns:

➤ That another health professional's conduct, knowledge, skill or judgement falls below the standard;

➤ A health professional is not suitable to be registered;

➤ That an impairment affects a health professional's professional practice;

➤ A health professional has contravened the law or conditions imposed on their professional practice; or

➤ A health professional has given false information to the Board (s 144).

Protections

If a nurse or midwife makes a mandatory or voluntary report in good faith, the Act protects that person from legal proceedings (civil, criminal and administrative proceedings, including proceedings in defamation) (s 237). 'Good faith' is a legal term that means the report was made reasonably, sincerely and honestly with no malicious or fraudulent intent.

Fitness to practise

Part of the social contract is the capacity for the professions to take action to protect the public from members whose competence or conduct threatens the public's safety. The fitness to practise sections of the Act gives the professions the legal authority to take action against individual health professionals to protect the public. New South Wales did not adopt the Act in its entirety so what is described in these sections does not apply in New South Wales. Queensland subsequently decided to also not adopt this aspect of the Act in its entirety. As health professionals are a valuable, and in some contexts a scarce, resource, the public has an interest in making sure that health professionals maintain their ability to practise so long as mechanisms are in place to ensure the safety of the public (McDonald 2018).

There are two layers of mechanisms in place: panels and discipline. Panels focus on remediation and discipline focuses on the most serious competence or conduct issues. The fitness to practise mechanisms can be triggered by investigations by the Boards into mandatory, voluntary or self-reports, complaints, or other sources of information. These mechanisms are available in all jurisdictions but are administered at the state level in New South Wales.

To protect the public the Board has powers to suspend a professional from practice or impose conditions as an interim measure pending a full investigation (s 156). It also may take immediate action in a variety of other circumstances, including a suspicion that a person improperly obtained registration (ss 156, 178).

New South Wales

The New South Wales government elected to retain its pre-existing fitness to practise and disciplinary mechanisms. In that state the independent Health Complaints Commission retains primary responsibility for complaint investigation and commencing disciplinary proceedings in consultation with the professional boards. The professional boards administer the other fitness to practise processes.

Queensland

Queensland decided to adopt an hybrid model combining the national approach and New South Wales approaches. The Health Ombudsman retains primary responsibility for receipt of complaints. It must retain, investigate and bring proceedings in respect of the most serious cases and has discretion to refer the other less serious matters to the National Boards to address.

Health Panel

A person's health may affect his or her ability to practise safely. If the Board has a reasonable belief that a nurse or a midwife has an impairment (see definition at p. 72) which detrimentally affects their ability to practise it may order that person undergo a health assessment (ss 160, 169) and refer the case to a Health Panel (a panel established by the Board to assess professionals with impairments). A Health Panel examines the report by the assessors and any other evidence and may impose a programme to ensure the nurse or midwife will practise safely – for example, create a treatment plan, require supervision, or place conditions on practice (such as regular drug testing). In the most serious cases a Health Panel may impose conditions on a person's registration, suspend them or refer the matter for disciplinary action. The case discussed below is an example of how the process works.

Health Care Complaints Commission v Thompson [2008] NSWNMT 14 (22 August 2008)

Thompson was a registered midwife. She had been diagnosed with post-traumatic stress disorder, anti-depressant-induced hypomania and Substance Dependence Disorder. The hospital reported Thompson to the Board raising behavioural and performance problems and questioning her ability to practise safely and competently as they believed she was an impaired practitioner.

The Board imposed conditions on Thompson's practice requiring her to attend a medical assessment and only work under supervision. A medical assessment was undertaken by two psychiatrists. Thompson refused blood tests, provided an unclear or incomplete history in respect of current alcohol consumption and was uncooperative. The psychiatrists independently concluded that it was not possible to reach a conclusion about the impact of alcohol abuse or whether she was alcohol dependent but it was also not possible to say she was a safe practitioner.

As a consequence a disciplinary proceeding occurred. The Tribunal imposed additional conditions on Thompson's registration – that she undertake blood analysis tests and a neuropsychological assessment. She was seen by a psychologist who conducted a neuropsychological assessment but she was also uncooperative during this process. The psychologist concluded that she had some cognitive deficits consistent with organic brain damage which would impact on work efficiency and indicated reservations about Thompson's ability to practise safely even under supervision.

In respect of the particular complaints levelled against her in respect of omissions in midwifery care the Tribunal found she had committed unsatisfactory professional misconduct. The Tribunal was satisfied that Thompson lacked sufficient mental capacity to practise midwifery due to cognitive deficits, problems with higher order functioning and a lack of insight. The Tribunal also found that she had breached conditions imposed on her practice as she refused blood tests. The Tribunal found 'nurses and midwives who choose to ignore conditions and have no reasonable excuse for doing so, do so at their peril' (para 107) as it constituted professional misconduct (the most serious charge). Thompson was de-registered and not permitted to reapply for two years.

Performance and Standards Panel

If the Board reasonably believes that a nurse's or midwife's performance is or may be unsatisfactory it may order that the professional must submit to a performance assessment (ss 160, 170). A performance assessment is an external assessment of the health professional's performance and conduct. A report that raises concerns may be referred to a Performance and Standards Panel. The Panel will consider the report, and any other evidence, and if it considers the nurse's or midwife's performance is unsatisfactory the Panel may counsel the professional, impose conditions on registration, caution the professional, reprimand them or refer the matter for disciplinary proceedings.

Discipline

The primary purpose of disciplinary proceedings is to protect the public, not to punish the individual (this is the responsibility of the criminal law) or compensate the person who is harmed (this is the responsibility of civil law). The secondary purpose is to maintain standards within the profession (*Health Care Complaints Commission v Litchfield* [1997] NSWSC 297). The Board brings proceedings against professionals and matters are heard by an independent Tribunal. There are three charges: unsatisfactory professional performance (least serious); unprofessional conduct and professional misconduct (most serious). If the Tribunal makes an adverse; finding the nurse or midwife may be cautioned, reprimanded, fined, suspended or de-registered (s 196). An aggravating factor making the matter more serious will be if the health professional has lied to the Tribunal or to APHRA (*Nursing and Midwifery Board of Australia v Highet* [2016] SAHPT 11).

Disciplinary proceedings may be in relation to clinical practice and professional conduct but also may arise when a nurse or midwife is working in a different, although associated role, for example as a health researcher or health manager.

Kahler v Nurses Registration Board and Anor (Unreported, Supreme Court of New South Wales, 21 February 1995)

Kahler was a registered nurse working as an administrator of a complex providing a hostel and a nursing home for ex-service personnel. An elderly patient required a transfer from the hostel to the nursing home as he had dementia, hypertension and was regularly falling but the transfer was delayed by three months. He died two weeks after he was finally transfered, having been admitted with dehydration and multiple bedsores and lesions. Kahler was de-registered for not arranging the transfer in a timely way and for not ensuring the patient received adequate nursing care before transfer. Kahler appealed this verdict, arguing she was acting purely as an

▶

◄

administrator and not a nurse or a nursing administrator, therefore the Tribunal had no jurisdiction to censure her. The court upheld the de-registration, finding a direct nurse–patient relationship was not required for someone to be practising as a nurse. It found that the actions of a registered nurse acting as an administrator of such a complex were sufficiently related to nursing to amount to nursing practice.

Whistle-blowing

Public employees' willingness to blow the whistle or report concerns about organisational or individual wrong-doing is important to ensure the accountability of publicly funded agencies, organisations or pro-grammes, in addition to the ethical arguments outlined above. The legal system in Australia recognises that whistle-blowers have generally suf-fered both official and unofficial retribution for making these types of reports. Hence most Australian jurisdictions have passed legislation pro-tecting whistle-blowers from official repercussions as the result of their decision to report. The act of whistle-blowing raises complex legal and ethical issues as, by reporting, one is of necessity often divulging confi-dential information, sometimes outside of the organisation to which it relates. This can create tension between a perceived ethical obligation to disclose concerns about serious issues and the need to protect confidenti-ality, which is often protected by the law. The whistle-blower legislation also attempts to direct potential whistle-blowers to make disclosures to certain appropriate authorities, in part to manage issues in relation to confidentiality.

In some jurisdictions the legislation in this area is complicated. Before making a public interest or protected disclosure, check the local legisla-tion to ensure you comply with its specific rules (Tables 4.1 and 4.2).

Table 4.1 Whistle-blowing legislation

Whistle-blowing Legislation – Australia 1 July 2018	
Australian Capital Territory	*Public Interest Disclosure Act 2012*
New South Wales	*Public Interest Disclosures Act 1994*
Northern Territory	*Public Interest Disclosure Act 2008*
Queensland	*Public Interest Disclosure Act 2010*
South Australia	*Whistleblowers Protection Act 1993*
Tasmania	*Public Interest Disclosures Act 2002*
Victoria	*Protected Disclosure Act 2012*
Western Australia	*Public Interest Disclosure Act 2003*

Table 4.2 Key provisions: Public interest disclosure legislation 2018

Jurisdiction	Who can make a disclosure?	To whom?	About what?
Australian Capital Territory	Any person (s 14)	Disclosure officer; Minister; if the discloser is a public official their manager, a board member or the person in that organisation responsible for receiving disclosures (s 15). If no action after a disclosure or if nothing is heard for 3 months a secondary disclosure to a MP or journalist is permissible (s 27(3)).	Disclosable conduct (criminal offences, grounds for disciplinary action, maladministration by a public official, substantial misuse of public funds, substantial and specific danger to public health or safety or the environment) (s 8).
New South Wales	Public officials (s 8) which include those working for the government	Investigation authority; principal officer of a public authority, investigating authority; if about a MP the principal officer of the Department of Legislative Assembly, Parliamentary Services or Legislative Council. If no action after a disclosure or if nothing is heard for 6 months a secondary disclosure to a MP or journalist is permissible (s 8).	Corrupt conduct, maladministration, serious and substantial waste of resources, government information contravention, local government pecuniary interest contravention (ss 10–14).
Northern Territory	An individual (s 10)	If it relates to a member of the legislative assembly the Speaker, otherwise the Commissioner for Public Interest Disclosures or the responsible Chief Executive (s 11).	Improper conduct (s 5) (includes reprisal, dishonesty, receiving bribes, bias, breach of public trust, misuse of confidential information, substantial misuse of public resources, substantial risk to health and/or safety or the environment, substantial maladministration that adversely affects a specific person's interests).
Queensland	Any person (s 12) or any public official (s 13) (depending on what is reported)	Proper authority (the relevant public sector organisation, other entities that can investigate (i.e. Crime and	Any person may report: danger to the health and safety of a person with a disability, danger to the environment, reprisals. A public official may report: official

Table 4.2 *Continued*

Jurisdiction	Who can make a disclosure?	To whom?	About what?
		Misconduct Commission) or an MP (s 14). If no action after a disclosure or if nothing is heard for 6 months a secondary disclosure to a journalist is permissible (s 20).	misconduct, maladministration, misuse of public resources or danger to health and/or safety or the environment (s 12).
South Australia	A person (s 5)	Appropriate authority (as defined in s 5(4)).	Illegal activity; or an irregular and unauthorised use of public money; or substantial mismanagement of public resources; or conduct that causes a substantial risk to public health or safety, or to the environment; or maladministration (s 4).
Tasmania	Public officer or contractor (s 6) which include those working for the government	Ombudsman; relevant public body; Integrity Commission; if about a State Service Agency the State Services Commission; if about a police officer the Commissioner of Police; if MP to the President of the Legislative Council or House of Assembly; and otherwise as specified in s 7(1)).	Improper conduct (illegal or unlawful activity, corrupt conduct, maladministration, professional misconduct, wasting public resources, conduct that is a danger to public health and/or safety or the environment, misconduct, reprisals against people who made a public interest disclosure) (ss 4(a), 6).
Victoria	A natural person (s 9) (i.e. not a company)	The Independent Broad-based Anti-corruption Commission or an investigating body. A disclosure about a public service body, a council or a prescribed public body may be made to that agency (s 13). Or for some types of disclosures to other agencies (ss 14–19).	Improper conduct (corrupt conduct; or a substantial mismanagement of public resources; or conduct involving substantial risk to public health or safety of the environment – that would, if proved, constitute a criminal offence; or reasonable grounds for dismissing the person (ss 4, 9)) and reprisals against person who made a disclosure (s 9).
Western Australia	Any person (s 5)	Proper authority (as defined in s 5).	Criminal offences; substantial, unauthorised or irregular use or substantial mismanagement of public resources; administration (s 5).

For the disclosure to be protected, all jurisdictions require that the disclosure is made with good intentions – in other words it must be made in good faith, it must be honest and reasonable and not false or misleading. All of the Acts provide protection for a person who makes a disclosure in accordance with the specific rules set out in that Act. In all jurisdictions the person who makes a disclosure is protected from criminal and civil liability and in all jurisdictions, but South Australia, a discloser is protected from any administrative processes (i.e. discipline).

In all jurisdictions, it is a criminal offence for a person to take reprisals or detrimental action against a person who made a disclosure that is protected by the Act, except in South Australia where reprisals are grounds for a civil action by the person who has been victimised or the basis of a claim under the Equal Opportunities Act. (*Public Interest Disclosure Act 2012* (ACT) ss 35, 36, 40; *Public Interest Disclosures Act 1994* (NSW) ss 20, 21; *Public Interest Disclosure Act 2008* (NT) ss 14, 15; *Public Interest Disclosure Act 2010* (Qld) ss 36, 37, 41; *Whistleblowers Protection Act 1993* (SA) ss 5(1), 9; *Public Interest Disclosures Act 2002* (Tas) ss 10, 16; *Protected Disclosure Act 2012* (Vic) s 45; *Public Interest Disclosure Act 2003* (WA) ss 13, 14).

When Whistle-blowing and Confidentiality Collide

Case note 2049 [1996] NZPrivCmr 7 – Nurse Discloses Psychiatric Patient Details to Opposition MP.

In New Zealand, in the 1990s, a registered mental health nurse was concerned about changes to New Zealand's Mental Health Act that saw the release of some patients from a secure psychiatric unit into the community. The nurse wrote to the Minister of Health (cc'd to the Minister of Police and the National Director of Mental Health) expressing concerns about the release of a particular patient. In the letter the nurse identified the patient and provided information about the patient's condition, history and associated risks. The nurse did not have the patient's permission to release the information. No action was taken. Several months later the nurse sent a copy of the letter to an opposition Member of Parliament (MP) who had publicly raised concerns about changes to the Mental Health Act after another patient, who had been released under the same changes to the Act as the patient the nurse raised concerns about, sexually violated a child. The nurse believed that the patient he identified in the letter posed a serious and imminent threat to the public and was an example of why the amendments to the Act were misconceived. The letter was made public by the MP. New Zealand's Privacy Commissioner investigated whether the patient's privacy

▶

◄

had been violated by the nurse when he sent the letter to the opposition MP. The Commissioner concluded:

1. Given the perceived risk to the public the patient's permission to release the information to an appropriate authority was not required.

2. Given the nurse's long involvement with the patient's care and his expertise and experience the nurse had reasonable grounds to believe that the patient posed a serious and imminent threat to the public at the time the disclosure was made.

3. An opposition MP was not an appropriate authority to release such information to as he was powerless to manage the risk posed by this patient (however, note in some Australian jurisdictions the legislation states that any MP is an appropriate authority).

4. Even if there were reasonable grounds to believe it was necessary to disclose information to the MP, the nurse disclosed more personal health information than was necessary for the purpose of managing the risk posed by the individual.

The Privacy Commissioner did not bring proceedings against the nurse being satisfied that the nurse had been subject to considerable stress because of extensive publicity, did not intend for the MP to disclose the personal information and was not likely to breach the Privacy Code in future.

Overview

This chapter highlights that the ethical principles, professional ethics and legal rules relating to the professions of nursing and midwifery or that affect those professions emphasise that the professions have responsibilities to society for the manner in which nurses practise their profession. The professions also have responsibilities arising from the nature of those professions and the access they have to information about the systems within which they often work. The law emphasises professional obligations to protect the public from harm and this is particularly evident in the registration and reporting requirements and the mandatory reporting requirements imposed on nurses and midwives around the country. The ethical frameworks and the legal frameworks also emphasise that nurses and midwives must be accountable to their profession and through that profession to the public for their actions.

Figure 4.1 highlights the interactions between the ethical principles and the legal principles relevant to nursing practice.

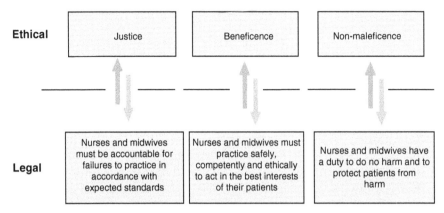

Figure 4.1   Ethical and legal principles relevant to nursing and midwifery practice

Further reading

Baca, M. 2011, 'Professional boundaries and dual relationships in clinical practice', *The Journal for Nurse Practitioners*, 7: 3, 195–200.
Wilmot, S. 2000, 'Nurses and whistleblowing: The ethical issues', *Journal of Advanced Nursing*, 32: 5, 1051–1057.

Questions

It is now a requirement to report health professionals for a significant departure from professional standards that places the public at risk of harm.

1. Discuss what the phrase 'significant departure' means to you in the context of your professional practice.

2. Discuss the ethical and professional issues you believe are associated with reporting a colleague.

Do you think having a sexual relationship with a past patient could ever be ethically appropriate? Explain your reasoning.

Is it ever appropriate to accept a gift from a patient?

Scenarios

1. Debbie, a registered nurse managing a private rehabilitation centre, initiated the withdrawal of $20,000 belonging to Patrick, a patient of the centre, which Debbie then had deposited into her personal account. Shortly afterwards she organised for Patrick (who had no close family) to appoint her as his Enduring Power of Attorney (financial). Debbie knew that Patrick had an acquired brain injury that affected his decision-making and therefore he did not have legal capacity to make an Enduring Power of Attorney. She then initiated a further withdrawal of money from Patrick's account again depositing it into her personal account.

Apply the decision-making framework to this problem.

2. Ben is a registered midwife. He provided care to Annie who was admitted for one night mid-pregnancy. She drew pictures while she was on the ward. The day after Annie was discharged Ben sent a message to Annie's Facebook page from a Facebook account set up in the name of his dog. It said 'My name is Humphrey. I just wanted to thank you for drawing my picture and making me look as beautiful as I am in real life. My human thinks you are a very talented young lady and so do I. So many people have said how amazing my picture is which is hanging in the lounge. My feeder, the silly grey cat (Muffy) and I hope all is going well with you. Thanks for making me a happy dog. Love Humphrey.' This was followed a few days later by another Facebook message from Ben's account 'First – I'm sorry to bug you but I just really wanted to tell you something and it's fine if you don't reply. That picture you drew of my little dog Humphrey. As you already know I love it and am so grateful to you. But so many people have called over and seen it at my house. I said a special friend drew it for me and they are amazed at how good it is. I know I could find friends who would love their pets drawn at some stage. But it's whatever suits you. Your needs are of course priority. We (staff) think of you and we hope things are going well for you and of course your family. You touched a lot of people – other patients included. I already knew you were a gifted artist but hearing my friends comment just made me ... well really proud. That picture is one of the loveliest gifts I've ever received. I wish you and your family a beautiful Christmas, take care and please just know how special we think you are.' Annie responded and a series of Facebook messages were subsequently exchanged between them dealing with suggested prices for paintings, draft pamphlets, marketing possibilities and the like.

Apply the decision-making framework to this problem.

5

Adult patients – Consent and refusal of consent

Introduction

The need for patients to consent before nursing or midwifery care or treatment is provided is a fundamental legal and ethical principle that respects the right of patients to make decisions about what health care they do and do not receive. The giving, or refusal, of consent by a patient shapes the nurse–patient or midwife–patient relationship and is linked to the need for nurses and midwives to provide patients with appropriate information, be willing to answer questions and, where necessary, assist patients in their decision-making. The notion of consent – or 'informed consent' as it is often referred to – is intrinsically linked to the recognition of the human rights of all individuals and notions of dignity and respect for all members of humanity. These principles are recognised in international documents such as the *Universal Declaration of Human Rights* and the *United Nations Convention on the Rights of Persons with Disabilities* as well as the Nursing and Midwifery Codes.

In this chapter, we examine the ethical importance of patient consent or refusal of consent and the recognition of this in the Codes of Ethics and the Australian Codes of Conduct. (The issues of consent and refusal of consent in relation to patients are dealt with in Chapter 6.) Also, the ethical issues relevant to when responsibility is placed with another person to make a health care decision on behalf of an adult patient who does not have the capacity to make the relevant health care decision will be considered. This chapter also describes the law relating to patient consent and refusal of consent. The law recognises that where a patient has the capacity to consent or refuse consent, this needs to be respected. However, the law also provides mechanisms for others (that is, 'substitute decision-makers') to provide consent where adult patients lack the ability to do so themselves.

Ethical importance of consent

The principles approach

Autonomy

The requirement for patients to provide consent before any health care is provided is a way in which the principle of autonomy manifests in a health care setting. The need for consent before providing a patient with health care, and the requirement to respect a refusal by an adult patient who has sufficient capacity, represents the fact that each of us has the right to determine what happens to our own bodies. We have a right to choose what health care we receive. If we were not asked before health care was provided, or had our refusals ignored, generally, this would constitute a violation of our right to self-determination (autonomy) and interfere with our right to bodily integrity (the right to decide what happens to our bodies). There would also be a failure to recognise that each of us as individuals may make different decisions. By ignoring individual choice, there is a failure to respect that each patient has their own views, values, culture and ideals. It must be remembered that some individuals may not agree with some forms of treatment or health care.

As noted by Beauchamp and Childress, health professionals such as nurses and midwives also have obligations to assist patients to make autonomous decisions (Beauchamp and Childress 2009, pp. 103–105). This may be realised by having positive attitudes towards patients' rights to make decisions, helping them to overcome fears, confusion or lack of information that may impair their ability to make autonomous decisions and assisting them, when requested, in the process of making decisions. This also encompasses recognising that some patients can be 'supported' to make decisions, and will sometimes have a trusted friend, relative or support person who helps them in the decision-making process (often called 'supported decision-making'). Prioritising patient autonomy in this context includes allowing patients the time and space as well as accessing the support needed to make decisions for themselves.

Within the concept of autonomy is the implicit recognition that decisions made by patients will be made voluntarily. Where patients are pressured or coerced by others (whether by health professionals, family or others) to make certain decisions, such decisions are unlikely to be truly autonomous.

Autonomy is also a relevant ethical principle in circumstances where an adult – who previously could make decisions and expressed wishes as to what should happen to them if they lost capacity – now lacks the ability to make decisions for themselves. Acknowledging and respecting the previously expressed wishes of the adult, who now lacks decision-making capacity, is another way that individual autonomy can be recognised.

Despite the priority given to autonomy in most western societies, this perspective is not reflected within all communities or individuals within a diverse country such as Australia. Cultural perspectives of different minority groups within Australia may mean that autonomy is not considered to be as important as other ethical principles, and individuals who hold different views or values may also not place prominence on the notion of autonomy. While in some Asian cultures (for example, Japanese and Chinese), and among some Aboriginal and/or Torres Strait Islanders, there may be a tendency not to prioritise autonomy to the same extent, it goes without saying that great variation exists within cultures and peoples and that assumptions should not be made about the ethical perspective likely to be held by a patient. For some, family or community decision-making may be preferred over individual decision-making. See the box below for a discussion of how the notion of consent may be influenced by some different cultural or religious perspectives.

Sometimes there may be a conflict between respecting the autonomy of a patient and what some nurses and midwives consider to be in their best medical interests – particularly where a refusal of health care or treatment results in a decline in their health status. There may also be a perceived conflict between nurses and midwives respecting autonomy and adhering to non-maleficence (the duty to do no harm), if the choice made by a patient will lead to what some may see to be preventable pain, suffering and/or a shorter life. In this circumstance, the principle that supports maintaining life – the 'sanctity of life principle' – also conflicts with autonomy. See Chapter 11 for more discussion of the sanctity of life principle.

Some cultural and religious perspectives of the notion of consent

Aboriginal and/or Torres Strait Islander peoples – While not all Aboriginal and/or Torres Strait Islander peoples will share the same views, understanding the potential range of perspectives about what 'consent' means is important. McGrath and Phillips suggest that the following five issues need to be understood and considered in relation to consent:

- Some Aboriginal and/or Torres Strait Islander peoples may place importance on consent being given by a person other than the patient (e.g. authority figures in

▶

◀

the community). Disrespect for traditional practices can lead to 'payback' for the patient or their families.

- Cultural differences exist in relation to concepts of time. Western approaches to medicine often require urgent decisions to be made. As such, there is a tendency for western medicine to view the process of attempting to obtain 'community consent' as a waste of time.

- Practical problems exist in obtaining community consent given the distances between communities and the time taken to reach the correct authority figure in the community.

- A lack of understanding (e.g. about side effects, pain, distress or consequences where the patient will need to be located for treatment) may exist even in circumstances where it was thought that a patient had already consented.

- Language barriers may exist between patients and health professionals (McGrath and Phillips 2008).

Chinese – While many western Chinese patients identify strongly with western values and the notion of consent understood in Australia, some may hold more traditional Chinese views. These traditional views may include:

- Less prominence attached to the notion of an individual's right to choice and self-determination.

- Chinese patients giving the family or community members the 'right to receive and disclose information, to make decisions and to coordinate patient care, even when they themselves are competent' (Bowman and Hui 2000).

Islam – A variety of Islamic views are likely to exist with different Muslim people adhering to different levels of religious observance. Generally, however, the notion of consent is viewed quite similarly by those who practise Islam as that generally accepted in western society. Often patients may wish to consult with family members before consenting to some procedures. Like in other cultures, female patients may prefer to deal with female health professionals (Daar and Khitamy 2001).

Beneficence

Respecting patients' decisions to receive or not receive particular treatment or care generally accords with the ethical principle of beneficence. Usually, respecting a patient's choice will be most consistent with maintaining their overall wellbeing (that is, be in their 'best interests'). Even in circumstances where a patient refuses health care, potentially resulting in a decline in a patient's medical wellbeing, respecting a patient's wishes may still be consistent with the patient's overall wellbeing through providing the patient with control (over what happens to their body), dignity (in being given a choice and having that choice respected) and respect for their individual cultural or personal values. Where an adult lacks capacity to consent, and previously did not give an indication as to their preferred treatment options, often the best interests principle (the application of the ethical principle of beneficence) will assist others to make decisions on behalf of the adult.

Conflicts between autonomy and beneficence will exist in some circumstances where a refusal of consent by a patient will lead them to suffer avoidable medical decline – for example, where a patient refuses life-sustaining treatment which means their life will inevitably end soon.

Non-maleficence

Not providing patients with a choice, or failure to respect patients' wishes as to whether to receive health care, may also cause patients harm. The lack of respect for patients' right to self-determination and bodily integrity may be viewed as an affront to the notion of individual choice and dignity. Where a patient's wishes are not respected this could lead to harm in the form of psychological consequences or emotional distress experienced by the patient. A failure to involve patients in the decision-making process for health care or treatment they are about to receive would also fall foul of the principle of non-maleficence. Such actions assume an inability by individual patients to contribute or participate in the decision-making process in any way, which may not be correct and does not respect their inherent dignity and worth. Historically, those with disabilities had assumptions made – often wrongly – about their ability to participate in decision-making.

In adults who lack the ability to make decisions for themselves, the duty to do no harm (non-maleficence), along with acting in the patient's best interests (beneficence), will usually be significant principles that influence decision-making by others on their behalf.

Similar conflicts between autonomy and non-maleficence (as have already been discussed in relation to autonomy and beneficence) can arise in circumstances where a patient's decision leads to an avoidable deterioration in health or even death. However, it is clear that, in Australia, our society prioritises individual choice in health care decision-making over the possible non-beneficial consequences of those choices. In Australia it is considered very important, in an ethical sense, to respect the decisions of competent adults, whatever those decisions may entail. This is reflected in the legal position (discussed in the section 'Competent adult patients have the right to refuse health care'), which requires that a competent adult's decision be respected regardless of concerns about potential harms to that patient (non-maleficence) and what might be considered to be in the best medical interests of that patient (beneficence).

Justice

The concept of justice is clearly important to the notion of consent as it relates to a key right of competent patients to consent to or refuse treatment within the health care system. Justice is also important for those adults who may have trouble making decisions by themselves or communicating their decisions to others. Some adults will be fully capable of making decisions but use alternative means of communicating (e.g. sign language) which must be recognised and respected. Others may be able to make decisions but require some support or assistance from others (supported decision-making). It is important that the rights of those individuals are respected and assumptions not made about those individuals lacking capacity simply on the basis that they have a disability. This respectful approach is consistent with the principles contained in the widely adopted and internationally recognised *United Nations Convention on the Rights of Persons with Disabilities*. Australia is a signatory to this *Convention* that recognises the right to make decisions and the right to receive support for decision-making by those with disabilities.

There is also an obligation under justice for society to safeguard the interests of vulnerable adults and, where necessary, to act to protect adults from abuse and exploitation. Some adult patients may lack literacy skills, English language skills or have lower health literacy levels which require approaches to obtaining consent to be modified to ensure understanding (e.g. verbal explanations of all written documents to those lacking English literacy skills). Without appropriate modification in approach these adults may be denied their right to make informed decisions regarding their own health care.

The nursing and midwifery codes

Both the Nursing and Midwifery International Codes of Ethics recognise the importance of a patient's right to make decisions about their own health care. As part of this, the Codes emphasise the corresponding rights of patients to participate in decisions regarding their own health care, be informed about treatment options, be able to ask questions and be given information when requested. The Codes also recognise the potential contribution of other people to informed decision-making. These reflect the human right of respect for individual autonomy when receiving health care.

Patients' rights to make decisions

A patient's right to make decisions is recognised as coming within the scope of human rights that nurses and midwives must recognise and respect.

Both international Codes of Ethics importantly refer to the concept of 'informed decision-making' which highlights the importance of health professionals, such as nurses and midwives, disclosing adequate and timely information to patients so that they have sufficient understanding of the choices available to them and so that the decision made by them is ultimately an informed one (see ICM Code of Ethics, I(a); ICN Code of Ethics, Element 1). This recognition of a patient's right to make a decision implicitly recognises that a decision ought to be made voluntarily and not under undue pressure or coercion from health professionals or anyone else.

The Australian Nursing and Midwifery Codes of Conduct offer more specific guidance relating to informed consent. Principle 2.3 of both Codes of Conduct states that informed consent is 'a person's voluntary agreement to healthcare, which is made with knowledge and understanding of the potential benefits and risks involved'. It goes on to provide a list of actions that nurses and midwives can take to support a patient's right to informed consent including:

➢ The provision of information in a way they can understand;

➢ Giving a patient time to ask questions and make decisions;

➢ Acting in accordance with a patient's capacity for decision-making and consent; and

➢ Obtaining informed consent or consent from a 'valid authority' (e.g. substitute decision-maker) where needed before providing health care.

Assisting with and sharing decision-making

As well as recognising a patient's right to informed decision-making, both Codes of Conduct also recognise that decision-making can be a shared responsibility. It recognises that some patients may wish to involve partners, friends and family together with nursing, midwifery and other health professionals in the process of shared decision-making (at 2.2). Principle 3.3 in both Codes of Conduct addresses the need to consider effective communication that is respectful, kind, compassionate and honest. There is recognition that there are different levels of health literacy in the community and, for some patients, arrangements may need to be made to meet their communication needs (2.3(a), 3.3(a)–(b)). The need for additional aids for effective communication can impact on a patient's understanding and their ability to make decisions. Communicating in an appropriate way allows patients and their families to fully participate, thus maximising a patient's autonomy.

There is also an acknowledgement that nurses and midwives have an obligation to 'advocate on behalf of the person/woman where necessary, and recognise when substitute decision-makers are needed' (2.2(b)). The patient advocacy role of midwives and nurses on behalf of their patients is an important one; the case below provides an example of a situation where an enrolled nurse failed to act in accordance with this principle, resulting in disciplinary action.

Awareness of culture

The ICN Code of Ethics (at 1) and the Nursing and Midwifery Codes of Conduct (at 3.1–3.2) remind nurses and midwives to be aware of the

---

Nursing and Midwifery Board of Australia v George [2015] VCAT 1878

In this case an enrolled nurse was reprimanded for, among other things, failing to advocate for her patient. The patient was a woman who underwent a late termination of pregnancy at a private hospital in Melbourne. Prior to attending the hospital the nurse was informed that the patient had been difficult to rouse and was unresponsive. When the patient arrived at the hospital she was brought to theatre. There the opinion of the doctors and another nurse present was that the patient was unconscious and a decision was made to provide no anaesthetic or pain relief medication prior to the procedure. However, the enrolled nurse had formed the opinion that the patient was not unconscious but merely drowsy and saw her open her eyes. The enrolled nurse did not communicate her observations or opinion to those in the operating theatre or query the decision to proceed without anaesthetic or pain relief.

This failure to communicate her observations and opinions to others in theatre was found to fall within unprofessional conduct and led to the enrolled nurse being reprimanded. The Victorian Civil and Administrative Tribunal in that case noted that: 'It is essential that both enrolled and registered nurses discharge their responsibilities as advocates for patients, including in the operating theatre where the patient is particularly vulnerable.'

various cultural influences that may affect how decisions are made by a patient regarding their care and treatment. Some patients will feel that the choice regarding whether to receive health care is not an individual decision but one that must be made with close or extended family and community members. Importantly, at 3.1(c) of the Nursing and Midwifery Codes of Conduct, it states that nurses and midwives must:

> … recognise the importance of family, community, partnership and collaboration in the healthcare decision-making of Aboriginal and/or Torres Strait Islander peoples, for … care delivery.

Some (but not all) Aboriginal and/or Torres Strait Islander patients may wish to communicate with family and others in the community before providing consent (see McGrath and Phillips 2008). Other patients will make decisions to accept or reject offered medical treatment based on other personal, cultural or religious reasons which also ought to be respected. As noted at 3.2(a) of the Nursing and Midwifery Codes of Conduct, it must be understood that only the patient (and/or their family) 'can determine whether or not care is culturally safe and respectful'.

The law relating to consent and refusal of consent

The legal principles in relation to consent are fundamental to how health professionals interact with patients. Usually consent is obtained from, or on behalf of, every patient for every health care intervention. As such, an understanding of the legal principles of consent and the consequences of not following the law in this area is crucial for every health professional, including nurses and midwives.

In this section of the chapter we will examine the legal principles that apply to adults (18 years and over) who have capacity to make decisions and also those who lack the capacity to make decisions for themselves. For a discussion of the legal principles of consent in relation to children, refer to Chapter 6.

Adults with capacity to consent

The law generally provides that adults will be presumed to have capacity to make decisions in relation to health care unless shown to be incapable (see the case of *Re B (adult: refusal of medical treatment)* [2002] 2 All ER 449 discussed at p. 97). The situation where an adult is found to lack the necessary capacity to make a health care decision is also considered (see the section on Adult patients lacking capacity to make decisions about their health care).

Here we consider what constitutes a legally valid decision by a competent adult to consent to or refuse consent.

What constitutes valid consent or refusal?

A valid consent or refusal can be communicated in writing or orally. Just because a patient signs a consent form does not mean that it automatically constitutes legally valid consent (although it may help to prove that consent was validly given). A person may sign a consent form without reading it or without understanding what the form says (for example, if they do not understand English well), so there is still a need to consider if the questions set out below have been satisfied.

Consent may also be express or implied. Express consent may be written or in the form of a statement from the patient saying, 'yes, I consent'. An example of an implied consent is where a health professional requests to take a sample of blood from a patient and the patient responds by rolling up their sleeve and presenting their arm for the needle to withdraw blood. In this case it can be assumed that the patient has consented, even if they have not said anything.

In order for a consent or refusal of consent to be legally valid, the following questions need to be asked and the answer to each should be 'yes':

➢ Does the adult have capacity to make this health care decision?

➢ Was sufficient information given to the patient about the proposed health care intervention?

➢ Has the decision been made voluntarily and without coercion?

➢ Was the consent or refusal of consent given in relation to the specific health care intervention in question?

The law provides guidance as to how we answer these questions in practice.

Does the adult patient have capacity to make the health care decision?

Both the common law and the legislation in some jurisdictions in Australia provide guidance as to what is relevant when deciding whether or not an adult patient has capacity to make a specific decision. While a determination about whether a patient has capacity will usually be made by a medical practitioner, in circumstances where nurses (such as nurse practitioners in rural areas) or midwives practise independently the initial assessment of capacity, or a determination of whether a referral for capacity assessment needs to be made, may be done by nurses or midwives. Practical assistance in making determinations of capacity has been recognised as a problematic area for health professionals and others; however, some practical guidelines are available (see Attorney General's Department of New South Wales 2008).

The law tells us that in order for a person to have capacity to make health care decisions they must be able to 'comprehend and retain the information' that is important to the decision (that is, the consequences of having or not having the treatment) and be able 'to use the information and weigh it in the balance as part of the process of arriving at a decision'. This test was made clear in the English case of *Re B* (discussed at p. 97). A person must also be able to communicate their decision in some way.

As discussed later (see the section on Adult patients lacking capacity to make decisions about their health care), these principles are also reflected in legislative definitions of capacity and incapacity.

Was sufficient information given to the patient about the proposed health care intervention?

In order for a consent or refusal of consent to be legally valid, the patient must have sufficient information about the proposed health care to make the decision. The type of information that needs to be provided to a patient about the proposed intervention need not be very detailed and specific.

The High Court of Australia made clear in *Rogers v Whitaker* (1992) 175 CLR 479 'the patient's consent to the treatment may be valid once he or she is informed in broad terms of the nature of the procedure which is intended'. (In contrast, health professionals *can* be held legally liable where specific risks were not discussed under a civil action of negligence; see Chapter 8 on 'Patient safety and negligence'.)

However, in practice, information should be given to the patient to assist with their understanding to the greatest extent. For example, health professionals should try to use plain English, avoid overly technical language or unnecessary jargon and tailor the information to the patient's level of knowledge and their intellectual abilities.

Has the decision been made voluntarily and without coercion?

Another legal requirement is that the decision must be made voluntarily by the patient. If the decision was made under undue pressure or the patient was coerced then this can invalidate their decision. While this is a common law principle, the legislation in Queensland also includes this principle within the legislative definition of 'capacity' (*Guardianship and Administration Act 2000* (Qld), sch 4).

While fairly old, the Canadian case in the box below provides a useful example of when a decision made by a patient was considered by a court to not have been made voluntarily and, as such, was not valid.

Beausoleil v La Communaute des Soeurs de la Charite de la Providence (1965) 53 DLR (2d) 65

This Canadian case was brought by a woman who had suffered paralysis from the waist down following a procedure on her back. The patient had suffered backaches and was admitted to hospital for planned surgery on her back. The patient had wanted to have a general anaesthetic for this procedure and had discussed this with her surgeon and with the assistant anaesthetist prior to the operation. However, she ended up with a spinal anaesthetic administered instead, as the chief anaesthetist, after she had been sedated, convinced her to change her mind just prior to surgery. As part of her case against the defendant doctor and hospital it was alleged that the consent she gave to a spinal anaesthetic was not valid. The court heard conflicting evidence from the patient and the defendant doctor regarding whether or not she had consented. The court also received evidence from a nurse present during the conversation between the patient and the chief anaesthetist who stated that 'she did not want that type of anaesthetic, she refused and they continued to offer it to her; finally she became tired and said "You do as you wish" or something like that.' The patient's alleged consent to the spinal anaesthetic was obtained by a doctor she had not previously met 30 minutes prior to the procedure while the patient was under the influence of sedatives. One of the judges of the court noted that the words of the patient, 'Do as you like', were words that denoted 'defeat, exhaustion, and an abandonment of will power'.

In relation to this aspect of the case the majority of the court found that the patient did not validly consent to the spinal anaesthetic.

Was the consent or refusal of consent given in relation to the specific health care in question?

The final component of a legally valid consent or refusal is that it must have been given in relation to the specific health care intervention in question. For example, a surgeon cannot rely on consent given for surgery on a patient's left toe to carry out a 'spinal fusion' operation on the patient's back (as happened in the Canadian case of *Schweizer v Central Hospital* (1974) 53 DLR (3d) 494). Specific consent is needed for each intervention.

Competent adult patients have the right to refuse health care

Where all these questions are answered positively, legally valid consent or refusal of consent exists and must be respected. Competent adults have the absolute right to refuse health care that has been offered; even if this means they will suffer serious harm or die from lack of treatment. While ethically this presents a challenge between the principles of respecting autonomy, beneficence and non-maleficence, the law is clear that it respects competent adults' decisions first and foremost. The cases below illustrate this very clearly.

Re B (adult: refusal of medical treatment) [2002] 2 All ER 449

This English case concerned 'Ms B', a 43-year-old woman who at the age of 41 suffered complete tetraplegia (paralysis from the neck down). At the time the case came before the courts, Ms B was on an artificial ventilator. The case was brought to the courts by Ms B who sought a declaration that the artificial ventilation she was being given – and which she did not want – was unlawful. Ms B was totally reliant on carers to feed, clothe, wash and assist with bodily functions. She found 'the idea of living like this intolerable' and had made requests to hospital staff that her ventilator be switched off. The main issue for the court was to determine whether Ms B had capacity to make her own decision about her treatment in hospital.

The court stated the following principles:

• There is a presumption that every person has capacity to consent or to refuse medical treatment unless and until proven otherwise.

• Where a person has capacity to make decisions, their decision must be respected (even if the reason for their decision is 'rational, irrational, unknown or even non-existent').

• A person lacks capacity if a person is 'unable to comprehend and retain the information' that is important to the decision (that is, the consequences of having or not having the treatment) and the patient is 'unable to use the information and weigh it in the balance as part of the process of arriving at a decision'.

▶

◄

The judge in this case found Ms B to be 'an exceptional witness', demonstrating 'a very high standard of mental competence, intelligence and ability'. This view was supported by evidence from some doctors. As such, the court found that Ms B *did* have capacity to make all relevant decisions about her medical treatment, including the decision regarding whether to withdraw artificial ventilation. As such, the artificial ventilation given to Ms B against her expressed wishes was unlawful and Ms B could decide whether to have the ventilation withdrawn.

Brightwater Care Group (Inc) v Rossiter (2009) 40 WAR 84

The principles in the English case of *Re B* were confirmed and applied in the Western Australian case of *Brightwater* where a patient with capacity requested that artificial nutrition and hydration via a PEG tube be ceased. Similar to *Re B*, the Supreme Court of Western Australia made a declaration that Mr Rossiter had the ability to make this decision regarding his future treatment regardless of the fact that it would ultimately result in his death.

Adult patients with variable capacity to make decisions about their health care

Some patients will experience variable capacity to make decisions about their health. This is because a determination of capacity or incapacity is not 'black and white'. It is possible for a person to lose decision-making capacity temporarily, or regain capacity if their condition improves, or to have capacity in respect of some relatively uncomplicated health treatments but not more complex interventions. It is also possible that a person – if unsupported – might be considered to lack decision-making capacity but, if provided with the correct support, may be assessed as having capacity for a particular decision. Indeed, determining if a patient has capacity to consent or refuse should be *time-* and *decision-*specific (Stewart and Biegler 2004). The law looks at the specific time a decision needs to be made to determine if the patient can make the decision themselves (is competent) or if they require someone else to make the decision on their behalf (i.e. the patient lacks decision-making capacity). However, just because a person cannot make a decision at 10 a.m. on one day, does not mean that they will necessarily be considered incompetent at 8 p.m. the following day. Indeed, for some conditions, like early onset dementia and some mental health conditions (e.g. those where temporary psychotic episodes may occur), fluctuations in capacity are quite common. In these circumstances it would be contrary to a patient's human rights to simply assume they lack capacity because they were assessed to lack capacity at a previous time. Reassessment of decision-making capacity for health care decisions is likely to be needed as a patient's condition changes.

Summary of the law: Adults with variable capacity

- Assessing whether a person legally has capacity to consent or refuse is *time*- and *decision*-specific.

- The law looks at the specific time a decision needs to be made to determine if the adult can make the decision herself (i.e. the patient is competent to make that decision) or if she requires some other mechanism for a decision to be made on her behalf (i.e. the patient lacks capacity to make that decision).

- Some legislation in Australia recognises that a patient can be supported by another person to make decisions (see, for example, *Medical Treatment Planning and Decisions Act 2016* (Vic)). Those decisions are considered to be made by the patient, not the supporter.

Next we consider what happens in circumstances where, for the particular health care decision in question, the patient is found to lack decision-making capacity.

Adult patients lacking capacity to make decisions about their health care

There are many circumstances where an adult patient may be incapable of making a decision regarding their health care and treatment. This might be because the patient is unconscious, has severe dementia, or an acquired brain injury or an intellectual disability of such severity that it affects a patient's ability to make decisions. In all these circumstances if the person is found to lack capacity to make a decision the law requires that consent on behalf of the patient be obtained through another mechanism. The laws that provide authority for substitute decision-making are sometimes referred to as a type of 'guardianship law'.

This section describes the laws that give power, usually to other people, to make decisions on behalf of adults lacking the ability to consent or refuse consent themselves. A person who makes a decision on behalf of a patient who lacks decision-making capacity can be given many titles but will be referred to generally as a 'substitute decision-maker' in this section of the chapter.

The threshold at which the law gives power to substitute decision-makers to make health care decisions on behalf of adults lacking the ability to make decisions depends on a finding of incapacity. Earlier in this chapter we discussed how to determine if a patient has capacity. If an adult patient cannot fulfil the requirements and give a valid consent or refusal of consent, they will be considered as lacking the capacity to make the decision (i.e. be considered 'incompetent'). In general, the legislation in New South Wales, the Northern Territory, Queensland, Tasmania, South Australia and Victoria largely reflects this definition of capacity and incapacity discussed earlier. In the Australian Capital Territory, and in some circumstances in South Australia, the legislation provides that in order for others to make decisions on behalf of adult patients, the patient must be found to be lacking capacity due to a particular medical condition (e.g. the patient suffers from some illness, disorder or intellectual condition which has led to their incapacity). In Western Australia the approach is different, with others being able to make decisions on behalf of adult patients where it is considered the patient is 'unable to make reasonable judgments in respect of any treatment proposed to be provided'.

How do decisions get made if an adult patient lacks the capacity to make a health care decision?

Legislation in the different States and Territories around Australia tells us how health care decisions can be made on behalf of a patient who lacks the capacity to consent or refuse consent. The legal position around Australia is not identical, but generally legislation will provide for a number of ways in which decisions can lawfully be made. Usually there are options for health professionals to rely on:

➤ An advance directive;

➤ The decision of a person appointed by the patient (before they lost capacity) to make health care decisions on behalf of the patient;

➤ The decision of a person appointed by a court or tribunal to make health care decisions on behalf of the patient;

➤ The decision of a person who is identified under legislation as being the appropriate substitute decision-maker when none of the other situations apply; or

➤ The decision of a court or tribunal as to what treatment should or should not occur.

What is an 'Advance Directive'?

These are generally written documents known as 'advance health directives' (in Western Australia and Queensland), 'health directions' (in the Australian Capital Territory), 'advance personal plans' (in the Northern Territory) and 'advance care directives' (in South Australia and Victoria). These documents are recognised in legislation as a way for a person with capacity to record their wishes as to what treatment they want or do not want if they lose the capacity to make health care decisions. While New South Wales and Tasmania do not mention advance directives in its legislation, it is recognised that these types of directions as to future care still exist and apply. The legislation in different States and Territories describes how these written documents need to be executed. These documents will generally apply at a later time when the patient has lost decision-making capacity, as long as the instructions contained within the document are not ambiguous, apply to the decision that needs to be made and have not been superseded.

Who are substitute decision-makers appointed by the patient (prior to a loss of decision-making capacity)?

These are persons appointed by the patient via a written document (e.g. an enduring power of attorney or an advance directive) that is executed before the patient loses decision-making capacity. Those appointed are known as 'enduring guardians' (in New South Wales, Tasmania, Victoria and Western Australia), 'enduring attorneys' (in the Australian Capital Territory and Queensland), a 'substitute decision-maker' (in South Australia) and a 'decision-maker' (in the Northern Territory). The document appointing the person can specify the types of decisions that can be made by those appointed, so can include health care decisions. Similar to an advance directive, usually the appointed person will only be allowed to make decisions on behalf of a patient once the patient loses the ability to make health decisions. Those appointed act as a substitute decision-maker.

Who is an appointed 'guardian'?

Courts and tribunals in Australia have power to appoint a person to make decisions on behalf of an adult who cannot make decisions for themselves. The person appointed by the court or tribunal with power to make health care decisions for an adult who lacks decision-making capacity is called a 'guardian'. Appointed guardians are a type of substitute decision-maker.

This area of guardianship law has been undergoing legal reform in recent years and further changes are likely to take place in the near future. The current situation in each State and Territory in Australia is discussed in more detail next.

However, some types of 'special' or 'prescribed' health care are considered so serious that only a tribunal or court can authorise an adult patient who lacks capacity to undergo such procedures. These procedures include sterilisation, termination of pregnancy and tissue transplantation from an adult lacking decision-making capacity. They remain outside the normal decision-making processes due to their invasive nature and the serious consequences that result for the adult patient.

The Australian Capital Territory

In the Australian Capital Territory the three relevant pieces of legislation are the *Guardianship and Management of Property Act 1991* (ACT), the *Powers of Attorney Act 2006* (ACT) and the *Medical Treatment (Health Directions) Act 2006* (ACT). The Australian Capital Territory has a version of an advance directive called a 'health direction' but it only applies to future 'refusals'. Also, unlike most other advance directives, a 'health direction' can be written or oral. Where an adult has a health direction that applies in the circumstances, generally the refusal in that document must be followed. However, if the patient has an appointed enduring power of attorney for health care decisions, where there is an inconsistency in directions, whichever was executed later – the health direction or the enduring power of attorney document – will apply. In the absence of such a direction, or one that applies in the circumstances, the legislation in the Australian Capital Territory provides a range of ways in which decisions may be made on behalf of adult patients who lack decision-making capacity for health decisions:

➢ An enduring power of attorney that was appointed by the patient (for health care decisions) before they lost capacity;

➢ A guardian appointed by the ACT Civil and Administrative Tribunal who has power to make decisions about health care;

➢ A 'health attorney', who is the first of the following to apply:

  – The patient's domestic partner – where the relationship is close and continuing;

  – The person who cares for the patient (without being paid);

  – A close relative or friend of the patient.

The courts in the Australian Capital Territory may also provide authorisation for health care interventions to take place. (See *Guardianship and Management of Property Act 1991* (ACT), pt 2A; *Powers of Attorney Act 2006* (ACT), ss 12, 13(2), 32, 46; *Medical Treatment (Health Directions) Act 2006* (ACT), pts 2–4.)

New South Wales and Tasmania

The situation in New South Wales and Tasmania is similar. The Tasmanian *Guardianship and Administration Act 1995* (Tas) and the New South Wales *Guardianship Act 1987* (NSW) provide a hierarchy of persons who may provide consent on behalf of an adult patient who lacks decision-making capacity for a health care decision. The first of the following persons who can be identified is known as the 'person responsible' and they can then consent on behalf of the patient:

➢ A guardian that has been appointed with power to make decisions about health care by the relevant Tribunal (the Guardianship and Administration Board in Tasmania and the NSW Civil and Administrative Tribunal in New South Wales) or an 'enduring guardian' that was appointed by the patient (for health care decisions) before they lost capacity;

➢ The patient's spouse – where the relationship is close and continuing;

➢ The person who cares for the patient (without being paid); or

➢ A close friend or relative of the patient.

While the legislation in New South Wales and Tasmania does not mention advance directives, these would be recognised under the common law. The tribunals or the courts in either State may also provide authorisation for health care interventions to take place. (See *Guardianship and Administration Act 1995* (Tas), s 4, pt 6; *Guardianship Act 1987* (NSW), pt 5.)

The Northern Territory

In the Northern Territory a form of advance directive exists known as an 'advance personal plan'. This document can be executed by a person with decision-making capacity to provide for future consents or refusals of consent to treatment at a later time when they lack capacity. The *Guardianship of Adults* (NT) and *Advance Personal Planning Act* (NT) provide that, for health care decisions to be made on behalf of an adult who lacks capacity, health professionals must rely on one of the following:

➢ An advance directive (known as an 'advance consent decision' contained in an 'advance personal plan') – where one exists, was completed by the patient before losing capacity, and which applies to this health care decision;

➢ A 'decision-maker' appointed by the patient under their 'advance personal plan'; or

➢ A 'guardian' appointed by the Northern Territory Civil and Administrative Tribunal with power to make decisions about health care.

The Northern Territory Civil and Administrative Tribunal or the courts may also provide authorisation for health care interventions. (See *Guardianship of Adults* (NT), s 23; *Advance Personal Planning Act* (NT), pt 4, div 2.)

Queensland

In Queensland the *Guardianship and Administration Act 2000* (Qld) and *Powers of Attorney Act 1998* (Qld) provide a priority list of ways in which decisions can lawfully be made where a patient lacks capacity to make health care decisions. Health professionals move down this list until an option that applies can be relied on for the patient lacking decision-making capacity:

➢ An advance directive (known as an 'advance health directive') – where one exists, was completed by the patient before losing capacity, and which applies to this health care decision;

➢ A 'guardian' has been appointed by the Queensland Civil and Administrative Tribunal for health care decisions;

➢ An 'attorney' has been appointed by the patient for health care decisions under an advance directive or under an enduring power of attorney; or

➢ A 'statutory health attorney' who is the first of the following to apply:

  – The patient's spouse – where the relationship is close and continuing;

  – The person who cares for the patient (without being paid);

  – A close friend or relative of the patient; or

  – The Public Guardian (an independent statutory office in Queensland).

The Queensland Civil and Administrative Tribunal or the courts may also provide authorisation for health care interventions. (See *Guardianship and Administration Act 2000* (Qld), s 66; *Powers of Attorney Act 1998* (Qld), ch 3, pts 2–3, ch 4.)

South Australia

In South Australia the *Advance Care Directives Act 2013* (SA) and the *Consent to Medical Treatment and Palliative Care Act 1995* (SA) outline the legal mechanisms for decision-making on behalf of adult patients who lack the ability to make health decisions. South Australian advance directives are known as 'Advance Care Directives', which can be executed by a person at a time when they have decision-making capacity. While these documents can contain directions as to advance refusals and consents to treatment, only the *refusals* will be considered legally binding. The legislation provides that one of the following may be the appropriate decision-making mechanism for an adult patient who lacks decision-making capacity:

➢ An advance directive (known as an 'advance care directive') – where one exists, was completed by the patient before losing capacity, and which applies to this health care decision;

➢ A 'substitute decision-maker' appointed by the patient through an 'advance care directive', before the patient lost capacity to make the health care decision;

➢ A 'person responsible' who is the first of the following to apply:

– A guardian appointed by the South Australian Civil and Administrative Tribunal who has power to make decisions about health care;

– A relative of the patient (i.e. spouse; domestic partner; adult related by blood, marriage or adoption; and, for an Aboriginal or Torres Strait Islander patient, a person related according to their kinship rules);

– An adult friend of the patient; or

– An adult who is charged with the patient's care and wellbeing.

The South Australian Civil and Administrative Tribunal or the courts may also provide authorisation for health care interventions to take place. (See *Guardianship and Administration Act 1993* (SA), pt 4, div 2; *Consent to Medical Treatment and Palliative Care Act 1995* (SA), pt 2A; *Advance Care Directives Act 2013* (SA), pt 3.)

Victoria

The relevant Victorian legislation is the *Medical Treatment Planning and Decisions Act 2016* (Vic) and the *Guardianship and Administration Act 1986* (Vic). The Victorian version of an advance directive is called an 'advance care directive' and applies in relation to future consents and refusals of consent to treatment.

Where an adult has a valid 'advance care directive' that applies in the circumstances, the decision in the directive must be followed. In the absence of an advance care directive, the first of the following persons who can be identified is known as the 'medical treatment decision maker'. They can make a health care decision on behalf of the adult patient who lacks decision-making capacity:

➤ A person appointed by the patient as a 'medical treatment decision maker', before the patient lost capacity to make the health care decision;

➤ A 'guardian' appointed by the Victorian Civil and Administrative Tribunal with power to make decisions in relation to health care;

➤ The patient's spouse or domestic partner – where the relationship is close and continuing;

➤ The person who cares for the patient (without being paid); or

➤ The patient's relative (being the first of the following who are adults – child of the patient; parent of the patient; or sibling of the patient).

The Victorian Civil and Administrative Tribunal or the courts may also provide authorisation for health care interventions to take place.

Victoria is unique in providing a way for a patient – who has capacity if supported – to appoint a legally recognised 'support person' – whose role is to 'support the person to make, communicate and give effect' to a patient's decisions regarding health care. The support person does not make the decision for the patient but is recognised as being someone chosen by the patient to assist them in that task. (See *Guardianship and Administration Act 1986* (Vic), pt 4; *Medical Treatment Planning and Decisions Act 2016* (Vic), pts 2–4.)

Western Australia

The *Guardianship and Administration Act 1990* (WA) provides a hierarchy of persons who may provide consent on behalf of an adult patient who lacks decision-making capacity for a health care decision in Western Australia. The first of the following mechanisms that can be identified will provide a means of determining what health care decision gets made for the patient:

➤ An advance directive (known as an 'advance health directive') – where one exists, was completed by the patient before losing capacity, and which applies to this health care decision;

➤ An 'enduring guardian' that was appointed by the patient (for health care decisions) before they lost capacity;

➤ A 'guardian' appointed by the State Administrative Tribunal with power to make decisions about health care; or

➤ A 'person responsible' who is the first of the following to apply:

  – The patient's spouse or de facto partner – where they live with the patient;

- The patient's nearest relative who is an adult (spouse, child, parent or sibling) and who maintains a close relationship with the patient;

- The person who is the primary carer for the patient (without being paid); or

- Any other person who maintains a close personal relationship with the patient.

The Supreme Court in Western Australia may also provide authorisation for health care interventions to take place. (See *Guardianship and Administration Act 1990* (WA), pts 5, 9A–9D).

Obligations on substitute decision-makers acting on behalf of adult patients lacking capacity

Substitute decision-makers making health care decisions on behalf of adult patients lacking capacity are required by the legislation (identified above) to consider certain factors or apply certain principles in making their decisions. In the majority of jurisdictions a substitute decision-maker acting on behalf of an adult patient lacking capacity should:

➢ Take into account the patient's wishes;

➢ Adopt the least restrictive approach; and

➢ Consider the patient's best interests or their interests and welfare (White, Willmott and Then 2018).

In some States and Territories there may also be the obligation for those acting on behalf of the adult to consult with others before making a decision. If a person acting on behalf of an adult patient needs advice about making a decision, the legislation in most States and Territories provides that they can approach the relevant tribunal to seek advice or directions.

Resolving disputes about decision-making on behalf of adults lacking capacity

Occasionally there will be disagreements about decisions made on behalf of adults lacking capacity. This may be because a family member or the treating team does not agree with the decision made by the person who has the legal power to make decisions on behalf of the adult patient. Alternatively, more than one person may have the legal power to consent (for example, where there are two guardians who can make decisions about health care for the adult) and those people cannot agree on whether a health care intervention should take place. In these circumstances the legislation in each State and Territory provides ways of resolving such disputes.

Approach the tribunal or court

In all Australian States and Territories, a dispute can be resolved by approaching a court (usually the Supreme Court) or the relevant tribunal. Applications to courts or tribunals can be made and issues resolved quickly in urgent cases. However, for non-urgent cases, it may take some time for a decision to be made. Lawyers and hospital administration would most likely need to be involved in any application to a court or tribunal.

Other ways of resolving disputes

In the Australian Capital Territory

In the Australian Capital Territory the *Guardianship and Managements of Property Act 1991* (ACT) has provisions that allow matters to be referred to the Public Trustee and Guardian (a public official) in the following circumstances:

➤ If a 'health attorney' refuses to give consent for medical treatment proposed by a health professional and that refusal appears to be inconsistent with a 'health direction' (s 32H *Guardianship and Management of Property Act 1991* (ACT)).

➤ If there is more than one 'health attorney' and they do not agree on whether treatment should be consented to (s 32I *Guardianship and Management of Property Act 1991* (ACT)) (see p. 101 for the terms 'health attorney', 'enduring attorney' and 'health direction').

The Public Trustee and Guardian can decide whether to apply to the ACT Civil and Administrative Tribunal to be appointed as the guardian of the patient in both situations. In the second circumstance the Public Trustee and Guardian also has the option of trying to help the health attorneys reach agreement.

In Queensland

In Queensland an independent statutory body exists called the Office of the Public Guardian. In some circumstances, the Public Guardian may be able to resolve disputes without the need to approach a court or the Queensland

Civil and Administrative Tribunal. In the following situations the Public Guardian can be contacted to make the relevant health care decision:

➢ Where there is a disagreement between substitute decision-makers (who both have legal power to make health care decisions on behalf of an adult patient) about a health care decision and this cannot be solved through mediation (s 42 *Guardianship and Administration Act 2000* (Qld)).

➢ Where the substitute decision-maker acting on behalf of the adult patient makes a decision that others consider to be contrary to the principles that a substitute decision-maker is obliged to follow (i.e. taking into account the patient's wishes, adopting an approach least restrictive of the patient's rights, and considering the best interests of the adult patient) (s 43 *Guardianship and Administration Act 2000* (Qld)).

In South Australia

The *Advance Care Directives Act 2013* (SA) provides that the South Australian Public Guardian (a public official) has power to mediate disputes, make declarations or refer matters to the South Australian Civil and Administrative Tribunal in relation to issues arising from advance care directives. This would include disputes about the role or decision made by a substitute decision-maker appointed through an advance care directive (*Advance Care Directives Act 2013* (SA), pt 7, div 2).

In Victoria

The legislation in Victoria has particular safeguards in place for when a substitute decision-maker (known as a 'medical treatment decision maker' in Victoria) refuses medical treatment known as 'significant treatment' (i.e. it involves a significant degree of bodily intrusion; risk; side effects; or distress to the patient). If a doctor believes that the wishes of the person are not known in relation to the treatment, the doctor must notify the Victorian Public Advocate (a public official), who can decide whether or not the refusal is 'not unreasonable in the circumstances'. The Victorian Public Advocate can choose to take the matter to the Victorian Civil and Administrative Tribunal if they think the refusal of treatment by the substitute decision-maker is unreasonable (*Medical Treatment Planning and Decisions Act 2016* (Vic), ss 62, 67).

Legal consequences of not having consent

Where no legally valid consent has been obtained and none of the legal exceptions (discussed below at 'Legal exceptions to the need for consent') apply, there will be consequences for those health professionals that proceed to provide health care and administer treatment. In these circumstances a health professional may be liable for the civil action of the tort of trespass (sometimes called civil 'assault' or 'battery') – which can be brought by the patient themselves – or a criminal action of assault or battery.

Civil trespass

The action of trespass is likely to come about where there is actual physical contact with a patient in providing health care that has not been consented to by the patient. For the action to succeed, it must be shown that the act of physically touching the patient (e.g. in providing nursing care that has been refused) was *intended* by the nurse. It is irrelevant that the nurse's motivation in touching the patient and providing such care was to act in the patient's best interests. It is also irrelevant that the patient suffers no harm from the touching. In fact, even if the patient could be said to benefit from the care that was given this will not make any difference.

Criminal assault

The criminal law in all States and Territories could potentially apply and give rise to criminal actions against a health professional for physically touching a patient without consent. While the criminal laws around Australia differ, in each jurisdiction there is a criminal action (variously called common or aggravated assault, battery, grievous bodily harm or wounding) that would potentially be available in this circumstance. In practice, it would be unlikely that a health professional would be criminally prosecuted for physical touching without consent, unless this was accompanied by more sinister intentions or malicious intent.

There are also offence provisions contained in the various guardianship legislation that may be breached by providing treatment – in the absence of consent or other lawful authority – to adult patients lacking capacity.

Legal exceptions to the need for consent

The law does provide for certain circumstances where consent from the patient, or those acting on behalf of a patient lacking capacity, is not necessary. Although there are potentially a range of specific exceptions (found in various legislation) here, the main legal exceptions are briefly discussed.

Emergency and necessity

The provision of medical treatment without consent can also be justified on what has been called the 'emergency principle' or the 'principle of necessity'. As noted in *Rogers v Whitaker* (1992) 175 CLR 479 where a person is unable to consent and medical intervention is considered necessary and reasonable then no consent is needed. This principle is most commonly applied when an unconscious patient is brought into the emergency department of a hospital following trauma; in this circumstance the treating team can rely on this legal principle to administer urgent treatment without the need to obtain consent for the intervention. While this is a common law principle, it is also given legislative backing in some of the States around Australia.

Court order

In circumstances where a court order has been obtained authorising particular health care or treatment to be provided to a patient, then no further consent needs to be obtained. This will usually only happen where there is a dispute over what health care decision should be made for an adult who lacks decision-making capacity.

Mental health

In some circumstances mental health legislation allows treatment to be administered without consent. These circumstances are considered in Chapter 9.

Overview

This chapter has demonstrated the ethical and legal importance of patients participating in decisions affecting their health care. A patient's right to choose what happens to their body is a fundamental human right that must be respected. The prominence given to the ethical principle of autonomy is reflected in the legal principles applicable in Australia which absolutely respect a competent adult's right to choose whether to submit to health care and treatment. The law has also developed other mechanisms for decision-making, including allowing others close to the patient to make decisions on their behalf should they lose the ability to make decisions themselves.

Figure 5.1 highlights the interactions between the ethical principles and the legal principles relevant to consent and refusal of consent.

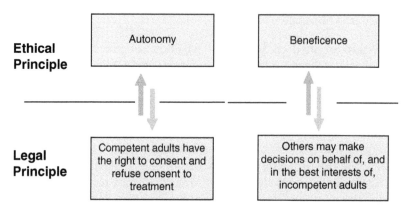

Figure 5.1   Ethical and legal principles relevant to consent and refusal of consent

Further reading

➤ McGrath, P. & Phillips E. 2008, 'Western notions of informed consent and indigenous cultures: Australian findings at the interface', *Journal of Bioethical Inquiry*, 5: 21–31.

➤ Attorney General's Department of New South Wales. 2008, Capacity Toolkit, www.justice.nsw.gov.au/diversityservices/Documents/capacity_toolkit0609.pdf.

Questions

1. Consider the legal, ethical and practical challenges in treating a patient with variable capacity. What approach should be taken to decision-making about treatment for such a patient?

2. Discuss how the principles of beneficence and non-maleficence come into conflict when a competent person decides to refuse life-saving treatment.

Scenario

Juliet is a 48-year-old woman diagnosed with carcinoma of the colon. She was a university lecturer in biochemistry and presented as alert, oriented and intelligent. She understood her diagnosis and agreed to the recommended surgery to remove the tumour and whatever else could be done for her. Following the surgery she experienced multiple complications and remained in ICU. During that time she experienced cardiac failure, renal failure, sepsis and required multiple surgical procedures and experienced significant pain. One day, she was asked to sign a consent form for revision of her colostomy and removal of scar tissue. She refused saying she did not want to suffer any more pain, did not want further procedures and wanted to be left alone. The nurse taking care of her told the junior medical officer the patient's wishes. He ordered that Juliet be sedated. Forty minutes later the senior medical officer visited the patient and had her sign a consent form.

Apply the decision-making framework to this scenario.

6

Children as patients

Introduction

Children hold a special place in our society. The innocence and vulnerability of the young mean that we regard them as a special group worthy of specific treatment, rules and attention. While the legal definition of children is generally accepted in Australia as being those under 18 years of age (and this is the definition we adopt for this chapter), it is recognised that this legal definition may differ from country to country. In addition, the terms child and adult may generally be used by some in recognition that an individual is of a certain maturity or exhibits a certain level of independence, regardless of their chronological age.

Children's vulnerability comes about through their young age, lack of understanding and power, and reliance on others for care. However, the diversity of children as a group – that encompasses infants through to teenagers – means that different issues arise depending on the age and maturity of the child patient being dealt with. Studies examining children's understanding at various ages show that they often have a greater capacity for understanding than might otherwise be attributed to them (see, for example, Weithorn 1982). As children age and develop we particularly see notions of dependence and vulnerability being challenged when teenagers mature before reaching adulthood.

These issues in relation to children present themselves in particular ways in the health care context. While paediatric patients make up a smaller proportion of patients nationwide, studies have shown that they require additional time, effort and skill from hospital staff caring for them compared with adult patients (Hanson et al. 1998). In particular, the cost of caring for child patients is often greater due to the increased level of nursing care they receive (Hanson et al. 1998), demonstrating the importance of nurses in paediatric care. Nurses and midwives have particular responsibilities, both ethically and legally, towards child patients which they must understand and act in accordance with.

In this chapter we examine the ethical issues surrounding consent and refusal of consent on behalf of children and by mature children. Nurses and midwives also have ethical responsibilities to ensure the welfare of children whom they see. This chapter also describes how the law deals with these issues of decision-making by, and on behalf of, children and the mandatory reporting of child abuse and neglect.

Ethical importance of children

The principles approach

Autonomy

The principle of autonomy, which is so highly respected when dealing with adult patients, is not given such prominence when dealing with children. More influential is the principle of beneficence discussed below. Unsurprisingly, in the health care setting, we do not always respect the wishes of children; to do so would present problems. For example, a 6-year-old who says that he or she does not want to receive an injection (because of the pain associated with the needle), will not have their wishes respected if their parents and medical team consider that the injection will be in their best interests. However, this does not mean that the principle of autonomy is irrelevant to children. Today, the participation of children in decision-making is very important in the health care context (Donnelly and Kilkelly 2011). Respecting the right of children to be involved in decisions affecting their health care – whether through age-appropriate explanation of health care or health care professionals addressing the child patient and not just parents – is another way autonomy can be recognised. There has also been increasing recognition that some children, particularly those with chronic conditions, have good insight and understanding into their own conditions and may be able to legitimately participate in decisions affecting them, even if they appear quite young.

    The issue of whether to respect the autonomy of older, more mature children is a difficult one. Teenagers who are mature or are close to adulthood often make major decisions in other aspects of their lives. Some may be living independently, supporting themselves and may even have children themselves. Clearly these children deserve to have their autonomy respected more than infants and younger children. However, the extent they should be allowed to make decisions for themselves – particularly when those decisions may not be considered by others to be in their best interests – is still debated.

The decision-making autonomy of parents, who generally make decisions on behalf of their children, can also be an ethically challenging area. This may arise when parents are faced with difficult decisions regarding treatment of their children – particularly at the end of life (Gillam and Sullivan (2011) – or when health professionals disagree with the decision made by parents (see, for example, the case of *Children's Health Queensland Hospital v AT* discussed at p. 123). Parents making decisions on behalf of their children are entitled to sufficient information and support to allow them to make decisions on the best available information.

Beneficence

The principle of beneficence or the need to act in the best interests of children is one of the main ethical principles that governs how health professionals deal with children. Maintaining and supporting the welfare of children is generally acknowledged to be an aim of our society and, as such, acting in the best interests of children in a health care context mirrors this societal concern.

Acting in the best interests of children will generally override the need to respect their autonomy (although, as discussed above in the situation involving older, more mature children, the interaction between these two principles becomes more complicated). The need to act in the best interests of a child patient may also override the autonomy of the parents of the child. While rare, situations may arise where parents make decisions that others, including health professionals, do not consider to be in the best interests of children (see, for example, the case of *Children's Health Queensland Hospital v AT* discussed at p. 123). In these circumstances parental decision-making may be superseded.

Sometimes there may be legitimate debate over what course of action is in the best interests of a child patient. In these circumstances dialogue and discussion – between the child, where they are old enough to communicate and participate (regardless of whether they are considered the legal decision-maker), parents and health professionals (and sometimes ethics committees) – will be used to investigate the options and reach agreement as to what course of action to take.

As noted in Chapter 2 the principle of beneficence applies to society as a whole, so supports public health-related programmes that benefit the broader community. This is particularly relevant in relation to public health initiatives in childhood, such as vaccination of children. Children as a group benefit greatly when vaccination programmes are supported within the community and promoted by health professionals in accordance with the best available evidence. This is also the case in Australia where childhood vaccination programmes are supported by the Nursing and Midwifery Board of Australia (see section on 'Health advocacy for children').

Non-maleficence

The duty to 'do no harm' and to prevent harm under the principle of non-maleficence also strongly influences our actions towards children. Many steps are taken by health professionals to try to minimise the pain and suffering of children who are patients. Most hospitals decorate their paediatrics wards in bright colours, have play therapists, music therapists and child-focused activities to try to minimise the pain and discomfort of child patients who require uncomfortable or painful treatment. This is consistent with the principle of non-maleficence.

This principle also becomes particularly relevant when considering health professionals' obligations to prevent abuse or harm of child patients. Health professionals will often be in a position to assess the physical and psychological state of child patients and this may lead to suspicions or knowledge that a child has been intentionally harmed by others. There is also an obligation to advocate against practices that can harm – such as female genital mutilation (also recognised as unlawful). The principle of non-maleficence places moral obligations on health professionals to take action to try and prevent a child from being exposed to harm. This moral obligation is also reflected in a legal obligation (see section on 'The law relating to child protection').

Justice

The principle of justice, and in particular rights-based justice, is important in interacting with children. Today, there is increasing recognition at an international level that children have certain rights. The *United Nations Convention on the Rights of the Child* recognises a range of rights, including children's rights to access health care, their right to communicate their views and participate, and their right to protection from abuse and neglect. These are all very important in the health care context where children are patients. In addition, the obligation for nurses and midwives to follow morally just laws – such as the requirements for mandatory reporting discussed later in the chapter – also comes within the ambit of justice.

Nurses and midwifery codes

The Australian Codes of Conduct of both professions explicitly recognise the legal and ethical obligations on Australian nurses and midwives to act and report where children may be at risk of harm, and provide guidance in relation to decision-making by and for children. In addition, both the ICN and ICM Codes of Ethics touch on issues relating to children as patients.

Participation of children in health care decisions

Principle 2.2(b) in both professions' Code of Conduct, relevantly states that nurses must 'advocate on behalf of the [patient] where necessary, and recognise when substitute decision-makers are needed'. Children are vulnerable patients, by virtue of their lack of power and, often, their lack of understanding. Where necessary, nurses and midwives may have to act as an advocate for child patients, particularly in circumstances where it appears others tasked with this role are not acting appropriately.

This statement implicitly recognises that with children the capacity for decision-making and participation in decision-making will differ depending on the child, their stage of development and their understanding. As already mentioned, the range of abilities, maturity and understanding present within children – from newborns to adolescents – is hugely variable. As such, consideration always needs to be made in relation to the current child patient and their current situation. Even though children may not have the legal ability to make decisions regarding their health care and treatment, their views cannot be ignored. Children, like other patients, are entitled to participate in decisions affecting them to the extent possible given their age and understanding.

Both Codes of Conduct at Principle 2.2 refer to 'shared decision-making'. This is relevant in recognising that nurses and midwives should assist in facilitating family members and, in the case of children, particularly parents, to make decisions, where relevant, together with the child patient.

At 2.3(c) of both Codes of Conduct, it states that nurses and midwives must:

> act according to the person's capacity for decision-making and consent, including when caring for children and young people, based on their maturity and capacity to understand, and the nature of the proposed care.

Principle 3.2(d) in both Codes of Conduct also notes that nurses and midwives 'adopt practices that ... avoid bias ... and challenge belief based upon assumption (for example, based on ... age ...)'. The preamble to the ICN Code of Ethics for Nurses also notes that nursing care is 'respectful of and unrestricted by considerations of age'. These statements remind us that nurses and midwives have to keep in mind not to treat patients who are children in a prejudicial fashion simply because of their age – for example, by assuming that all children cannot make decisions for themselves.

Protection from harm and mandatory reporting

The ICM Code of Ethics for Midwives, at III(e), states that 'Midwives understand the adverse consequences that ethical and human rights violations have on the health of women and infants, and will work to eliminate these violations'. Perhaps one of the greatest human rights violations that children can experience is suffering abuse from those who are meant to be caring from them.

The national Codes of Conduct recognise the significance of nurses' and midwives' roles in protecting children, clearly outlining the ethical and legal responsibility of the professions in relation to mandatory reporting of suspected abuse. This is also reflected in the ICN Code of Ethics, which notes at Element 1, that a nurse 'shares with society the responsibility for initiating and supporting action to meet the health and social needs of the public, in particular those of vulnerable populations'. Nurses and midwives, along with other health professionals, are often in a unique trusted position when they come into contact with paediatric patients. This raises particular ethical obligations to consider the welfare of this vulnerable group. Principle 1.3 in both professions' Codes of Conduct also relevantly states:

> Caring for those who are vulnerable brings legislative responsibilities for midwives, including the need to abide by relevant mandatory reporting requirements as they apply across individual states and territories. [Nurses and midwives] must:
>
> a. abide by the relevant mandatory reporting legislation that is imposed to protect groups that are particularly at risk, including reporting obligations about … child abuse and neglect and remaining alert to the newborn and infants who may be at risk.

More generally, at 1.1 and 1.2, both Codes of Conduct recognise the need for nurses and midwives to act in accordance with the law. In this context, this relates to the law regarding decision-making by and on behalf of children and also to the laws regarding mandatory reporting of suspected child abuse (discussed further at 'The law relating to decision-making for and by children' and 'The law relating to child protection').

Also relevant to nurses' and midwives' ethical obligations to children is Principle 3.2(c) which acknowledges 'the social, economic, cultural, historical and behavioural factors' that can influence health. Children will not often be in control of their domestic circumstances but this can influence their wellbeing and, where relevant, their recovery. As such this is something for nurses and midwives to be mindful of in providing care and support to child patients and their families.

Health advocacy for children

Both the nursing and midwifery Codes of Conduct deal with health advocacy of broader populations (7.2) and this has specific relevance to children in the community due to the impact of vaccination programmes in preventing outbreaks of harmful disease. Principles 7.2(c) relevantly states that nurses and midwives must 'participate in efforts to promote the health of communities and meet their obligations with respect to disease prevention including vaccination'. It references the Nursing and Midwifery Board's position statement on nurses, midwives and vaccination (NMBA 2016) which supports the provision of the best available evidence to the public about the safe and effective use of vaccines and the public health benefits associated with vaccination programmes. Principle 7.1(a) of both professions' Codes of Conduct reinforces this by stating that nurses and midwives must 'understand and promote the principles of public health, such as … vaccination'.

The law relating to decision-making for and by children

Here we consider what legal principles nurses and midwives must be familiar with in dealing with decision-making by and for child patients.

Consent and refusal of consent on behalf of young children – Parental decision-making

Where children are patients in a health care setting, there is a presumption that the child does not have capacity to make health care decisions, unless there is evidence that they can. For a discussion of when a child will have capacity to make health care decisions, see the section on 'Consent and refusal of consent by mature children'.

For most babies, infants and young children it is clear that they do not have sufficient communication skills or understanding to make decisions about their own health care. In this circumstance, generally parents are recognised by law to be the correct person(s) to make decisions for their children.

Who can make decisions on behalf of a child patient

Normally the natural parents of a child will have the ability to legally make decisions on behalf of their child (*Family Law Act 1975* (Cth) s 61C; *Marion's case*). However, circumstances can arise where the natural parents are no longer alive, or other adults have taken on the role of caring for the child. In these circumstances it can be more difficult to determine who has the ability to make decisions on behalf of child patients.

Where children have been adopted, then the adopted parents have the same ability to make decisions as if they were the natural parents of the child. If the parents of a child patient are under 18 years of age themselves, then in order to make decisions on behalf of their children they must be considered competent (see discussion of *Gillick*-competence at 'Gillick-competent children and consent'). If the parents are not considered competent, then relevant government departments need to be contacted to have a legal guardian appointed for the child patient.

Sometimes, orders may be made by the Family Court that give another person (who is not a natural parent) the power to make health care decisions on behalf of a child. Step-parents and de factos do not generally have power to consent unless the child has been adopted or the person is the child's legal guardian. One exception is in South Australia where legislation specifically includes in the definition of 'parent' someone 'in loco parentis', that is, someone 'standing in the shoes of the parents' to make decisions on behalf of child patients (*Consent to Medical Treatment and Palliative Care Act 1995* (SA), s 4). So in South Australia someone 'standing in the shoes' of the parent would have legal authority to make decisions for a child patient (*Consent to Medical Treatment and Palliative Care Act 1995* (SA), s 12).

In some cases if children are under the protection of the State then the relevant State department dealing with child protection may need to be contacted to establish who has the legal ability to make decisions on behalf of a child patient.

For the purposes of this chapter, where we refer to 'parental' decision-making, this includes whoever has legal authority to make decisions on behalf of a child patient.

Limits on parental decision-making

While ordinarily parents, or the person exercising responsibility for the child, will be able to consent or refuse consent to treatment and health care on behalf of a child patient, there are limits to their decision-making ability.

Best interests of the child

The first limitation on parental decision-making is that the decision made must be considered to be in the 'best interests' of the child. While usually the fact that parents will be acting in the best interests of their child will not be in question, sometimes there is disagreement between the treating team and the parents, or between the parents, as to what is in the best interests of the child. In these circumstances a court may be asked to decide what is in the best interests of the child.

The courts have made clear that assessing the best interests of a child includes consideration of medical factors – including physical, psychological and emotional wellbeing – and social and welfare factors. It therefore includes an assessment of a child's welfare from a medical and non-medical perspective. One case which demonstrates the broad factors that need to be applied in determining the best interests test was the New South Wales case of *TS & DS v Sydney Children's Hospital Network* discussed below.

TS & DS v Sydney Children's Hospital Network [2012] NSWSC 1609

The child patient in this case had experienced health problems since the age of 2 months. He had elevated blood lactate levels, daily seizures, profound developmental delay, severe reflux and was deaf and almost blind. His treating team believed he had a fatal metabolic disorder and had, at most, months left to live. At the time of the application to the court he was 9 months old. The treating team considered that further treatment was not in the child's best interests and wanted to provide palliative care. The child's parents disagreed and applied to the Court for an order that he be treated by mechanical ventilation. The question for the Court was whether that treatment was in Mohammed's best interests. In doing so it considered the risks and benefits of ventilation. It was found that the child would need to be sedated, have a catheter inserted (with associated pain and discomfort) and be suctioned regularly. He was also at risk of suffering an airway injury through the ventilator. Placing him on a ventilator would not improve his underlying condition, his seizures, sight or hearing.

As the child had a short life expectancy and a ventilator would provide only temporary benefit and not improve his underlying condition, the Court decided he should not be subjected to pain and discomfort for the remainder of his life. Ventilation was not considered to be in his best interests and the Court did not grant the order sought by his parents.

Where a court (a State or Territory Supreme Court or the Commonwealth Family Court) decides particular treatment is in the best interests of the child, that treatment will be lawful even though a parent continues to voice an objection. The cases discussed below provide further examples of this.

Children's Health Queensland Hospital and Health Service v AT & Anor [2018] QSC 147

In this Queensland case, an 11-month-old boy – 'K' – was diagnosed with cortical dysplasia in the left hemisphere of his brain. This meant he suffered from frequent and severe seizures as a result of refractory epilepsy which did not respond to medication. The Supreme Court found that K's parents loved him very much, and were devoted to him. Over a period of time, a number of conventional and experimental medical interventions were tried by the treating team, together with traditional remedies and religious ceremonies requested by K's parents. However, all of these were considered to be largely ineffective. The treating team considered that the only way to ensure that K had the best possible chance of a future life, was to perform an invasive operation called a functional hemispherectomy – where the two sides of the brain are 'disconnected', in an attempt to preserve the 'good' side of the brain.

K's parents refused consent to that operation, as they retained hope, 'in accordance with their sincerely held religious and cultural beliefs' that 'traditional remedies might provide ... a miracle cure'. The Court considered all the options, including the parents' wish that the child be treated by alternative means, but ultimately it was decided that there was an 'urgent need' for the operation to prevent K's condition from deteriorating further. The hemispherectomy was also considered to give K the 'best chance to reach his potential' and without it he would never be able to walk or converse. As such it was in the best interest of K to undergo the operation and the Court authorised it, despite the wishes of the parents.

Re Heather [2003] NSWSC 532

In this New South Wales case an 11-year-old girl, 'Heather', had been diagnosed with a malignant tumour of the ovary when she was 10 years old. At that time she was operated on and part of the tumour was removed. Following this the treating team advised that ongoing chemotherapy was needed, and if this was given she was assessed as having an 85% chance of cure. Over the next six months (and prior to the court hearing), the medical team continued to advise that chemotherapy should commence but had trouble getting in touch with the family. During this time Heather's parents sought alternative opinions from a number of health professionals

▶

◄

and commenced Heather on non-conventional cancer treatment. Heather's parents wished to find an alternative to chemotherapy for their daughter. Two weeks before the court hearing, Heather was assessed in hospital and found to have a recurrence of cancer in her spleen and groin. It was the opinion of specialists at that point that it was 'imperative to begin chemotherapy within the next week' as there was a risk the mass in her spleen could bleed into her abdominal cavity and threaten her life. The parents remained reluctant to start chemotherapy and wished to undertake more research and obtain more opinions on alternative treatments. Proceedings were commenced in court by the Department of Community Services.

The Court found that while there were serious side effects and risks in undergoing chemotherapy, the consequences of inaction were likely to result in the death of Heather. The Court stated that the 'fundamental test must be what is in the best interests of the child'. As such, the Court authorised the medical team to carry out chemotherapy and other associated tests and procedures, in spite of the parents' wishes.

Special medical procedures

Another limitation on parents making decisions on behalf of children in a health care context relates to 'special' medical procedures which are considered to be so serious as to place them outside the scope of ordinary parental decision-making. The types of procedures that are within this limited category of special procedures on children include sterilisation, abortion and some gender-reassignment procedures. When decisions must be made regarding whether or not a child undergoes these types of procedures, generally a court or tribunal is given the task of deciding and they will authorise such a procedure where they consider it to be in the best interests of the child.

The legal principles relevant to these types of 'special' medical procedures were outlined in the famous Australian High Court case known as *Marion's case*.

Secretary, Department of Health and Community Services v JWB and SMB (1992) 175 CLR 218 (known as *Marion's case*)

Marion was a 14-year-old girl who had an intellectual disability, deafness and epilepsy, as well as other conditions, and was not able to care for herself. Her parents applied to the Family Court for an order authorising Marion to have a sterilisation procedure (procedures the court referred to as hysterectomy and ovariectomy) to prevent pregnancy, menstruation and to stabilise hormonal fluxes with the aim of helping to

►

> ◀
>
> eliminate psychological and behavioural consequences. Once the matter was before the High Court, the judges had to decide whether the parents of Marion were able to consent to such a procedure.
>
> The Court decided that sterilisation was one of a number of 'special' medical procedures which were outside the scope of parental decision-making. The reasons for this were the:
>
> - **significant risk that the wrong decision could be made**: due to the complex issue of consent, the potential conflict of interest held by parents and the fact that not all medical staff might act appropriately; and
>
> - **the grave consequences if the wrong decision is made**: due to the invasive and irreversible nature of the procedure and the long-term consequences for the child.
>
> As such, the High Court stated that for 'special' medical procedures authorisation from a court was required as a 'procedural safeguard' to ensure that the proposed procedure was in the best interests of the child. (Note, that some tribunals have the power to provide authorisation for special medical procedures in some children.)

Gillick-competent children

A third limit on parental decision-making is when older, mature children may be able to make decisions themselves. Where children are considered *Gillick*-competent, they can generally give consent themselves and parental consent is not required.

Consent and refusal of consent by mature children

The legal principles applicable to older, mature children who have an understanding of their condition and the treatment proposed for them differ from those applicable to younger children. The law has recognised that some children have matured to the extent that they should be able to make some health care decisions independently of their parents. Here we discuss these legal principles.

Gillick-competent children and consent

In the well-known English case, the Court in *Gillick v West Norfolk and Wisbech Area Health Authority and Department of Health and Social Security* [1986] AC 112 (known as *Gillick's case*) found that children who were sufficiently intelligent and mature and had an understanding of the proposed treatment could consent to treatment themselves. While the

High Court in *Marion's case* (discussed in the section on 'Special medical procedures') was dealing with a child with an intellectual disability,
in their judgment the majority of the Court made clear that the principles in *Gillick's case* should be accepted and adopted in Australia. As such
the *Gillick* test is applicable law in Australia. A description of *Gillick's case*
is set out below. You may hear people refer to mature children as '*Gillick*-
competent' children – meaning they are deemed capable of making
some health care decisions by themselves.

**Gillick and West Norfolk and Wisbech Area Health Authority
and Department of Health and Social Security [1986] AC 112
(known as *Gillick's case*)**

In this case Mrs Gillick objected to advice given by the Department of Health to
health authorities that suggested in exceptional cases doctors could decide whether
to prescribe contraception for girls under 16 years old without the knowledge of their
parents. Mrs Gillick, who had five daughters, sought a declaration from the court that
the advice was unlawful.

This case stated that a child would have capacity to consent to medical examination
and treatment, including contraceptive treatment, if the child had:

  sufficient maturity and intelligence to understand the nature and implications of the
  proposed treatment.

Where a child is assessed as satisfying this test, parental consent is not required and
the consent provided by the Gillick-competent child will be legally valid.

Practically, the treating health professional will make the assessment of
whether a child is *Gillick*-competent. Nurse practitioners, or nurses who
are part of a treating team for a child, may have to assess or may be asked
their opinion on whether child patients are *Gillick*-competent and capable
of consenting to health care.

South Australia

In South Australia some of these legal principles have been reflected in
legislation. Section 12 of the *Consent to Medical Treatment and Palliative
Care Act 1995* (SA) states that a medical practitioner can provide medical
treatment to a child if they believe the child is 'capable of understanding
the nature, consequences and risks of the treatment' and it is in the 'best
interest of the child's health and well-being'. In addition, the legislation

also provides (at Section 6) that 'A person of or over 16 years of age may make decisions about his or her own medical treatment as validly and effectively as an adult'. So in South Australia children aged 16 and above will be treated the same as adults for the purpose of consenting to medical treatment.

Refusal of consent by *Gillick*-competent children

While the law recognises that *Gillick*-competent children may consent to health care, this does not necessarily extend to a *Gillick*-competent child's refusal of recommended health care being respected. While the decision made by a *Gillick*-competent child cannot be overridden by the treating team or parents, in Australia it is clear that a decision made by a *Gillick*-competent child may be overridden by a court (a Supreme Court or the Family Court). Therefore, where the treating team or parents have concerns that the decision made by a child patient is not in their best interests, they may approach a court to make a decision. The court will decide based on its view of what is in the child's best interest. This occurred in the cases described below.

Minister for Health v AS (2004) 33 Fam **LR 223**

The patient in this Western Australian case was a 15-year-old boy diagnosed with atypical Burkitt's lymphoma. Treatment of this condition involved chemotherapy and treatment of the side effects of chemotherapy through blood transfusions. The patient and his parents were Jehovah's Witnesses. The patient accepted chemotherapy but refused blood transfusions. An application was made to the Supreme Court of Western Australia by the Minister for Health. The Court in outlining the relevant legal principles stated:

> [T]he fact that the child refusing to consent to treatment may be of sufficient maturity and intelligence to understand the nature and implications of the proposed treatment, so as to be '*Gillick* competent', while relevant and important does not prevent the court from authorising medical treatment where the best interest of the child require.

While the treating team declared it would use all strategies other than blood transfusions which were reasonably available and clinically appropriate, in this case the Court also made an order authorising blood transfusions to be given if certain tests indicated that blood transfusions were necessary for the medical wellbeing of the patient.

▶

X v The Sydney Children's Hospitals Network [2013] NSWCA 320

In this case the child patient – 'X' – suffered from an aggressive cancer (Hodgkin's disease). X was aged 17 years 8 months when he appealed a previous Court's decision to authorise health professionals to give him a blood transfusion. X and his parents were Jehovah's Witnesses and he had previously refused a transfusion, a decision supported by his parents.

X had previously had courses of low-dose chemotherapy to avoid the need for a blood transfusion. However, when the matter came before the Court, X was severely anaemic. The treating team were concerned that when chemotherapy was restarted, the anaemia would worsen and could result in death. X had threatened to remove the intravenous tube if blood was administered in an emergency.

The Court considered that X was a highly intelligent and mature minor. Despite this, the Court decided that providing treatment was in X's best interests. The Court ordered that the hospital was authorised to carry out the treatment. (Note, in other jurisdictions, there is specific legislation that allows blood transfusions to be given in the absence of consent, see discussion below).

Despite overriding the children's refusal in these cases, courts today are increasingly likely to give older children's views more weight in assessing what is in their best interest.

Legal exceptions to the need for consent

Some legal exceptions exist which allow certain treatment to be given without the need to obtain consent for, or from, a child patient. Here we consider some of the major legal exceptions.

Blood transfusions

In the Australian Capital Territory, Northern Territory, Queensland, Tasmania, Victoria and Western Australia, legislation exists which allows blood transfusions to be given to children either without the need for consent (which would normally be provided by parents or by *Gillick*-competent children themselves) or in the face of a refusal. The legislation in these States and Territories generally allows blood transfusions to be given if two doctors are of the opinion that a blood transfusion is necessary to prevent the death of a child and a parent (or other authorised person) has either refused consent or it is not practical to contact them in the circumstances. (See *Transplantation and Anatomy Act 1978* (ACT), s 23; *Emergency Medical Operations Act* (NT), ss 2–3; *Transplantation and Anatomy Act 1979* (Qld), s 20; *Human Tissue Act 1985* (Tas), s 21; *Human Tissue Act 1982* (Vic), s 24; *Human Tissue and Transplant Act 1982* (WA), s 21.)

In New South Wales and South Australia health professionals who wish to administer an urgent blood transfusion may be able to rely on other legislation (described next) which allows for treatment to be given in circumstances of emergency.

Emergencies

Similar to the position in relation to adults, providing medical treatment to children without consent can also be justified on the 'emergency principle' or the 'principle of necessity' (see Chapter 5). So if a child is brought into a hospital requiring urgent and immediate treatment, the treating team can rely on this legal principle to administer urgent treatment without the need to obtain consent for the intervention.

In some jurisdictions, like the Northern Territory, New South Wales and South Australia, this principle has been included in legislation. In the Northern Territory section 3 of the *Emergency Medical Operations Act* (NT) provides that where two doctors consider the child patient is 'in danger of dying or of suffering a serious permanent disability; and … the performance of an operation on the patient is desirable in order to prevent the death of the patient or the occurrence of the disability' consent does not need to be obtained. In New South Wales section 174 of the *Children and Young Person's (Care and Protection) Act 1998* (NSW) provides that where a doctor considers that as a matter of urgency treatment needs to be given to save a child's life or prevent serious damage to their health, then that treatment can be given without the need for consent from the child's parent or the child themselves. In South Australia section 13 of the *Consent to Medical Treatment and Palliative Care Act 1995* (SA) provides that in emergency situations, while consent to treatment ought to be sought from parents, 'the child's health and well-being are paramount' and as such treatment can be administered despite a refusal 'if it is in the best interests of the child's health and well-being'.

Court order

As shown in the cases discussed above (in 'Best interest of the child' and 'Refusal of consent by *Gillick*-competent children'), where a court makes an order authorising treatment there is no need for parental or child consent. The order of a court is sufficient authority for health professionals to administer treatment in accordance with the order.

The law relating to child protection

As emphasised by the nursing and midwifery Codes of Conduct, another aspect of the law that nurses and midwives must be familiar with regarding child patients are laws that attempt to address the issue of harm against children – including child abuse and neglect and female genital mutilation.

Mandatory reporting obligations of health professionals

All States and Territories in Australia place obligations on nurses and midwives to report known or reasonably suspected cases of child abuse to local authorities. The purpose of these laws is to protect children from harm and also enable State departments to initiate processes to help families in need of assistance. Mandatory reports are immediately assessed by staff in the relevant government department dealing with child safety and protection. Staff there will decide what course of action needs to be taken in relation to the child. At this initial assessment sometimes it is decided that no action needs to be taken or that support should be offered to the family via government agencies or non-governmental organisations. However, if this initial assessment indicates that it is necessary, a formal assessment and investigation will begin into the safety of the child. Where intervention is justified, children may be moved to the care of others for their own protection.

It is crucial that nurses and midwives understand their obligations in relation to reporting child abuse and neglect. Indeed, in the majority of States and Territories a failure to make a mandatory report when required results in an offence being committed (*Children and Young People Act 2008* (ACT), s 356; *Care and Protection of Children Act* (NT), s 26; *Children and Young People (Safety) Act 2017* (SA), s 31; *Children, Young Persons and Their Families Act 1997* (Tas), s 14; *Children, Youth and Families Act 2005* (VIC), s 184; *Children and Community Services Act 2004* (WA), s 124B).

The legislation in the Australian Capital Territory, New South Wales, the Northern Territory, Queensland, South Australia and Victoria also makes clear that the person who makes the report in good faith will be protected against disciplinary action and, in most cases, legal liability. In most of these jurisdictions, their identity will be protected (*Children and Young People Act 2008* (ACT), s 874; *Children and Young Persons (Care and Protection) Act 1998* (NSW), s 29; *Care and Protection of Children Act* (NT), s 27; *Child Protection Act 1999* (Qld), s 197A; *Children and Young People (Safety) Act 2017* (SA), ss 163, 166; *Children, Young Persons and Their Families Act 1997*

(Tas), ss 16, 101A; *Children, Youth and Families Act 2005* (Vic), ss 189, 191; *Children and Community Services Act 2004* (WA), ss 124F, 129).

Where there has been a failure to make a mandatory report in circumstances that justify it, this can result in disciplinary proceedings against health professionals. This occurred against a doctor in the New South Wales case of *Health Care Complaints Commission v Dunstan* [2018] NSW-CATOD 102.

Table 6.1 summarises the circumstances that nurses and midwives are *required* by law to report circumstances of child abuse to government departments. Unless stated otherwise, these mandatory reporting requirements apply to all children aged below 18 years. While the requirements are similar, each jurisdiction has specific provisions relating to what needs to be reported in what circumstances.

It should also be noted that members of the public, including nurses and midwives, can also make voluntary reports to relevant government departments where they have concerns about the welfare of a child.

In relation to prenatal reports regarding concerns about the safety of an unborn child, see Chapter 12.

Offences relating to female genital mutilation

Female genital mutilation (FGM) is the practice of 'intentional, non-therapeutic physical modification of female genitalia' (Mathews 2011). It is predominately a cultural and historical practice within Africa and some Asian countries and has been experienced by millions of girls and women worldwide. As Australia is a multicultural nation, there will be some people who have experienced or are familiar with the practice of FGM. There are various forms of FGM but all forms are non-therapeutic and physically harmful and this practice is unlawful in Australia. Those that assist in the practice of FGM are liable for offences in all States and Territories in Australia (*Crimes Act 1900* (ACT) pt 4; *Crimes Act 1900* (NSW) s 45; *Criminal Code Act* (NT) pt VI, div 4A; *Criminal Code* (Qld) s 323A; *Criminal Law Consolidation Act 1935* (SA) pt 3, div 8; *Criminal Code Act 1924* (Tas) s 178A; *Crimes Act 1958* (Vic) s 32; *Criminal Code* (WA) s 306).

In some jurisdictions, for example South Australia, child protection officers and courts are empowered to take action to protect children at risk of FGM *(Children and Young People (Safety) Act 2017* (SA), ss 53, 149).

Unfortunately, the first group of individuals convicted by a jury for FGM offences in Australia included a person who was a registered nurse and midwife.

Table 6.1 Summary of mandatory reporting duties in each Australian jurisdiction

Jurisdiction	Legislation	When to report	Types of harm
Australian Capital Territory	*Children and Young People Act 2008* (ACT), s 356.	Nurses, enrolled nurses and midwives must report, as soon as possible, to the director general where they believe on reasonable grounds that a child has experienced, or is experiencing **sexual abuse** or **non-accidental physical injury** and this belief arises from information obtained during the course of their work.	**'Non-accidental physical injury'** **'Sexual abuse'**
New South Wales	*Children and Young Persons (Care and Protection) Act 1998* (NSW), ss 23, 27, 27A.	A person who delivers health care (e.g. nurses, enrolled nurses, midwives) must report, as soon as possible, to the Secretary of the Department if, during the course of their work, they have reasonable grounds to suspect that a child* is at '**risk of significant harm**'. *Only applicable to children aged 16 years and under.	**'Risk of significant harm'** means where concerns exist for the safety, welfare or wellbeing of the child due to the any of the following being present to a significant extent: (a) the child's basic physical or psychological needs are not being met or are at risk of not being met, (b) the parents or other caregivers have not arranged and are unable or unwilling to arrange for the child to receive necessary medical care, (b1) in the case of a child who is required to attend school, the parents or other caregivers have not arranged and are unable or unwilling to arrange for the child to receive an education, (c) the child has been, or is at risk of being, physically or sexually abused or ill-treated, (d) the child is living in a household where there have been incidents of domestic violence and, as a consequence, the child or young person is at risk of serious physical or psychological harm, (e) a parent or other caregiver has behaved in such a way towards the child that the child or young person has suffered or is at risk of suffering serious psychological harm.

Jurisdiction	Legislation	When to report	Types of harm
Northern Territory	Care and Protection of Children Act (NT), ss 15, 16, 26.	Any person (including nurses and midwives) who believes on reasonable grounds that: • A child has suffered or is likely to suffer **harm** or **exploitation**; • A child less than 14 years has been or is likely to be a victim of a sexual offence; • A child over 16 has been the victim of a sexual offence by a person who is in a special position of care for that child; must report to the CEO or a police officer as soon as possible. AND Nurses, enrolled nurses and midwives who believe on reasonable grounds that a child aged 14 or 15 years has been or is likely to be a victim of a sexual offence and that the difference in age between the child and alleged sexual offender is more than 2 years, must report to the CEO or a police officer as soon as possible.	'**Harm**' to a child is any significant detrimental effect caused by any act, omission or circumstance on: (a) the physical, psychological or emotional wellbeing of the child; or (b) the physical, psychological or emotional development of the child. It can be caused by physical, psychological or emotional abuse or neglect, sexual abuse or other exploitation, or exposure of the child to physical violence. '**Exploitation**' of a child includes sexual and any other forms of exploitation of the child such as: (a) sexual abuse of the child; (b) involving the child as a participant or a spectator in an act of a sexual nature, prostitution or a pornographic performance.

Table 6.1 *Continued*

Jurisdiction	Legislation	When to report	Types of harm
Queensland	*Child Protection Act 1999* (Qld) ss 9, 13E.	If a nurse or midwife forms a **reportable suspicion** about a child, in the course of their work, they must give a written report to the chief executive.	'**Reportable suspicion**' about a child is a reasonable suspicion that the child: (a) has suffered, is suffering, or is at unreasonable risk of suffering, significant **harm** caused by physical or sexual abuse; and (b) may not have a parent able and willing to protect the child from harm. '**Harm**', to a child, is any detrimental effect of a significant nature on the child's physical, psychological or emotional wellbeing. Harm can be caused by – (a) physical, psychological or emotional abuse or neglect; or (b) sexual abuse or exploitation.
South Australia	*Children and Young People (Safety) Act 2017* (SA) ss 17, 18, 30, 31.	If a nurse, enrolled nurse or midwife suspects on reasonable grounds that a child is, or may be, at risk and the suspicion is formed in the course of their work, they must report to the Minister as soon as possible.	'**Harm**' will be taken to be a reference to physical harm or psychological harm (whether caused by an act or omission) and, without limiting the generality of this subsection, includes such harm caused by sexual, physical, mental or emotional abuse or neglect. However, psychological harm does not include emotional reactions such as distress, grief, fear or anger that are a response to the ordinary vicissitudes of life. A child will be taken to be '**at risk**' if— (a) the child has suffered harm (being harm of a kind against which a child is ordinarily protected); or (b) there is a likelihood that the child will suffer harm (being harm of a kind against which a child is ordinarily protected); or (c) there is a likelihood that the child will be removed from the State (whether by their parent or guardian or by some other person) for the purpose of— (i) being subjected to a medical or other procedure that would be unlawful if performed in this State (including, to avoid doubt, female genital mutilation); or (ii) taking part in a marriage ceremony that would be a void or invalid marriage, under the *Marriage Act 1961* of the Commonwealth; or

Jurisdiction	Legislation	When to report	Types of harm
			(iii) enabling the child to take part in an activity, or an action to be taken in respect of the child, that would, if it occurred in this State, constitute an offence; or
			(d) the parents or guardians of the child are unable or unwilling to care for the child; or have abandoned the child, or cannot, after reasonable inquiry, be found; or are dead; or
			(e) the child is of compulsory school age but has been persistently absent from school without satisfactory explanation of the absence; or
			(f) the child is of no fixed address; or
			(g) any other circumstances of a kind prescribed by the regulations exist in relation to the child.
Tasmania	*Children, Young Persons and Their Families Act 1997* (Tas) ss 3, 13, 14.	Any person (including nurses and midwives) who knows, believes or suspects on reasonable grounds that a child is suffering, has suffered or is likely to suffer **abuse or neglect** has a responsibility to take steps (i.e. inform the Secretary or a Community-Based Intake Service) to prevent the occurrence or further occurrence of the abuse or neglect. AND If a nurse, enrolled nurse or midwife during the course of	'**Abuse or neglect**' means – (a) sexual abuse; or (b) physical or emotional injury or other abuse, or neglect, to the extent that – • the injured, abused or neglected person has suffered, or is likely to suffer, physical or psychological harm detrimental to the person's wellbeing; or • the injured, abused or neglected person's physical or psychological development is in jeopardy.

Table 6.1 *Continued*

Jurisdiction	Legislation	When to report	Types of harm
		their work knows, believes or suspects on reasonable grounds that a child has been or is being **abused or neglected** or there is a reasonable likelihood of a child being killed, abused or neglected, they must report to the Secretary or a Community-Based Intake Service as soon as possible.	
Victoria	*Children, Youth and Families Act 2005* (Vic) ss 162, 184.	A nurse or midwife who in the course of their work or the practise of their profession forms a belief on reasonable grounds that **a child is in need of protection** must report to the Secretary as soon as possible.	'**A child is in need of protection**' if the child has suffered, or is likely to suffer, significant harm as a result of physical injury or sexual abuse and the child's parents have not protected, or are unlikely to protect, the child from harm of that type.
Western Australia	*Children and Community Services Act 2004* (WA) ss 124A, 124B.	A nurse or midwife who in the course of their work believes on reasonable grounds that a child has been the subject of **sexual abuse** or is the subject of ongoing sexual abuse must report to the CEO or person approved by the CEO as soon as possible.	'**Sexual abuse**' in relation to a child includes sexual behaviour in circumstances where – (a) the child is the subject of bribery, coercion, a threat, exploitation or violence; or (b) the child has less power than another person involved in the behaviour; or (c) there is a significant disparity in the developmental function or maturity of the child and another person involved in the behaviour.

R v Magennis [2016] NSWSC 282

In this criminal proceeding against three people for crimes associated with FGM, one of the accused – Magennis – was a registered nurse and midwife who had worked in the health system. In that case the jury found that two young girls were subjected to a procedure known as 'khatna' that resulted in a cut to the clitoris. 'Khatna' was described as 'a rite of passage for girls in this culture when they reach seven years of age'. Magennis was found to have performed the FGM with a metal instrument. The NSW Supreme Court noted that: 'Female members who seek to have "khatna" performed on their own children ... have themselves experienced "khatna" in their childhood ... The generational cycle involved in the practice of "khatna" has no doubt contributed to the difficulty in stamping out the practice.'

After the trial the jury found all three accused, including Magennis, guilty of offences under the *Crimes Act 1900* (NSW), related to FGM. The suggestion that the procedure performed on the girls was purely symbolic and inflicted no injury was rejected by the jury. In a summary of the case the NSW Supreme Court noted that Magennis had 'abused her professional vocation in performing the procedure'.

The three offenders were each sentenced to 15 months' imprisonment.

Overview

This chapter has highlighted that children, as a vulnerable cohort within the health care system, are considered 'special'. This has resulted in the development of certain ethical approaches and legal rules that only apply to child patients. The law in relation to children often emphasises the societal obligation to protect children from harm, and this is particularly evident in the mandatory reporting requirements imposed on nurses and midwives around the country. Legally and ethically, there is also increasing recognition of the need to allow child patients to participate in decisions affecting their health care.

Figure 6.1 highlights the interactions between the ethical principles and the legal principles relevant to children and child protection.

Further reading

➤ Gillam, L. & Sullivan, J. 2011, 'Ethics at the end of life: Who should make decisions about treatment limitation for young children with life-threatening or life-limiting conditions?', *Journal of Paediatrics and Child Health*, 47, 594–598.

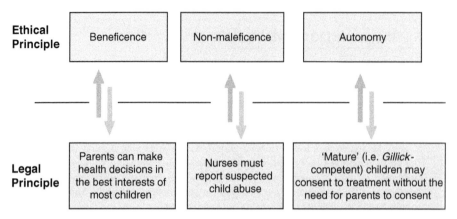

Figure 6.1 Ethical and legal principles relevant to children and child protection

➤ Mathews, B. & Smith, M. 2018, 'Children and consent to medical treatment', in B. White, F. McDonald, & L. Willmott (eds), *Health Law in Australia*, 3rd edn, Thomson Reuters: Sydney.

Questions

Discuss the difficulties in applying the ethical principles of beneficence and autonomy in a situation where a 13-year-old female patient with a chronic terminal illness expresses the wish to cease active treatment.

1. When should governments interfere in parental decision-making regarding treatment on behalf of child patients?

2. What are the arguments in favour of minimal intervention by governments?

Scenarios

1. Gary, an 8-year-old child, presents in the emergency department of a major hospital with his father, Wayne. Gary presents with limited mobility in his right arm, swelling and an open cut that looks to be a few days old. Wayne informs staff that the injury was sustained while Gary was playing and says he's been too busy to come in with Gary any earlier. JingYu, a registered nurse assigned to Gary, notes that the

child seems very withdrawn, does not engage when asked questions and has been crying.

The treating team recommend an x-ray to check if there are any broken bones. Wayne agrees to this. The x-ray shows no fractured bones. The treating team inform Wayne that the wound in Gary's arm is, however, showing signs of infection and that a course of antibiotics should be given to prevent it getting worse. Wayne refuses, saying that his son is just being a 'big cry baby' and that he will be fine.

Apply the ethical decision-making framework to this scenario.

2. Helena is a nurse who works as a paediatric nurse in a major tertiary children's hospital in Australia. Abul is a 15-year-old patient – well known to staff – who had previously suffered from a rare malignant blood condition. He is well liked by staff who know him and he is considered mature for this age. Abul is now back in hospital after recent tests showed a re-emergence of his condition. Abul attends the hospital with his parents and Helena is aware that the treating doctor has suggested that Abul receive a new treatment that has just been released. After meeting with the doctor, Abul finds Helena and asks to speak to her in confidence. He says that his parents are refusing to let him receive the treatment, saying the risks are too high. But he says to Helena, 'I know the risks, I want to do this, it's my best chance of a cure'.

Apply the ethical decision-making framework to this scenario.

7

Law, ethics and health information management

Introduction

The gathering of personal information is a critical part of the provision of health care and of maternity services. But the gathering of such information and its use raise a number of ethical and legal issues about how well, or poorly, that information is recorded, stored, used, shared and managed by health professionals. The clinical record is critically important to ensure continuity of care between health professionals and as a record of the patient's treatment. It also can be used as evidence in various types of legal proceedings.

Personal information involves two central concepts: confidentiality and privacy. These are often considered as interchangeable but they are distinct. The concept of confidentiality in health care has a long history; it was referred to in the Hippocratic Oath for doctors in ancient Greece from about 460 BCE to 370 BCE. Under this concept all health professionals have an obligation to keep information that was provided to them in confidence confidential or secret. The justification for confidentiality is that if patients do not believe that the health professional will keep their information confidential they may not be absolutely truthful with or provide complete information to health professionals. For example, they may not tell health professionals about their sexual practices or about illicit drug taking. In addition, if they do not trust that information will be kept confidential they may not come to a health professional at all, threatening that individual's health and safety and potentially the health and safety of the public as a whole. The obligation to keep information confidential is not absolute – there are exceptions that will be discussed in more detail below.

Privacy is a much broader and more recent concept, having been developed in the twentieth century. The concept of privacy implies that, as individuals, we have expectations that when we pass personal information to others, in particular the government, it will be kept private, even if we have not specifically or implicitly requested it. Privacy also encompasses physical privacy. While maintaining confidentiality and, increasingly, privacy has always been challenging, the introduction of electronic health records and social media, among other things, adds new complexities.

Electronic records address the difficulties associated with handwritten records and may have built-in systems for detecting errors, such as a health professional prescribing a medication to which the person is allergic; however, such systems are not fail-safe. Australia is currently rolling out a national electronic health record for all Australians, except those who opt out. The *Healthcare Identifiers Act 2010* (Cth), the *My Health Records Act 2012* (Cth) and the *My Health Records Rule 2016* (Cth) provide the legal framework for the electronic record. A variety of health professionals and administrators can access My Health Record. While this is a 'brave new world' for health services, national electronic health records raise important issues in respect of the maintenance of confidentiality and, especially, privacy.

Social media is more and more ubiquitous and raises issues for nurses and midwives about the maintenance of patient privacy and confidentiality, the maintenance of professional boundaries between nurses or midwives and their patients, and professionalism more generally. Some people argue that social media has led to people having fewer expectations around privacy and confidentiality; this may be so in terms of how comfortable some people are with self-disclosing information. But that does not mean they are comfortable with others disclosing information about them, especially sensitive information. It also does not change the obligations of health professionals in respect of confidentiality and privacy or the need to maintain boundaries.

Ethics and nursing practice

The principles approach

Justice

One relevant face of the principle of justice is rights-based justice – respect for patient rights. Privacy is increasingly recognised as a human right, a right arising from the right to be left alone by government. For example, article 12 of the *Universal Declaration of Human Rights* states that:

> No one shall be subjected to arbitrary interference with his privacy, family, home, or correspondence, nor to attacks upon his honour and reputation. Everyone has the right to the protection of the law against such interference or attacks.

Beneficence

Beneficence is the duty to benefit and assist others, to care for their welfare and to always act in the best interests of the patient. This duty extends to the need for nurses and midwives to keep good records. Good records benefit patients by fostering continuity of care between health providers and providing a history of that patient's care and treatment. The principle of beneficence also suggests that there may be some occasions where personal information should be disclosed to others in the best interests of the patient. For example, it is necessary for health professionals to share information in order to provide the best care to the patient.

Non-maleficence

Non-maleficence is the duty to do no harm and to protect others from harm. Patients might be harmed if records are poorly kept – for example, by being prescribed or administered medications they are allergic to. Patients and/or their families may also be harmed if their personal information is shared with others through their privacy or confidentiality being breached. The relationship between a nurse or a midwife and a patient and/or their family might be harmed if promises to keep information confidential are violated without a good reason.

New South Wales intimate photo case

A woman in New South Wales was admitted to a private hospital for gynaecological surgery. While the patient was anesthetised, a registered nurse used her phone to take a photograph of the patient's genitals. The nurse showed the photo to two other nurses who immediately reported her to management. The patient was told five weeks later by the surgeon during a follow-up call. The nurse was dismissed from the hospital. A Nursing and Midwifery Council investigation led to the nurse being reprimanded. The patient was terrified that the photo would end up on social media. A government-commissioned inquiry into privacy examined this case and recommended changing the law in New South Wales to provide protections against the sharing of intimate photographs without consent (Standing Committee on Law and Justice 2016 at p. 20).

Autonomy

Autonomy has been characterised in earlier chapters as the right for an individual to make choices as to what is in that person's best interest.

This would include a person being able to choose who can access their personal information and whether and how their personal information can be shared with others. It would also include individuals entering into agreements with others that personal information should not be shared outside that relationship in the expectation that those promises of confidentiality would be respected.

As discussed in earlier chapters, John Stuart Mill (1985) suggested that a legitimate restriction on autonomy was to protect others from serious harm. This would imply that personal information can be shared with appropriate others without an individual's consent if that information places others at serious risk of harm. An example of this could be if a patient is threatening to kill his or her family – this threat is against identifiable individuals and is a serious threat. An appropriate disclosure of this threat would be to an agency or a person from an agency, such as the police, that could prevent the threat manifesting. Many suggest that it also would be appropriate to warn the person or people who are threatened so they can take steps to protect themselves from harm. Another legitimate restriction on autonomy may be to protect the individual from harm. For example, if a patient was threatening to commit suicide there may be an argument that personal information can be released to prevent harm to that patient. But how far does this go? Competent adults have the right to take risks and make choices to put themselves at risk of harm – extreme sports, the choice to smoke and so on. So when does breaching confidentiality to protect an individual from harm slip over into paternalism? A further question of course is whether there are any limits on what information can be released and to whom.

The nursing and midwifery codes

Both the ICM and ICN Codes of Ethics and the Nursing and Midwifery Board of Australia's Codes of Conduct also have specific provisions in relation to information.

Confidentiality and privacy

The ICM states (at III a): 'Midwives hold in confidence client information in order to protect the right to privacy, and use judgement in sharing this information except when mandated by law.' The ICN Element 1 states: 'The nurse holds in confidence personal information and uses judgement in sharing this information.' The Codes of Conduct state at 3.5 that midwives and nurses 'have ethical and legal obligations to protect the privacy' of women and patients and (at 3.5.b) 'provide surroundings to enable private and confidential consultations and discussions, particularly when working with multiple people at the same time, or in a shared space'.

Access to records

Access to records relates both to a patient's ability to access records and to the ability of nurses and midwives to access patient records. In relation to the former, the Codes of Conduct also note at 3.5.f that nurses and midwives must 'recognise people's right to access information contained in health records, facilitate that access and promptly facilitate the transfer of health information when requested by people, in accordance with local policy'. In relation to the latter, the Codes of Conduct note at 3.5.d that nurses and midwives must 'access records only when professionally involved in the care of the person and authorised to do so'.

Information sharing with colleagues

The Codes of Conduct note with state at 3.3.d that nurses and midwives must 'clearly and accurately communicate relevant and timely information about the person to colleagues, within the bounds of relevant privacy requirements'.

Disclosure

The Codes of Conduct note at 3.5.a that nurses and midwives must 'respect the confidentiality and privacy of people by seeking informed consent before disclosing information, including formally documenting such consent where possible'.

Social media

The Codes of Conduct also note at 3.5.c that nurses and midwives must 'abide by the NMBA [Nursing and Midwifery Board of Australia] Social Media policy and relevant Standards for practice, to ensure use of social media is consistent with the [nurse's or midwife's] ethical or legal obligations to protect privacy'. The Codes of Conduct also state at 3.5.e that nurses and midwives must 'not transmit, share, reproduce or post any person's information or images, even if the person is not directly named or identified, without having first gained written and informed consent'.

The AHPRA (2014a) *Social Media Policy* was developed jointly by the Registration Boards and shows the seriousness with which they regard social media issues as they relate to the obligations of health professionals. It states:

Registered health practitioners should only post information that is not in breach of these obligations [Code of Ethics, Code of Conduct and the national law] by:

➤ complying with professional obligations

➤ complying with confidentiality and privacy obligations (such as by not discussing patients or posting pictures of procedures, case studies, patients, or sensitive material which may enable patients to be identified without having obtained consent in appropriate situations), presenting information in an unbiased, evidence-based context ...

The Policy also notes that when using social media, whether it is publicly available or limited to a group of people, professional standards need to be maintained. Information that is privately circulated can become public. It notes at 1: 'posting unauthorised photographs of patients in any medium is a breach of the patient's privacy and confidentiality, including on a personal Facebook site or group even if the privacy settings are set at the highest setting (such as for a closed, "invisible" group).'

Law and health information management

Access

If we as a society privilege the idea of autonomy and consider that individuals should be able to control access to personal information, it follows that individuals should be able to access information that is about them, specifically that they should have access to their clinical record. The High Court of Australia considered whether patients had a right in the common law to access their clinical records in the 1995 case of *Breen v Williams*.

Breen v Williams **[1995] HCA 63**

Ms Breen had tried for five years to access her clinical records that were held by her plastic surgeon. She wanted to access them to support her participation in a class action lawsuit in the United States over allegedly defective breast implants. Ms Breen

▶

◄

had sought an order from the Supreme Court of New South Wales to enable her to access those records, claiming that they contained information about her and she was entitled to access that information. The doctor argued that the record was for his private use. The High Court of Australia said that although a doctor may have a duty to provide personal information to a patient that does not amount to a duty to allow the patient to access clinical records specific to that patient or to copy them.

As a consequence of this ruling, the Commonwealth government created rules under the *Privacy Act 1988* (Cth) (sch. 1 APP 12.1) about the privacy of personal and health information. The Commonwealth government overruled the common law and created a legal right for individuals to access their personal information held by private sector health providers and other private agencies and Commonwealth public sector agencies. Patients also have a right to access under the legislation controlling electronic health records. Some states and territories have legislation granting patients access to their medical records. In jurisdictions without such legislation patients must rely on right to information legislation for access.

Privacy

As discussed, the concept of privacy is based on the presumption that individuals should be able to control their personal information. Privacy laws in Australia focus on the idea that there should be rules governing the collection and handling of personal information to protect the privacy of individuals. Privacy legislation has been passed by the Commonwealth government, as well as by some state and territorial governments (Table 7.1).

Table 7.1 Privacy legislation in Australia

	Public sector	Private sector
Commonwealth	*Privacy Act 1988* (Cth)	*Privacy Act 1988* (Cth)
Australian Capital Territory	*Health Records (Privacy and Access) Act 1997* (ACT)	*Privacy Act 1988* (Cth)
New South Wales	*Health Records and Information Privacy Act 2002* (NSW)	*Privacy Act 1988* (Cth)
Northern Territory	*Information Act* (NT)	*Privacy Act 1988* (Cth)
Queensland	*Information Privacy Act 2009* (Qld)	*Privacy Act 1988* (Cth)
Tasmania	*Personal Information Act 2004* (Tas)	*Privacy Act 1988* (Cth)
South Australia	*Information Privacy Principles Instruction* (SA)	*Privacy Act 1988* (Cth)
Victoria	*Health Records Act 2001* (Vic)	*Privacy Act 1988* (Cth)
Western Australia	*Freedom of Information Act 1992* (WA)	*Privacy Act 1988* (Cth)

Table 7.2   Overview of Australian Privacy Principles

Principle number	Australian Privacy Principles
1	Open and transparent management of personal information
2	Anonymity and pseudonyms
3	Collection of solicited personal information
4	Dealing with unsolicited personal information
5	Notification of the collection of personal information
6	Use or disclosure of personal information
7	Direct marketing
8	Cross-border disclosure of personal information
9	Adoption, use or disclosure of personal information
10	Quality of personal information
11	Security of personal information
12	Access to personal information
13	Correction of personal information

The *Privacy Act 1998* (Cth) created 13 Australian Privacy Principles (APP) (Table 7.2). These principles overlap with state and territory laws and so create a complex legal framework. In the event of a specific inconsistency where both Commonwealth and state legislation applies, the Commonwealth legislation prevails in respect of the inconsistency.

If a person believes that the APPs have been breached they may make a complaint to the Information Commissioner. The Commissioner may make a declaration that the complainant is entitled to a specified amount by way of compensation. Similar remedies are available at the state level.

My Health Records Act 2012 (Cth) ss 59–60 also sets out civil and criminal sanctions for the unauthorised collection, use and disclosure of patients' information from the My Health system.

Confidentiality

While a duty of confidentiality has long been recognised as an important ethical principle supporting the health professional–patient relationship, it has also been recognised as a legal duty. A legal duty can arise in the context of negligence, that is, if it would be reasonably foreseeable that release of one person's health information to another person without consent could cause harm to that person (generally psychological harm). See, for example, *Furniss v Fitchett* – a New Zealand case that has been accepted by the High Court as applying in Australia.

Furniss v Fitchett [1958] NZLR 396

Mr and Mrs Furniss were both patients of a doctor. The doctor knew that their marriage was in trouble. In the course of divorce proceedings Mr Furniss produced a
medical certificate from the doctor stating that Mrs Furniss had symptoms of paranoia.
Mrs Furniss had no knowledge that the certificate had been issued and the doctor
had not told her his views on her mental state. She suffered 'shock and injury to her
health'. She sued the doctor for negligence. The court found the doctor had a duty
of care to Mrs Furniss and he should have foreseen that disclosure of her supposed
medical condition in an open court without her prior knowledge could result in harm.

A legal duty can also arise in the context of a contract between a patient
and health professional, as there might be an explicit or implied term
in the contract that personal information will be kept confidential. Any
breach of that term could allow the patient to bring a civil proceeding
against the health professional seeking compensation for the breach of
contract.

But most commonly the duty arises in the context of an area of law
called equity. Equity focuses on the moral dimension of human relationships and in this context the importance of keeping promises. If
a promise to keep information confidential is broken, then the affected
person can bring a civil proceeding seeking compensation for that breach.
According to the common law (*Trevorrow v South Australia (No. 4)* (2006)
94 SASR 64), the affected individual would need to establish:

➤ The information is of a confidential nature (it is personal information
that is not in the public domain).

➤ It was disclosed when there was an expectation that it would be
kept confidential (this expectation can be presumed from a health
professional–patient relationship).

➤ There has been actual or threatened disclosure, which is or will negatively affect the affected person.

If all three of these factors can be established a successful claim for damages can be brought. This applies to intentional and unintended disclosure. Unintended disclosure could include where personal information
is being discussed by health professionals and is overheard by others, for
example a conversation in a lift (see Vigod et al. 2003), or it could include
nurses or midwives discussing details about their work day on social
media. If the person has consented to their personal information being

shared then proceedings will not be successful – a competent adult has the right to consent to information being disclosed.

Exceptions where disclosure is permitted

Ethical and legal difficulties often arise when considering whether there should be any situations where a health professional can release personal information about a patient, for example when that patient may be threatening harm to self or others, without fear of being sued in negligence, contract or for breach of confidence or face disciplinary or employment proceedings. Both the common law and legislation may require a health professional to breach confidentiality by providing personal information to a public agency. The common law and legislation may also establish an exception from the duty to keep information confidential so that a health professional may disclose personal information about a patient and be protected from any legal consequences. The most relevant exceptions are discussed below.

Disclosure to other health professionals

In the context of providing appropriate care and treatment to a patient, it is often required that health professionals share information between each other to enable continuity of care for that patient and to coordinate the provision of care and treatment. In general, such sharing of information proceeds with the explicit (for example, a referral letter is provided for a patient) or implicit consent of the patient (for example, when a patient is admitted into hospital they implicitly consent to personal information being passed from one nurse or midwife to another when shifts are being changed), and only where it is required for the care and treatment of the patient. The exception only allows disclosure in the context of what is necessary and required for the care and treatment of the patient.

Disclosure to substitute decision-maker or caregiver

Obviously, in an emergency situation or where a patient permanently or temporarily does not have the competence to consent to treatment, information must be communicated to the substitute decision-maker to enable informed decisions to be made by that person (see Chapter 5).

It is increasingly recognised that caregivers may need personal information about the person for whom they care in order to provide appropriate care and support to that person, and particularly if that information is pertinent to some risk to the caregiver (e.g. risk that the person might harm the caregiver) or the person (e.g. a risk of self-harm). In some circumstances, therefore, legislation recognises that otherwise confidential information may be shared with caregivers without the consent of the patient (see generally s 93(3)(c) *Health Care Act 2008* (SA); s 146 *Hospitals and Health Boards Act 2011* (Qld)).

A health service provider is not permitted to disclose a patient's health information to a patient's relative without careful consideration of whether the disclosure is appropriate. In *Dunne v Victorian Aboriginal Health Services Co-operative (Health and Privacy)* [2012] VCAT 1770 a doctor approached a woman in the clinic waiting room to offer condolences on the death of her sister. The doctor also mentioned that the woman's daughter was in hospital. The woman replied that she and her daughter were estranged. Later the doctor told the patient that she had not been aware that she and her mother were estranged and that she had told her mother about her being hospitalised. The Tribunal stated that the disclosure to the mother constituted a disclosure of health information contrary to the *Health Records Act 2001* (Vic).

Disclosure required by law

In some circumstances legislation has been passed to require that health professionals disclose otherwise confidential information to designated agencies. Obligations to mandatorily report suspected child abuse are discussed in Chapter 6, as are obligations for registered health professionals to mandatorily report other health professionals in Chapter 4. Other mandatory reporting requirements may include the requirement to report certain diseases, provide information to a coroner, tell the court about the presence of alcohol or drugs in the breath or blood of a car driver, and reporting births and deaths. It is expressly set out in legislation requiring reporting that those who report in good faith will be protected from having legal proceedings commenced against them for breaching confidentiality.

The law also states that confidential information, such as the clinical record, must be released in response to a court order (i.e. a search warrant or subpoena (summons to court)) – see the case discussion below.

Royal Women's Hospital v Medical Practitioners Board of Victoria (2006) 15 VR 22

In 2000 Mrs X sought a termination of pregnancy for her 32-week foetus after scans indicated that it might have dwarfism. After she received counselling and her mental state was assessed, the termination was performed. Later a Senator made a ▶

◄

complaint to the Medical Practitioners Board (MPB) about the termination, claiming that the foetus had subsequently been found to be normal. The MPB conducted a preliminary inquiry and sought Mrs X's clinical record to inform their deliberations. The MPB obtained a search warrant from the Magistrates' Court to obtain it and the records of an internal investigation. The Royal Women's Hospital opposed the search warrant claiming that laws relating to confidentiality prohibited disclosure of clinical records and that such a disclosure was contrary to the public interest as it undermined the trust patients had in health professionals. A breach of that trust might mean that people may not seek health services which would be detrimental to that individual and contrary to the public interest. The Magistrates' Court, the Supreme Court and the Victorian Court of Appeal all agreed that the hospital was required to provide the documents to the MPB. Some judges noted that, despite disclosure, women would still present to health facilities for health treatment and that confidentiality protections for health records are limited in the broader interest of enabling a robust justice system.

However, considerations of privacy still apply as can be seen in the *Cristobal* case (2017). Ms Cristobal, a registered nurse, was notified by New South Wales' Health Care Complaints Commission that her care of patient A was being investigated. The nurse copied patient B's medical records at the hospital and saved them onto a thumb drive to transfer to her personal computer. She then, as part of her response to the complaint about patient A, emailed patient B's medical records to the Commission without authorisation from the hospital or the consent of the patient. This act was found to constitute unsatisfactory professional conduct as the disclosure was improper and unethical.

Threats to an individual's health, life or safety or to public safety or health

An exception in both the common law and in legislation (*Health Care Act 2008* (SA) s 93(3)(e); *Hospital and Health Boards Act 2011* (Qld) s 147; *Health Services Act 1988* (Vic) s 141(3)) relating to privacy and confidentiality is if a person or organisation receives information that an individual's health, life or safety is at risk or there is a more general risk to public safety. There have been a number of cases that have discussed the circumstances and manner in which information can be disclosed. These cases may arise in the context of an investigation by a Privacy Commissioner of an alleged breach of the laws relating to privacy by a health professional (see case discussion in Chapter 4 'When Whistle-blowing and Confidentiality Collide').

These cases may also arise when a patient brings legal proceedings alleging a breach of confidentiality, trying to stop information being disclosed or seeking damages for harm caused (see *W v Egdell*).

W v Egdell [1990] All ER 385

The plaintiff (patient) brought a claim for damages for breach of confidence in relation to a disclosure of personal information made by a doctor. The patient had sought an assessment by an independent psychiatrist in the hope of getting a report to support his request for a transfer to a less secure forensic mental health facility. The patient had been diagnosed with schizophrenia after shooting seven people, five of whom had died. He had been compulsorily detained under the *Mental Health Act* since the shooting.

The psychiatrist concluded that the patient still posed a risk and did not support his transfer to a less secure facility. On receipt of the report the patient withdrew his application for transfer and did not provide the Tribunal with a copy of the report. The patient also refused permission for the psychiatrist to send the report to an appropriate authority. The psychiatrist sent a copy of the report to the Home Office (the government department responsible for forensic mental health patients). The appeal court held that when a patient has committed multiple killings when mentally ill, decisions that may eventually lead to his release must be made with full information. If a psychiatrist is aware that a decision may be made without full information and there is a risk to the public then disclosure may be made to appropriate authorities (i.e. the Home Office). Disclosure in this case was deemed to be justified in the interests of public safety.

Finally, these cases may also arise when disciplinary proceedings are being brought against a health professional by the professional regulator for a breach of confidentiality (see *Duncan v Medical Practitioners Disciplinary Committee*).

Duncan v Medical Practitioners Disciplinary Committee [1986] 1 NZLR 513

Duncan was a GP in a rural community. A patient, Henry, was the local bus driver. Henry underwent a triple bypass after two heart attacks. Henry's surgeon provided him with a medical certificate stating he was fit to drive. The GP disclosed Henry's health status to a bus passenger, reported it to the local police and tried to organise a petition to have Henry's driver's licence revoked. Henry complained to the Medical Council. The Disciplinary Committee of the Medical Council of New Zealand found the GP guilty of professional misconduct and censured him.

The GP then made statements to the media about Henry's condition. Henry made a further complaint to the Medical Council. The GP was again found to have committed professional misconduct and he was de-registered. On appeal the courts upheld the de-registration.

▶

◄

The Disciplinary Committee held that confidentiality can only be breached in exceptional circumstances where the public interest is paramount. Disclosure cannot be made to laypeople or the media but only to responsible authorities. Duncan's disclosure to the police was considered by the Committee, and the appeal courts, to be appropriate.

The cases discussed address the issues of disclosing confidential information to an appropriate authority. Can or should confidential information be disclosed to the individual who is identified as being at risk? A well-known case from the United States, *Tarasoff v Regents of the University of California* 17 Cal. 3d 425 (1976), suggests US health professionals have a duty to protect an identified victim through disclosure. In the Tarasoff case a patient threatened to kill an identifiable woman. The threat was reported to police but not to the intended victim or her family. The woman was subsequently murdered by the patient. Her family successfully sued the doctor for failing to disclose the threat. It is not clear what the legal position is in Australia.

Documentation

Clinical records are a critical mechanism to ensure quality and continuity of care. Good record-keeping provides a record of what care and treatment has been provided and the care plan for that particular patient and enable continuity of care. Poor record-keeping can cause errors and harm to a enables patient. For example, if a medication order or prescription is illegible the patient may be given the wrong dosage of medication. If the administration of a medication is not recorded the patient may be inadvertently given additional medication resulting in an overdose. Poor record-keeping may be indicative of poor-quality care.

Alleged deficiencies in record-keeping can be grounds for a performance review or disciplinary proceedings and provide evidence in civil negligence actions of poor practice. Three recent disciplinary cases consider record-keeping.

HCCC v Thompson (No 1) [2012] NSWNMT 13

In this case Thompson was a registered nurse who assisted in the caesarean delivery of baby and then acted as a recovery nurse. The patient began to bleed in recovery, was returned to theatre for a hysterectomy, but later died. There were a number of allegations in respect of Ms Thompson's performance, one of which related

►

to a failure to make legible and contemporaneous entries in the clinical record. Ms Thompson made her notes (some unsigned or untimed) immediately after the events as she was dealing with a potentially life-threatening emergency. The Tribunal concluded that the expected standard of practice was that notes could be written immediately after an event and would be considered contemporaneous.

Nursing and Midwifery Board of Australia v Faulkner [2017] QCAT 141

Ms Faulkner was a registered nurse. It was alleged that Ms Faulkner signed patient medication charts in advance of the medications having being administered (although she generally did administer them); failed to administer the prescribed dose of medication to a patient on one occasion, despite having signed the patient's medication chart to indicate she had administered the medication; orally advised another nurse that medication had been administered to that patient when it had not been administered according to the patient and analysis of the patient's blood and there was no equipment indicating IV antibiotics had been administered; and that she took the handbag of another nurse. She was found to have committed professional misconduct and conditions were imposed on her practice.

HCCC v MacGregor [2012] NSWNMPSC 3

MacGregor was a registered midwife practising independently and the proceeding related to a planned home birth. The allegation was that the midwife failed to adequately assess, monitor and document various observations of the patient and foetus during stages one and two of labour, as well as other matters. In stage one the allegation was that there was no documentation of the strength and regularity of the contractions, vaginal loss, position of the foetus, foetal descent, care provided to the patient and maternal observations, advice and decisions relating to management of labour. In stage two there was no documentation of foetal heart rate and maternal observations, the management plan and the reasons for decisions. The Committee concluded that her failure to document these matters was significantly below the standard expected of a practitioner of her training and experience. Ms MacGregor advanced the opinion that in a planned home birth it was not necessary for her to perform the same observations and examinations as a hospital midwife. The Committee was highly critical of this perspective. It noted that in an emergency care would need to be urgently transferred (as happened in this case) and full documentation would be essential to enable adequate and appropriate care to be provided. In addition, the Committee noted that all observations must be undertaken and documented in every clinical setting to ensure the ongoing wellbeing of the woman and the foetus.

The expected standard in regard to documentation requires that records be accurate, complete, contemporaneous, legible and objective. Paper records should also be signed, dated and timed. Any errors should have a line drawn through them and should be initialled – no attempt should be made to delete them. Records should be integrated; that is, records should not be made on scraps of paper.

Needless to say any attempt to alter records on being advised of a complaint or proceedings is a very serious matter and grounds for disciplinary proceedings. In *Nursing and Midwifery Board of Australia v Sanchez (Review and Regulation)* [2017] VCAT 574 and *Nursing and Midwifery Board of Australia v Condon (Review and Regulation)* [2017] VCAT 575 a resident of an aged care facility was found deceased face down in a fountain. One registered nurse, Condon, directed another registered nurse, Sanchez, to write an entry into the clinical record stating that the patient had been found dead of a suspected massive myocardial infarction and was not a suspected drowning after a possible trip or fall. Sanchez also did not disclose this information to the general practitioner, the family or the night staff. She was found to have committed professional misconduct and cautioned. Condon also gave inaccurate information or failed to disclose relevant information about the circumstances of the patient's death to one of the patient's sons, the Aged Care Complaints Investigations Scheme, the Regional Manager and Victoria Police. She was found to have committed professional misconduct and was reprimanded, suspended for three months and required to undertake an educational programme on ethics and record-keeping.

Social media

The Australian Nursing Federation recently warned nurses to be aware that increasing numbers of nurses (and midwives) in Australia and internationally are being reprimanded by employers for inappropriate use of social media (Australian Nursing Federation 2011). In some cases this has also resulted in health professionals facing disciplinary proceedings for breaching patient confidentially and boundary-related issues.

Kore v Chief Executive, Department of the Premier and Cabinet (on behalf of the Chief Executive, Department for Health and Ageing) [2017] SAIRComm 3 at 40

Ms Kore was a registered midwife. The midwife had been friends with Mr A for 12 years. Mr A had been in a relationship with Ms H. Mr A told Ms Kore that Ms H was

▶

◀

pregnant and due in February but they had broke up in November after having a volatile relationship. Ms H was not communicating with him. He also said that Ms H had a troubled past and Ms H was jealous of Ms Kore despite never having met her. In February Ms Kore checked the birth register at the nurses' station and saw Ms H had given birth the day before (this checking was common practice to enable midwives to follow up women they had cared for). Some hours later she sent a Facebook message to Mr A advising him that his son was born, the date and time of birth, the weight and that it was a forceps delivery. Mr A inquired about the baby's name and Ms Kore said she would try and find out. Ms Kore messaged the attending midwife through her Facebook page, stating that the father of Ms H's baby was a close friend and that Ms H had 'blocked him out for no reason'. She asked the midwife for the baby's name, stating that Mr A was 'distraught' and did not know that the baby had been born. Ms Kore included a comment that the baby was 'fucking huge'. Ms H was subsequently readmitted to the Ward noting she was reluctant due to information relating to the birth of her child having been disclosed to her estranged partner by a midwife in the Delivery Suite. Ms H said she was worried that her ex-partner would find out that the baby was in the Ward and that she was fearful for her baby's safety due to a past history of his aggressive behaviour in their relationship. A Safety Learning System report was filed, citing disclosure of patient information to a member of the public.

Ms Kore was suspended and then terminated from her employment (*Kore v Chief Executive, Department of the Premier and Cabinet (on behalf of the Chief Executive, Department for Health and Ageing)* [2017] SAIRComm 3 at 40). Her employer noted:

> This trust is particularly relevant for a Hospital providing obstetric care ..., given the evidence which highlights that pregnancy/childbirth is a high risk factor for intimate partner violence. One in five women is known to experience emotional and/or physical abuse by an intimate partner in the first twelve months post-partum. There are significant security considerations for women birthing at the Hospital given this. ... Accordingly, it is the woman's right to determine who receives information about her pregnancy and her childbirth, given the potential and known threat of harm to herself and her baby that can exist at this vulnerable time. Women do not always disclose such risk factors to Midwives, and therefore ensuring the confidentiality of the woman's healthcare information and security of information regarding her childbirth is imperative. Whilst no judgement is made about whether such concerns were in place in this patient's case, health professionals must be alert to this possibility when caring for pregnant women. Protecting the confidentiality of women's health information is integral to the requirement for trust and security in this relationship.

Ms Kore was reported to have been cautioned by her regulatory body and to have been required to undertake training on ethics and confidentiality.

Overview

The management of health information is a critical part of providing quality care and maintaining good relationships between health professionals, patients and the public. The chapter highlights the continuing

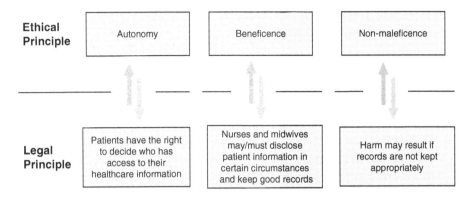

Figure 7.1 Ethical and legal principles relevant to the management of health information

relevance of the ancient concept of confidentiality and the emergence of the concept of privacy and its application to the health sector. Finally, the chapter also focuses on the importance of the maintenance of good documentation as a component of competent professional practice.

Figure 7.1 highlights the interactions between the ethical principles and the legal principles relevant to the management of health information.

Further reading

Green, J. 2017, 'Nurses' online behaviour: Lessons for the nursing profession', *Contemporary Nurse*, 53: 3, 355–367.

Siegler, M. 1982, 'Confidentiality in medicine: A decrepit concept', *New England Journal Medicine*, 307, 1518–1521.

Spector, N. & Kappel, D. 2012, 'Guidelines for using electronic and social media: The regulatory perspective', *The Online Journal of Issues in Nursing*, 17; 3.

Vigod, S., Bell, C. & Bohnen, J. 2003, 'Privacy of patients' information in hospital lifts: Observational study', *British Medical Journal*, 327, 1024–1025.

Questions

Is the protection of confidentiality and privacy still relevant in the age of social networking?

Are there different expectations for privacy and confidentiality in different settings (for example, between rural and urban contexts)?

What ethical and/or legal challenges do you see emerging with the movement to electronic records?

What are the ethical issues that were raised by the *Kore* case?

Scenarios

1. Stephanie Bateman is a 34-year-old woman who presents to the Emergency Department (ED) of a rural community hospital. She has a fractured arm and lacerations to her face and arms. There has been no loss of consciousness and Stephanie is orientated to time, place and person. While her injuries appear consistent with an assault having occurred, Stephanie provides the attending physician with a different account of how her injuries were sustained. The ED is extremely busy and understaffed, and the physician does not pursue the matter further. Simon Cartwright is the registered nurse in charge of Stephanie's care. He knows Stephanie socially as they live in a small community and over the coming hours he carefully asks a number of questions about her injuries. Simon suspects Stephanie has been the victim of domestic violence and Stephanie subsequently confirms this in confidence. Stephanie asks Simon to promise that he will not tell anyone about what her husband has done or she 'will cop it'. Stephanie tells Simon that she has tried to get away from her husband a number of times in the past and that he always manages to find her. She tells Simon that the last time her husband found her she was scared that he might actually kill her.

Apply the decision-making framework to this problem.

2. Kelly was a registered midwife. A famous celebrity was admitted to the birthing unit where Kelly worked to give birth to her second child. Kelly did not provide care to this person but used her access to look up the celebrity's complete medical record. She then told her husband the details but did not distribute the information any further.

Apply the decision-making framework to this issue.

After applying the decision-making framework, consider the following fact change: Kelly denied accessing the records during the internal investigation.

8

Patient safety and negligence

Introduction

Preventing adverse events is important for the many patients who could have been harmed (including most seriously killed) and/or inconvenienced by an adverse event, but also important for our health system and for Australia more generally. Research conducted into the quality of Australian health care (Wilson et al. 1996) established an adverse event rate in Australian hospitals of 16.6 per cent of patients, with 50 per cent of these events being preventable. In 1996 the direct costs, in terms of extra hospital days, of adverse events were calculated as being $867 million per year (Task Force on Quality in Australian Health Care 1996). In 2000 the costs to society (including lost income, lost household production, and disability and health care costs) were calculated at $2 billion per year (Australian Patient Safety Foundation 2000). A 2013 study suggests conditions acquired by patients during their stay amounted to 12–16 per cent of hospital expenditure (Health Policy Analysis 2013).

Some of our earliest surviving historical records raise issues of patient safety concerns. For example, the Babylonian *Code of Hammurabi*, the oldest surviving written legal code (dating from approximately 1750 BCE), states (in translation): 'If a physician make a large incision with the operating knife, and kill him, or open a tumor with the operating knife, and cut out the eye, his hands shall be cut off.' This legal principle is notable for the severity of the punishment imposed on the erring doctor – a punishment that would be inconceivable in modern Australia. However, it also illustrates that when we think about safety in a health context we have always tended to focus on assigning responsibility for acts or omissions to an individual health professional. This probably, at least in part, reflects the historical realities of health care in that, until relatively recently at least in historical terms, treatment and care were provided by individual health professionals or, at the most, small teams of health providers working in small organisations. As a consequence, patient safety was more directly the responsibility of the health professionals who were providing treatment. In addition, the individualised model of health care meant that individual health professionals had more autonomy in respect of the quality of the care and treatment they provided and the safety of their patients. There was little oversight by health professions or government actors and few expectations from patients about quality and safety – they were mostly grateful to be receiving health care of any form.

Recent research indicates that while individuals can and do make mistakes, if those individuals work within complex systems, any error may be a consequence, in whole, or in part, of that complexity (Reason 1990). To give an example, if a health professional makes a medication error by injecting a drug via an epidural rather than intravenously why did that occur? Was the mistake made because the person did not undertake a cross-check? Was it because the area was understaffed? Was it because the person had a heavy workload, or that the drug's name had recently changed, or because the medication was drawn into a syringe preparatory to injecting into an intravenous bag but the nurse was called away to an emergency before it could be injected? Was it all of these things? Did systems fail? Researchers in this area have argued that to prevent errors we must study the interrelationships between people, technology and their work environments (Reason 1990). They note that causally it may often be difficult to attribute an error to just one health professional.

In addition to studying interactions, those working in the area of patient safety and health care quality have advocated for the development of robust safety systems to try and prevent errors. They have also advocated for the development of systems to respond to adverse events (commonly called adverse event reporting systems) – for example, to identify when and in what circumstances adverse events have occurred, to analyse those events and learn from them and, as a result, to change systems or address identified issues in order to minimise the chance that a similar event will occur in the future. The effectiveness of these systems depends on the willingness of health professionals and managers to talk openly about errors and to learn from them. Patient safety advocates also argued for the development of systems to encourage the open disclosure of adverse events to patients. The Australian Commission on Safety and Quality in Health Care (2017) has issued a guidance document on the roles and responsibilities for nurses and midwives for clinical governance, emphasising their obligations to actively participate in patient safety and quality processes.

As a result of the research showing high rates of adverse events, Australian governments established policies and processes to require adverse event reporting, create quality assurance mechanisms and require open disclosure. A barrier to the development of these systems has been the traditional reluctance of health professionals to admit to making an error or being involved in an error. This may be because we have a culture orientated towards blame, and people are concerned that they might be blamed for their actions and omissions – by the affected person and their family and friends, by their colleagues, by their profession, by the courts, by the public and ultimately by themselves. Advocates have suggested the health system must give priority to the development of blame-free environments that treat errors as learning moments. After all, errors are involuntary – a person does not (usually) choose to make a mistake (Sharpe 2004). The difficulty with this has been that our legal system is still orientated towards finding fault.

Ethics and nursing and midwifery practice

The principles approach

Justice

A key element of the principle of justice is that health professionals should be accountable for their actions or omissions to act. Sharpe (2004) notes that, in this context, accountability is both prospective and retrospective. We are most familiar with the notion of retrospective accountability; that is, after an adverse event has occurred those involved, individuals and organisations, must be accountable for the acts and omissions that caused the adverse event. But when we think about accountability, it is often in the sense of accountability being imposed by external actors or processes. For example, accountability is imposed through an internal and/or external investigation and some type of legal proceeding during which a degree of fault may be attributed to individuals and/or organisations. However, retrospective accountability also involves an ethical element: that nurses and midwives accept responsibility for their actions and omissions. Accepting responsibility means to acknowledge to oneself that you or your colleagues or other health professionals did not provide safe care or treatment. It also involves acknowledging to your colleagues and/or your employer that safe care and treatment was not provided through participation in reporting processes and adverse event analysis. Most importantly, it involves taking responsibility in respect of the patient or groups of patients by providing the patient(s) with information about what has occurred (as far as is known), apologising or expressing regret, undertaking to participate in an investigation to determine what occurred and whether a change of personnel or organisational processes could prevent a similar event occurring in the future, and to implement those changes. It also involves not taking actions to subvert accountability, for example by not reporting an adverse event or by actively seeking to undermine accountability by changing clinical records.

What Sharpe (2004) terms 'prospective accountability' is as important. This concept relates to an individual nurse's or midwife's sense of commitment to their profession and their role. It is about taking responsibility for creating and implementing a plan as to how to fulfil the obligations inherent to that individual's professional role. In the patient safety context this may include how that individual proposes to act to promote the safety of their patients; assisting in the development of a safer environment within which care is provided; supporting colleagues to participate in patient safety processes; and participation in professional development and personal improvement processes to maintain professional competencies.

Beneficence and non-maleficence

Beneficence focuses on the positive intention to act in the best interests of others and non-maleficence on the negative obligation to refrain from causing needless harm. These principles are obviously centrally important when discussing patient safety. It is well established in the health care context that errors or mistakes in the provision of care and treatment can cause unnecessary harm (particularly physical harm, but also psychological, emotional and economic harm) to the patient – in the most serious cases the patient may die. Such events also affect the patient's friends and family. In addition, it is well established (see the introduction to this chapter) that adverse events harm the health system and that the economic costs to the nation are high.

We also should not disregard the harm adverse events may cause to health professionals. Many nurses, midwives and other health professionals report significant distress associated with adverse events (Wolf 2007; Kable et al. 2018) – guilt, emotional turmoil, feelings of failure, and having let themselves, their colleagues, their profession and their patient(s) down. If we accept the argument that if adverse events are reported and analysed then processes can be changed to minimise the chances of reoccurrence, this will benefit future patients, even if not the individual patient affected by the adverse event. It may also benefit health professionals by creating more rigorous safety-focused processes. The increased transparency associated with reporting and disclosure processes may also create a culture where there is greater willingness to provide more support to distressed health professionals. In this context, the ethical principles of non-maleficence and beneficence are consistent with the justice-related obligations regarding prospective accountability discussed above.

Autonomy

Enabling patients to exercise their autonomy through providing information to them is a key responsibility of nurses and midwives (see Chapter 2). In the context of patient safety, this would include being provided with information allowing patients to fully assess the risks and benefits associated with the proposed care and treatment (see Chapter 5). These risks are not just those associated with the procedure, but also arguably those risks associated with the skills and experience of the midwife or nurse who is providing care. For example, it would be a relevant consideration for an ordinary patient to know whether a midwife has had experience with managing breech births and the extent of that experience. It is established that a health professional's level of experience in relation to particular procedures is connected with the quality and safety of the health and/or maternity services provided (Bristol Royal Infirmary Inquiry 2001).

It is not just providing information about the risks and benefits associated with proposed care and treatment and the skills and expertise of the midwife or nurse providing care that recognises an individual's autonomy. Another facet of autonomy is that an individual has the right to know what has happened to them. This demonstrates respect for their dignity. This would include whether there has been an adverse event that has affected them. Some argue that it is not necessary to tell a patient about near misses (adverse events that do not cause harm), others that health professionals should exercise their discretion in disclosing near misses, while still others argue that respect for a patient indicates they should be told about near misses (Wu 2004). It is widely agreed that health professionals have an obligation to tell patients about adverse events that cause harm, not just because it respects patients' dignity, but also because it might impact on future decision-making about health and maternity care, and about the course of their life more generally.

The nursing and midwifery codes

Issues in relation to ensuring the safety of patients and maintaining the quality of services provided to patients are addressed in the ICN and ICM

Codes of Ethics and in the Nursing and Midwifery Board of Australia's Codes of Conduct for Nurses and for Midwives.

General

Generally, the ICN Code of Ethics in Element 2 states that: 'The nurse carries personal responsibility and accountability for nursing practice'; and in Element 3: 'the nurse assumes the major role in determining and implementing acceptable standards of clinical nursing practice.' The ICM Code of Ethics also notes at III b: 'midwives are responsible for their decisions and actions, and are accountable for the related outcomes in their care of women.'

In the Codes of Conduct domain 2 focuses on practising 'safely, effectively and collaboratively'. Both Codes note that nurses and midwives must 'practice in accordance with the standards of the profession and the broader health system (including the NMBA standards, codes and guidelines, the Australian Commission on Safety and Quality in Health Care' and for nurses the Standards for Aged Care (Principle 2.1.a). It also notes that midwives and nurses must 'provide leadership to ensure the delivery of safe and quality care and understand their professional responsibility to protect people, ensuring employees comply with their obligations' (Principle 2.1.b). These Codes speak to the importance of nurses and midwives placing safety and quality at the centre of their professional and ethical obligations to their patients.

Reporting and open disclosure

The ICN Code of Ethics notes that: 'The nurse takes appropriate action to safeguard individuals, families and communities when their health is endangered by a co-worker or any other person' (Element 4). The Codes of Conduct note nurses and midwives must 'document and report concerns if they believe the practice environment is compromising the health and safety of people receiving care' (Principle 2.1.c). The case *Nursing and Midwifery Board of Australia v George* [2015] VCAT 1878, discussed in Chapter 5, illustrates this.

Principle 2.4 of the Codes of Conduct extensively discusses nurses' and midwives' obligations in relation to reporting and open disclosure. They must recognise, reflect and report on adverse events, act to rectify the issue or intervene if needed, and abide by the principles of open disclosure and non-punitive incident management. Further their obligations to the patient are also set out and they must identify the most appropriate person to provide an apology and explanation to the patient, listen to the patient, acknowledge their distress and provide support and ensure people know how to make a complaint. Nurses and midwives should not allow a complaint made by that patient to negatively impact on that person's care.

Law relating to patient safety

There are a number of elements of the legal framework in Australia that address issues related to patient safety. These are discussed below.

Civil law

Although people can claim damages against health professionals for actions or omissions that have caused them harm by alleging a breach of contract, the most common cause of action is that they allege that a health professional(s) has been negligent and thus use a body of law known as tort law (the law of wrongs). The purpose of negligence is primarily to compensate a person who has been wrongfully harmed. The secondary purpose is to set standards.

The law of negligence was modernised in 1932 in the seminal case *Donoghue v Stevenson* [1932] AC 562, heard by the House of Lords in the United Kingdom (but the rules set out in this case also apply in Australia). This case related to a claim for damages against the manufacturer by a woman who had drunk a bottle of ginger beer made by that manufacturer. She had found a decomposing snail at the bottom of the bottle which had caused her to become ill. This case was important as the House of Lords created a general duty of care. Lord Atkin stated:

> You must take reasonable care to avoid acts or omissions which you can reasonably foresee would be likely to injure your neighbour. Who, then, in law, is my neighbour? The answer seems to be – persons who are so closely and directly affected by my act that I ought reasonably to have them in contemplation as being so affected when I am directing my mind to the acts or omissions which are called in question. (*Donoghue v Stevenson* at 580)

This rule is important because it clarifies that a person may have a duty to anyone whom they can reasonably foresee may be directly affected by their actions or omissions. Importantly, the rule also emphasises the concept of reasonableness – that the person's actions or omissions are going to be measured against what is judged as being reasonable in the circumstances. *Donoghue v. Stevenson* sets the general context for the law of negligence but how does it apply to nurses and midwives in Australia?

Negligence

The plaintiff must establish, on the balance of probabilities (see discussion in Chapter 3) the following three elements to advance a successful claim for negligence:

> Duty of care

> Breach of Duty

> Damage

It is important to note that although the tort of negligence comes from the common law, most states and territories have enacted legislation to modify it, especially in relation to the breach and damage elements.

Duty of care

It has been long recognised in law that all health professionals, including nurses and midwives, owe their patients a duty of care. Specifically, midwives and nurses owe patients in their care a duty to exercise reasonable care and skill, both when providing care and treatment and when providing information that patients use to make decisions about their care and treatment (*Rogers v Whitaker* (1992) 175 CLR 479).

Is there a broader duty of care for nurses and midwives? The neighbour test from *Donoghue v Stevenson* suggests that nurses and midwives may have a general duty of care to those who may be closely and directly affected by the nurse's or midwife's actions or omissions. This might include colleagues and, especially in the context of midwifery care, the patient's partner and/or family.

What about others less directly connected to the nurse or midwife – does a nurse or midwife have a duty of care to assist people in emergencies? There is no general common law duty for any person to assist in an emergency even if it is foreseeable that the person may be seriously injured or indeed die (*Sutherland Shire Council v Heyman* (1985) 157 CLR 424). But what of a nurse or midwife – does the fact that they are health professionals make a difference? One case, *Woods v Lowns* (1995) 36 NSWLR 344, considered whether a doctor had a duty of care in an emergency-type situation.

Woods v Lowns (1995) 36 NSWLR 344

A general practitioner was in his surgery when asked to attend a major life-threatening medical emergency occurring 300 metres from his premises. He refused. The affected

▶

◀

person, who was not a patient of the doctor's, was having a seizure and was left with brain damage and quadriplegia. The court, confirmed by the New South Wales Court of Appeal, determined that the doctor owed a duty of care to that person. In part they relied on the *Medical Practitioners Act 1938* (NSW) (this legislation has been repealed) which had a section relating to a doctor's obligations to attend and which, one judge believed, represented community expectations for health professionals. They also considered the doctor's physical proximity to the person in need of assistance and his capacity to assist.

This was a New South Wales case, decided by the New South Wales Court of Appeal. As discussed in Chapter 3, it is not certain whether this case would apply outside New South Wales. Nor is it certain whether the case might just apply to doctors or whether it might also apply to nurses and midwives. It is not certain even whether this case is limited to its facts – in other words it may not create a general duty. Finally, recent cases decided by the High Court of Australia (see Chapter 3) have changed the legal rules used to determine whether a general duty of care exists which might affect whether *Woods v Lowns* reflects current law on whether a doctor owes a duty in an emergency (Butler et al. 2010). At this time it appears unlikely that health professionals owe a duty of care to respond in an emergency. If they do respond they will be protected (see the discussion about Good Samaritan laws in the section 'Good Samaritans').

Breach of duty

Once a duty of care has been established, the next step is to determine whether the nurse or midwife has breached their duty of care. There are two parts to this. First, establish what the standard of care is and, second, consider whether it has been breached.

Standard of care

According to the common law, the standard of care for nurses and midwives is what an ordinary competent nurse in the circumstances would be reasonably expected to do in relation to the provision of professional advice and/or care and treatment (see, for example, *Rogers v Whitaker*; *Civil Liability Act 2002* (NSW) s 50(1); *Civil Liability Act 2003* (Qld) s 22(1); *Civil Liability Act 1936* (SA) s 41(1); *Civil Liability Act 2002* (Tas) s 22(1); *Wrongs Act 1958* (Vic) s 59(1); *Civil Liability Act 2002* (WA) s 5PB(1)).

The High Court of Australia in the seminal negligence case *Rogers v Whitaker* indicated that the standard of care applies to care and treatment and to the provision of information. The standard differs according to whether it is treatment- or information-related.

Information

The standards in relation to the provision of information are closely linked to the ethical value of autonomy (discussed in the context of information provision in Chapter 5). If a nurse or midwife advises a patient of the general nature of the proposed treatment before touching the patient then they will typically not be found to have committed the civil or criminal offence of battery, although if the touching is sexualised this will not apply.

For the purposes of determining whether there has been negligence, the High Court of Australia has stated the key issue is whether the patient has been advised of the risks associated with the care and treatment (*Rogers v Whitaker*). The High Court of Australia established in *Rogers v Whitaker* (see box titled '*Rogers v Whitaker*') that the patient must be advised of 'material risks' (see also *Civil Liability Act 2003* (Qld) s 21; *Civil Liability Act 2002* (Tas) s 21; *Wrongs Act 1958* (Vic) s 50). To determine whether a risk is material two factors must be considered:

➢ What a reasonable person in the patient's circumstances would consider important or material to their decision.

➢ What the particular patient would consider important or material to their decision.

Rogers v Whitaker (1992) 175 CLR 479

The plaintiff had been almost totally blind in her right eye since childhood. An ophthalmic surgeon advised her that a surgical procedure could remedy the appearance of her eye and restore sight. The plaintiff agreed to the surgery. The sight in her right eye did not change after the surgery and an inflammation meant she lost sight in her left eye leaving her blind. The surgeon was held to be negligent in not advising her of the 1 in 14,000 chance that the surgery could result in her losing sight in her other eye. Evidence was led that the surgeon did not advise his patients of that risk because of its remoteness and unlikelihood. The court held that this patient, given the condition of her sight, would attach significance to a risk that she might lose all her vision therefore it was a fact that was material to her decision-making and she should have been told of the risk.

Once the standard about information provision is determined the court must consider whether the nurse or midwife has fallen below the expected standard.

Recent cases have considered whether a health professional, a doctor in the cases that have been considered, has a duty to disclose their experience (*Chappel v Hart* (1998) 195 CLR 232) or performance data (personal failure rates in relation to the average) (*G, PA and C v Down* [2009] SASC 217) and have concluded that there is such a duty.

Treatment

The standard of care for treatment in the Australian context is set out in *Rogers v Whitaker*. As discussed, the standard of care is what the ordinary skilled person exercising that skill would have done. Traditionally, it has been determined by measuring what the health professional did against what a responsible body of professionals from that profession would have done. Interpreting this strictly would imply that a segment of the profession may determine the standard of care. This position was taken to ridiculous extremes in a Canadian disciplinary case against a doctor where the disciplinary tribunal applied the standard of care test used in negligence cases (Robinson 1999). In that case a doctor practised 'pelvic bonding', a so-called 'treatment' where patients were instructed to rub their faces against the doctor's genital area to 'treat' various psychological conditions. No doctor could be found to say that this practice accorded with the expected standard of care but the doctor used as witnesses other (non-medical and non-registered) practitioners who used this 'treatment' and gave evidence it was legitimate. This was accepted by the tribunal and the allegations against the doctor were dismissed. The case caused a public uproar; the public could recognise sexual abuse and a breach of the standard of care when they saw it.

The High Court of Australia in *Rogers v Whitaker* held that determining the standard of care is the responsibility of the court, not the profession. The court would offer a degree of deference to opinion coming from the profession, but the standard of care would not be determined solely or even primarily by the profession. The court was free to determine that the suggested standard was irrational. Once the standard has been established, the court must determine whether the nurse or midwife fell below the expected standard.

The common law applies in the Northern Territory. All the states have passed legislation setting out the law in relation to determining the standard of care in their jurisdiction. There are three stages:

1. The court considers whether the health professional has been negligent (using a similar rule to that established in *Rogers v Whitaker*).

2. The court considers whether the health professional has established a defence set out in legislation. The defence can be summarised as the defendant acted in a manner that, at the time the service was provided, was widely accepted in Australia by peer professional opinion as competent professional practice (*Civil Liability Act 2002* (NSW) s 50,

5P; *Civil Liability Act 2003* (Qld) s 22; *Civil Liability Act 1936* (SA) s 41; *Civil Liability Act 2002* (Tas) s 22; *Wrongs Act 1958* (Vic) ss 59, 60; *Civil Liability Act 2002* (WA) s 5PB).

3. If the health professional can establish the defence the court must make a determination regarding whether the standard established under the defence is irrational or, in Victoria and Western Australia, unreasonable (*Civil Liability Act 2002* (NSW) s 5O(2); *Civil Liability Act 2003* (Qld) s 22(2); *Civil Liability Act 1936* (SA) s 41(2); *Civil Liability Act 2002* (Tas) s 22(2); *Wrongs Act 1958* (Vic) s 59(2); *Civil Liability Act 2002* (WA) s 5PB(4) – note that the position in Western Australia is more complex).

Damage

When the plaintiff has established that the nurse or midwife had a duty of care to that person and had breached that duty of care they must also establish the third element – that the person has sustained damage. There are three sub-elements that must be worked through. First, the damage must be of a type recognised by law. Second, the damage must be caused by the defendant midwife or nurse's breach of their duty of care. Third, the damage must be a reasonably foreseeable consequence of the breach of the duty of care.

a) Damage recognised by law

Damage has been redefined as 'harm' in the legislative amendments to the common law. Harm is defined in most jurisdictions and can be summarised as including harm of any kind, including personal injury (including both physical and psychological injury) or death, damage to property, and economic loss (*Civil Law (Wrongs) Act 2002* (ACT) s 40; *Civil Liability Act 2002* (NSW) s 5; *Personal Injuries (Liabilities and Damages) Act* (NT) s 3; *Civil Liability Act 2003* (Qld) s 2; *Civil Liability Act 1936* (SA) s 3; *Civil Liability Act 2002* (Tas) s 9; *Wrongs Act 1958* (Vic) s 43; *Civil Liability Act 2002* (WA) s 3).

It is important to note that psychological injury requires a diagnosed psychological condition. In other words, generalised anxiety is insufficient to constitute harm or damage but an anxiety disorder may be sufficient. Economic loss relates to any financial loss; this might include such things as loss of income or transport costs associated with rehabilitation.

b) Damage caused by the breach of duty (causation)

The common law test for determining whether the defendant's breach of duty caused harm to the plaintiff is the 'but for' test – would the harm have occurred but for the negligence? The states and Australian

Capital Territory have passed legislation addressing causation which essentially restates the 'but for test' – that the negligence was a necessary condition or one of the main contributing factors for the occurrence of the harm (*Civil Law (Wrongs) Act 2002* (ACT) s 45; *Civil Liability Act 2002* (NSW) s 5D; *Civil Liability Act 2003* (Qld) s 11; *Civil Liability Act 1936* (SA) s 34; *Civil Liability Act 2002* (Tas) s 13; *Wrongs Act 1958* (Vic) s 51; *Civil Liability Act 2002* (WA) s 5C).

Barnett v Chelsea & Kensington Hospital Management Committee [1969] 1 QB 428

This case is the classic example of the common-law rule in relation to causation. An ill patient presented to a hospital. He was not treated and told to return home and see his general practitioner on the following day. Five hours later he died. On the face of this bare account it would seem that the failure to provide treatment led to the patient's death. However, the patient died of arsenic poisoning. Whether or not he had been kept in hospital or provided with treatment, he would have died anyway as there was no effective treatment for arsenic poisoning. Therefore the breach of the duty of care did not cause the harm to the patient.

It is more difficult to determine causation if something happened in between the negligence and the harm, an assessment would need to be made as to whether the subsequent act changed anything, or if something happened before the negligent act and whether that changed anything. It can also be difficult to determine whether the underlying condition, illness or injury led to the harm or whether the negligent act did – not all cases are as clear-cut as the *Barnett* case.

In respect of information cases, it is necessary to determine what the patient would have done had the patient received information about the material risks. Simply asking the patient is problematic due to the phenomenon of perfect hindsight – after you have been harmed you are always going to say you would have made a different decision had you known what you know now. The High Court of Australia (*Rosenberg v Percival* (2001) 205 CLR 434) states that the reliability of the plaintiff's evidence should be considered, including:

➤ The attitude and conduct of the plaintiff at the time

➤ The seriousness of the need for the procedure

➤ The extent of the risk (how remote it is)

➤ The plaintiff's knowledge

The common law test in relation to causation and information applies in the Australian Capital Territory, Northern Territory, South Australia and Victoria. In New South Wales, Queensland, Tasmania and Western Australia legislation has been passed (*Civil Liability Act 2002* (NSW) s 5D(3); *Civil Liability Act 2003* (Qld) s 11(3); *Civil Liability Act 2002* (Tas) s 13(3); *Civil Liability Act 2002* (WA) s 5C(3)). In those jurisdictions the matter is to be considered subjectively, but the person's statement about what that person would have done if they received information cannot be used. Cases that have interpreted these types of provisions (*KT v PLG* [2006] NSWSC 919; *Neal v Ambulance Services of New South Wales* [2008] NSWCA 346) consider very similar factors to those considered in common law jurisdictions, including:

➤ The attitude and conduct of the plaintiff at the time

➤ The evidence of others about what the plaintiff might have done

➤ The seriousness of the need for the procedure

➤ The extent of the risk (how remote it is)

➤ Previous and subsequent procedures or treatment

➤ The nature of the relationship between the health professional and the patient

c) Damage was a reasonably foreseeable consequence of the breach

This element really considers how remote the chance of the damage was. In other words the common law test is whether a reasonable person would consider the prospect of the type of damage that occurred due to the breach was a real prospect or whether it was far-fetched or fanciful (*Overseas Tankship (UK) Ltd v Miller Steamship Co Pty Ltd (No 2)* [1967] AC 617).

The legislative reforms have reframed this test to require the court to consider whether liability should be imposed on the negligent party (*Civil Law (Wrongs) Act 2002* (ACT) s 45; *Civil Liability Act 2002* (NSW) s 5D; *Civil Liability Act 2003* (Qld) s 11; *Civil Liability Act 1936* (SA) s 34; *Civil Liability Act 2002* (Tas) s 13; *Wrongs Act 1958* (Vic) s 51; *Civil Liability Act 2002* (WA) s 5C).

In order for a nurse or midwife to be found to be negligent they must:

➤ Owe a duty of care

➤ Have breached that duty

➤ Have caused damage of a sort recognised by law, caused by the breach of duty and it was reasonably foreseeable that the breach of duty could cause, harm

Harvey v PD (2004) 59 NSWLR 639

PD and her fiancé FH jointly consulted a general practitioner to be tested for sexually transmitted diseases. It was alleged that the doctor was negligent in not telling them that he could not release one person's test results to the other without consent due to confidentiality requirements. FH did not tell PD his tests showed that he was HIV-positive. They married, engaged in unprotected sex, and had a child. PD subsequently discovered she had contracted HIV. She subsequently had another child (by a different father). She claimed damages for, among other things, loss of capacity to care for both children (childcare costs). She established that if she had been told about the confidentiality issues she would have required FH to consent to disclosure of his test results or would have terminated her relationship with him (and would not have been in a position where she could be deceived by FH – a deceit that was foreseeable). Therefore she established that the damage she sustained was caused by the breach, at least in respect of caring for the child fathered by FH.

However, in relation to the second child the court accepted that the doctor had played a significant role in PD having to choose whether to have one child or if she had another to require childcare for that child (breach caused the damage). However, in relation to the test from the *Civil Liability Act 2002* (NSW) – whether the doctor should be held liable for damages from the harm – the court noted: she chose to become pregnant; she had a human right to procreate; she could have more children and make continual claims for childcare costs; parents have legal obligations to care for their children; and the overlap with her claim for loss of future earnings. It concluded that the doctor should not be held liable for damages associated with caring for the second child.

Vicarious liability

In relation to health services, vicarious liability means that an organisation or individual becomes liable for the negligence of another person (*Hollis v Vabu Pty Ltd* (2001) 207 CLR 21). In relation to health services, generally an employer becomes liable for the negligence of an employee, irrespective of whether the employer was actually at fault in any way. In order to establish vicarious liability it must be established that:

➢ There is an employer–employee relationship. Nurses and midwives are capable of being employees, but midwives in particular may work independently and would not generally be considered to be employees in these circumstances, even if they practise in association with an organisation.

➢ The employee has been negligent.

➤ That the negligence occurred in the course of that person's employment. An employer should not be liable for the negligence of an employee in situations where the negligent act occurred outside the course of employment. For example, if a hospital-based midwife drove negligently, the midwife's employing hospital should not be liable if he was driving to pick his daughter up from day care. On the other hand, if the midwife was driving to professional development training as required by his employer, this would be considered 'in the course of employment'.

Defences

There are several defences or partial defences to negligence. Three of the key defences are discussed in this section.

Voluntary assumption of risk

If the plaintiff after receiving full information accepts the risk of injury then they cannot receive any damages – they have voluntarily chosen to assume the risk. This is a very difficult defence to prove as the defendant nurse or midwife must establish that the plaintiff:

➤ knew that the risks existed (under the legislation listed below a health professional can assume that the plaintiff is aware of obvious risks);

➤ completely understood the risks; and

➤ freely and voluntarily accepted the risk.

(*Carey v Lake Macquarie City Council* [2007] NSWCA 4; *Civil Liability Act 2002* (NSW) s 5F; *Civil Liability Act 2003* (Qld) ss 13, 14; *Civil Liability Act 1936* (SA) ss 36, 37; *Civil Liability Act 2002* (Tas) ss 15, 16; *Wrongs Act 1958* (Vic) ss 53, 54; *Civil Liability Act 2002* (WA) ss 5F, 5N).

Contributory negligence

Contributory negligence is where the plaintiff's actions contributed to the damage they suffered. For example, the plaintiff discharged themselves from hospital, despite receiving advice they should not, which resulted in a greater physical injury; or the plaintiff did not adequately inform the midwife of her symptoms. To establish contributory negligence, the defendant nurse or midwife must show that:

➤ The plaintiff was negligent

➤ The negligence contributed to the harm sustained by the plaintiff

➤ The damage was a reasonably foreseeable consequence of the plaintiff's negligence.

(*Joslyn v Berryman* (2003) 214 CLR 552; *Civil Liability Act 2002* (NSW) s 5R; *Civil Liability Act 2003* (Qld) s 23; *Civil Liability Act 1936* (SA) s 5K; *Civil Liability Act 2002* (Tas) s 23; *Wrongs Act 1958* (Vic) s 44; *Civil Liability Act 2002* (WA) s 5K.)

However, it is important to note that contributory negligence is not a complete defence. If contributory negligence can be established it reduces the quantum of damages the defendant(s) owe to the plaintiff.

Good Samaritans

The name of this aspect of Australia's legal framework reflects its roots in Christian doctrine. The New Testament of the Bible tells the parable of the Good Samaritan. A traveller was beaten, robbed and left for dead on the side of the road. A priest and a Levite saw the man and crossed to the other side of the road to avoid him. Finally, a Samaritan (a group who were generally not respected) goes to his assistance – the Good Samaritan (Luke 10:29–37). As a society we want to encourage people to help others when they are in need of emergency assistance due to illness or injury. However, concerns were raised that some people, especially health professionals, may be reluctant to assist in an emergency due to a concern that they may face legal proceedings for any harm caused to the person they were assisting. Accordingly, all states and territories passed a 'Good Samaritan' law protecting them from liability. The provisions differ slightly across the states and territories (see Table 8.1).

Table 8.1 Good Samaritan laws across Australia

Jurisdiction	Law	Who is protected?	When are they protected from civil proceedings?
ACT	*Civil Law (Wrongs) Act 2002* s 5	Persons or a medically qualified person (doctor, registered health professional, paramedic or ambulance officer) providing advice over the phone, etc.	If emergency medical assistance or advice is provided to persons in need of such assistance honestly and not recklessly and without expectation of payment unless they are impaired (drug or alcohol).
NSW	*Civil Liability Act 2002* ss 56, 57	A person	If assistance in emergency is provided to persons in need of such assistance in good faith and without expectation of payment. Unless the person caused the accident in the first

Table 8.1 *Continued*

Jurisdiction	Law	Who is protected?	When are they protected from civil proceedings?
			place, was impaired by alcohol or drugs, failed to provide services with reasonable care and skill or was impersonating a health or emergency worker.
NT	*Personal Injuries (Liabilities and Damages) Act* s 8	Persons or a medically qualified person (doctor, registered health professional, paramedic or ambulance officer) providing advice over the phone, etc.	If emergency medical assistance or advice is provided to persons in need of such assistance honestly and not recklessly and without expectation of payment unless they are intoxicated.
Qld	*Law Reform Act* s 16	A medically qualified person (doctor, registered health professional, paramedic or ambulance officer)	If emergency assistance is provided to persons in need of such assistance at the scene in good faith and without gross negligence or expectation of payment.
SA	*Civil Liability Act 1936* s 74	A medically qualified person (doctor, registered health professional, paramedic or ambulance officer)	If emergency assistance or advice is provided to persons in need of such assistance in good faith and without recklessness or expectation of payment unless affected by drugs or alcohol.
Tas	*Civil Liability Act 2002* Pt 8A	A person	If assistance in an emergency or advice is provided to persons in need of such assistance in good faith and without recklessness or expectation of payment unless affected by drugs or alcohol or impersonating a health or emergency worker.
Vic	*Wrongs Act 1958* s 31B	A person	If assistance in emergency or advice is provided to persons in need of such assistance in good faith without expectation of payment.
WA	*Civil Liability Act 2002* s 5A, 5AD	Persons or a medically qualified person (doctor, registered health professional, paramedic or ambulance officer) providing advice over the phone, etc.	If assistance in emergency or advice is provided to persons in need of such assistance in good faith and without recklessness or expectation of payment.

Some explanation of certain terms may be required. The term 'good faith' essentially means doing something for the right reasons. 'Reckless-ness' essentially refers to doing an act disregarding or not giving any thought to the serious, substantial and unjustified risks arising from that course of action. The concept of gross negligence is discussed in the criminal law section of this chapter.

Protection from civil liability proceeding against 'Good Samaritans' appears lowest in New South Wales, which applies the normal negligence standard of reasonable care and skill. All other jurisdictions apply reck-lessness or gross negligence which are higher standards and which make allowance for the emergency situations that 'Good Samaritans' face.

Limitation on actions

Plaintiffs generally have a limited period of time within which they must bring civil proceedings. For most types of harm and in most jurisdictions the period is three years. The significant question is three years from when? In the Australian Capital Territory, the Northern Territory, Queens-land and South Australia the time begins to run from the moment when the three elements discussed below (duty of care, breach of duty and damage) are completed (*Limitation Act 1985* (ACT) s 16B(2); *Limitation Act 1981* (NT) s 12(1)(b); *Limitation of Actions Act 1974* (Qld) s 11; *Limitation of Actions Act 1936* (SA) s 36)). In New South Wales, Tasmania, Victoria and Western Australia the period begins when the plaintiff discovers the negligence (*Limitations Act 1969* (NSW) ss 18A, 50C; *Limitation Act 1974* (Tas) s 5(1); *Limitations of Action Act 1958* (Vic) s 5(1AA); *Limitation Act 2005* (WA) s 13(1)).

Apology laws

Both anecdote and research suggest that patients want an explanation of what happened to them, an apology, and an assurance that steps are being taken to ensure that the same adverse event will not occur again (Massó Guijarro et al. 2010). In the past legal advice has been provided to health professionals that they should not apologise or express regret as this could be taken as an admission of liability with consequences for civil and other types of legal proceedings. In order to facilitate apologies, changes were made to the legislative framework in Australian states and territories to enable health professionals to apologise or express regret without it being taken as an admission of liability and used as evidence of fault in legal proceedings (see Table 8.2). An apology is an expres-sion of sorrow, sympathy or regret. Apology laws essentially state that

Table 8.2 Summary of Apology laws

	Legislation	Summary of relevant sections
ACT	Civil Law (Wrongs) Act 2002 Pt 2.3	Apology does not constitute an express or implied admission of fault or liability and is not relevant to determination of fault or liability. An apology is not admissible as evidence in civil proceedings.
NSW	Civil Liability Act 2002 Pt. 10	An apology does not constitute an express or implied admission of fault or liability and is not relevant to the determination of fault/liability.
NT	Personal Injuries Liabilities and Damages) Act Pt. 2 div 2	An expression of regret does not amount to an admission of fault and is not admissible as evidence in civil proceedings.
Qld	Civil Liability Act 2003 Ch. 4 Pt 1	If made before proceedings commence an apology does not constitute an express or implied admission of fault or liability and is not relevant to determination of fault or liability. An apology is not admissible as evidence in civil proceedings unless proceeding relates to defamation, intentional acts or sexual assault.
SA	Civil Liability Act 1936 s 75	No liability or fault can be inferred from an expression of regret for the incident.
Tas	Civil Liability Act 2002 ss 6A–7	Apology does not constitute an express or implied admission of fault or liability and is not relevant to determination of fault or liability. An apology is not admissible as evidence in civil proceedings.
Vic	Wrongs Act 1958 s 14I, 14J	An apology does not constitute an admission of liability in respect of civil proceedings or an admission of unprofessional conduct etc in respect of professional regulation.
WA	Civil Liability Act 2002 ss 5AF–5AH	Apology does not constitute an express or implied admission of fault or liability and is not relevant to determination of fault or liability. An apology is not admissible as evidence in civil proceedings.

if a person or someone on behalf of that person expresses regret and/ or apologises that expression of regret/apology cannot be used in most types of civil proceedings in most circumstances as evidence of fault or liability.

Criminal law

The Code of Hammurabi (discussed in the introduction to this chapter) was a very early example of the criminal law being used against health professionals when they were negligent. The common law has also adopted the view that in certain circumstances it is appropriate for the weight of the criminal law, through convictions for manslaughter if the patient dies (or grievous bodily harm if the patient is severely injured), to be imposed on health professionals for certain levels of negligent acts or omissions (*R v Adamoko* [1994] 3WLR 288).

The test in the common law is whether the health professional is grossly negligent and that gross negligence caused the patient's death (*R v Adamoko* [1994] 3WLR 288). Jurisdictions with a codified or partially codified criminal law also have manslaughter offences. The High Court of Australia considered one of Western Australia's manslaughter provisions and determined that the test to determine whether someone who was negligent had committed manslaughter should be the same as the common-test – whether the person was grossly negligent (*Callaghan v R* [1952] 87 CLR 115). What does this mean? The Victorian Supreme Court in *Nydam v R* [1977] VR 430, a decision affirmed by the High Court of Australia (*Wilson v R* (1992) 107 ALR 257), states that death must be caused by the accused 'in circumstances which involved such a great falling short of the standard of care which a reasonable man would have exercised and which involved such a high risk that death or grievous bodily harm would follow that the doing of the act merited criminal punishment'. It is very rare in Australia that a health professional is charged with manslaughter due to criminal negligence and rarer still that they are convicted. While several nurses have been charged with criminally negligent manslaughter, none have been convicted (see, for example, Gregory 2008). Dr Pearce, a Queensland general practitioner, was one of the very few health professionals who have been convicted of manslaughter for negligence in Australia after she administered 10 times the lethal dose of morphine by mistake to a young child who had been burned (*R v Pearce* (Unreported, Supreme Court of Queensland, Holmes J, 15 November 2000)).

Overview

This chapter highlights the ethical principles, professional ethics and legal rules relating to patient safety and negligence. The ethical and legal frameworks also emphasise that nurses and midwives must be prospectively and retrospectively accountable to patients for their actions or omissions to act. The law sets out a framework to enable patients who have sustained harm to bring legal proceedings to attempt to receive compensation. The legal framework also allows the criminal law to be used to punish erring health professionals in certain very limited circumstances (Figure 8.1).

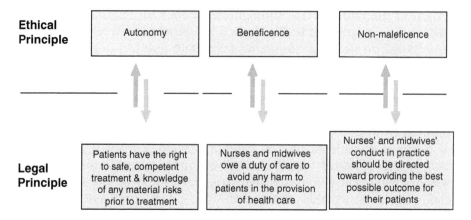

Figure 8.1 The ethical and legal principles relevant to patient safety and clinical negligence

Further reading

Australian Commission on Safety and Quality in Health Care. 2017, *Clinical Governance for Nurses and Midwives,* Australian Commission on Safety and Quality in Health Care, Sydney (www.safetyandquality.gov.au/wp-content/uploads/2017/12/Clinical-governance-for-nurses-and-midwives.pdf).

Leape, L. 2005, 'Ethical issues in patient safety', *Thoracic Surgery Clinics,* 15, 493–501.

Questions

How does autonomy apply to negligence and a nurse's or midwife's duty of care?

Should nurses and midwives have a duty (ethical and/or legal) to assist in emergencies?

Should we allow patients to bring legal actions for negligence against health professionals?

Scenarios

1. Amy Taylor is a night duty nurse in a private hospital. Over the past couple of weeks she has been working a series of double-shifts as a number of the nursing staff have been absent due to illness. In addition to the long working hours, Amy also cares for her disabled son

and elderly mother at home and is usually extremely fatigued when she arrives for her shift. One evening during a particularly busy shift on the ward, Amy accidentally administers the wrong medication to one patient, Bob. After realising her mistake, Amy immediately checks Bob's medical history and is certain Bob won't suffer any adverse reaction from her error. Bob is a particularly anxious patient and has previously been given incorrect medication. On that occasion he suffered no adverse reaction to the medication. However, he was so upset after hearing of the error that he decided to initiate legal action against the RN concerned. Amy discusses the matter with a colleague who suggests that, given Bob's history, it is probably in Bob's best interests if he is not told of the error as knowing about the error will only exacerbate his anxiety. The colleague adds, 'We're doing the best we can here. You just made a mistake.'

Apply the decision-making framework to this scenario.

After applying the decision-making framework, consider the following fact change:

If Bob is allergic to the medication and suffers disability or death as a result, what legal avenue/s may be open to Bob or his family in the circumstances?

2. Fatima was admitted to a private hospital for an induction as her baby was one week overdue. On arrival she was attached to a foetal heart rate monitor. Martin, a registered midwife was assigned to her care. Within 20 minutes abnormalities were apparent to Martin in the baby's heart activity and there were further episodes of bradycardia. Martin did not call the obstetrician for a further 1 hour and 15 minutes. The baby (Tariq) was born after a difficult birth with significant impairments that require 24-hour care. Fatima is now taking large quantities of medication and reports feeling despair, depression and hopelessness.

Apply the decision-making framework to this scenario.

9

Ethics, law and mental health

Introduction

About one in five Australians will experience mental illness and most people will have a mental health problem at some point in their life (Australian Bureau of Statistics 2008). For many people their experience with mental illness will be short-lived, with the illness responding rapidly to treatment and not reoccurring. However, some people will experience mental illness as a chronic disabling condition. This chapter focuses primarily on the legal and ethical issues arising from the care and treatment provided to people experiencing acute or serious chronic mental health conditions.

It is important to specifically discuss the care and treatment provided to people experiencing mental illness because of the impact of coercive legal mechanisms on patient rights, the history of abuse of persons experiencing mental illness within the legal and health systems, the potentially invasive and irreversible impact of, or side effects from, certain forms of treatment and the ongoing discrimination against them.

The way in which mental health law is structured in Australia enables patients to be detained and treated without their consent and, indeed, in the face of their express refusal. This means they lose their fundamental right to liberty, reasonable force may be used against them to compel treatment and they lose their right to make choices about their healthcare treatment. The gravity of these incursions into an individual's human rights has been widely recognised at the international level with the enactment of the *United Nations Convention on Rights of Persons with Disabilities*. Article 12 of the Convention appears not to permit compulsory detention and treatment and emphasises creating mechanisms to maximise the human rights of persons experiencing mental illness, including not taking away a person's ability to make decisions. Australia is a signatory to the Convention but has declared it may not comply with Article 12 so Australia can continue to detain and treat people with serious mental illnesses without their consent and in the face of their refusal.

The use of legislative powers to detain and treat persons with mental illness has a sorry history of misuse and abuse throughout the world. Misuse in that sometimes people have been assessed as having a mental illness, have been detained, and have been subjected to unwarranted and at times quite invasive treatment (for example, irreversible brain surgery) when they did not in fact have a mental illness or when they displayed behaviour that was at variance with the social norms at that time. For example, history shows us that some women were considered to be mentally ill if they were considered to be 'promiscuous' and homosexuality was, in the past, considered in Australia to be a mental illness warranting treatment. As noted by President Kirby then of the New South Wales Court of Appeal, 'Many reports of official bodies, in Australia and overseas, have demonstrated the way in which mental health law can sometimes be used to control the behaviour of individuals merely to relieve family, neighbours and acquaintances from their embarrassment' (*Harry v Mental Health Review Board* (1994) 33 NSWLR 315 at 322).

Persons experiencing mental illness have also sometimes been abused by the health professionals who were supposed to care for them, including physical, sexual and psychological abuse or exploitation. Others have been abused by other patients, with health professionals taking no action to stop the abuse or responding inappropriately to it. A recent small survey conducted by the Victorian Mental Illness Awareness Council (2013) found that 45 per cent of respondents reported being sexually assaulted during their time in a Victorian mental health facility, 61 per cent reported the assault to nurses or doctors, and 82 per cent reported that the nurses or doctors were not at all helpful. Respondents reported that they were not believed, or were subject to seclusion as a consequence of reporting, and that they had gained the impression, as one respondent put it, that 'crazy women don't matter'.

For a patient's perspective of involuntary mental health treatment read Jones, C. 2012, 'Life in a public mental ward: Enough to drive you insane', *Sydney Morning Herald*, 15 March 2012.

'I have been in a ward where electroconvulsive therapy was used as a threat; where a dirty look at a nurse could result in a "code" being called, a bashing by hospital security and hours in a padded cell; where psychological abuse and verbal insults from nurses and doctors were par for the course.'

Mental health law has also at certain times and places been used as a tool by repressive regimes to control and manage dissent with the complicity of health professionals. In Soviet Russia, for example, between 1960 and 1986 prominent dissidents were diagnosed with mental illnesses, detained and 'treated'. Such a diagnosis served multiple purposes: discrediting the person; removing them from the public eye; detaining them indefinitely, and treating them to try and 'cure' them so that they would no longer express dissenting views and, indeed, would henceforth support the regime. In Nazi Germany views about the so-called superiority of the Aryan race led to the enactment of eugenics laws, which targeted people experiencing mental illness and intellectual disability, among other conditions, to be forcibly sterilised so that they would not procreate. The sterilisation of these groups in Nazi Germany expanded to some health professionals being involved in the mass involuntary euthanasia (murder) of their mentally or intellectually disabled patients (and those with severe physical disabilities) in the name of racial 'purity'.

Some treatments for mental illnesses are particularly invasive and irreversible. Psychosurgery, for example, although rarely performed, removes brain tissue intending to reduce symptoms. Another example of the extreme consequences of some forms of 'treatment' for mental illness is set out in the box on 'Chelmsford Private Hospital, Sydney'.

Chelmsford Private Hospital, Sydney

A Royal Commission of Inquiry into Deep Sleep Therapy (1990) investigated the practices of a psychiatrist and other health professionals, including nurses, who admitted patients experiencing mental illness into Chelmsford private hospital. The patients received 'special treatment' which involved placing them in a barbiturate-induced coma lasting up to 35 days – so called 'deep-sleep therapy' – often supplemented with electro-convulsive therapy. During the 16-year period (1963–1979) during which the 'therapy' was provided at least 24 people died as a direct result of the 'deep-sleep therapy'.

There is a long history of discrimination against persons experiencing mental illness and they have been stigmatised and discriminated against in all aspects of their life. For example, individuals have been unable to access accommodation or employment and have been denied access to their children. At a societal level there has also traditionally been discrimination against persons experiencing mental illness. For example, communities have refused the placement of supported living in their neighbourhood – the not in my back yard (NIMBY) syndrome. Persons experiencing mental illness may not be believed when they report abuse or maltreatment. At the governmental level, mental health has traditionally attracted less funding proportionately to other areas of health. Even within the health system, health professionals, including nurses, have discriminated against persons experiencing mental illness (Ross and Goldner 2009).

Anti-discrimination law in the Commonwealth and the states and territories includes health status (i.e. mental illness) as a prohibited ground of discrimination (*Discrimination Act 1991* (ACT); *Anti-Discrimination Act 1977* (NSW); *Anti-Discrimination Act* (NT); *Anti-Discrimination Act 1991* (Qld); *Equal Opportunity Act 1984* (SA); *Anti-Discrimination Act 1988* (Tas); *Equal Opportunity Act 2010* (Vic); *Equal Opportunity Act 1984* (WA); *Disability Discrimination Act 1992* (Cth)). In addition, much progress has been made in educating the public about mental illness and attempting to eliminate stigma and discrimination.

Ethics and nursing practice

The principles approach

Autonomy

The concept of autonomy is important when considering the rights of persons experiencing mental illness. As a starting point it should be presumed that everyone is competent unless there is good reason to believe otherwise. Just because someone is experiencing mental illness does not mean that they are unable to make informed decisions about matters affecting them. Some of the stigma attached to mental illness is because of conscious or unconscious assumptions that a diagnosis of mental illness automatically means that a person is not capable of making decisions or indeed of looking after themselves. For the majority of persons experiencing mental illness or a mental health problem this is not the case. Even those experiencing the most serious and acute forms of mental illness may be competent to consent or refuse consent to treatment or may be able to do so with appropriate supports.

It is generally accepted that a person's ability to exercise their autonomy may vary depending on the severity of their illness and the type of decision that needs to be made. Some people experiencing mental illness, or with intellectual or cognitive impairments more generally, may not be considered by some people to have the capacity to make decisions about how to manage their financial affairs but may be considered capable in respect of making decisions about the activities of daily life or to make health care decisions. Some may be considered to lack capacity in relation to both finances and health care. Others would dispute this and say everyone has the capacity to make decisions with the appropriate supports.

Under current Australian law, a substitute decision-maker would make choices for an incompetent adult patient (see Chapter 5).

In Australia, at times the state may use its powers under mental health legislation to require both the detention of individuals and their treatment, irrespective of whether they have the capacity to make decisions about care and treatment (the rationale for this is discussed briefly in the next paragraph and in more detail under the concept of beneficence). In other words, the law in Australia can be used to override the rights of a competent adult patient to refuse or to consent to treatment and care.

Even if a person experiencing mental illness is considered under current Australian law not to have the capacity to make decisions about their treatment or about their life in general, and decisions are made by the substitute decision-maker or by mental health professionals pursuant to the powers given to them by the state, patients should still be treated with respect. This is because the concept of autonomy also has broader connotations associated with respecting an individual's inherent personhood, or respecting their dignity as a person. This would include engaging persons who are considered to lack the capacity to make decisions for themselves in the caring and treatment process to the greatest extent possible, and treating them in a manner and form that acknowledges and respects their inherent personal dignity as a human being.

A more controversial approach to the concept of autonomy in the context of mental illness is the idea of 'authentic autonomy'. Briefly put, 'authentic autonomy' is the idea that treatment should be provided to a person experiencing mental illness, irrespective of their consent or refusal of consent, as the illness has corrupted their ability to exercise their autonomy in a way that is a reflection of, or consistent with, their 'true' or 'authentic' self. Their 'authentic' self would not, it is argued, want to be floridly or acutely mentally ill, therefore it is justifiable to intervene to, in effect, save them from themselves by treating the biochemical imbalance in their brain, so stabilising their condition and bringing them back to authenticity. But what if a person considers that the mental illness is central to their sense of who and what they are – their authentic self? What if the illness defines their identity?

Starson v Swayze 2003 SCCC 32 (the 'Beautiful Mind' case)

The Canadian legal case involving Mr Starson illustrates the dilemma set out in the discussion on 'Autonomy'. Please note that Canadian legislation permits the detention of persons experiencing serious mental illness if they fit the defined criteria; however, it does not authorise compulsory treatment. In Canadian jurisdictions if the ▶

◀

patient is considered competent they make decisions about health care. If they are not then their substitute decision-maker makes the decisions.

Mr Starson had been diagnosed with bipolar disorder. He was a self-taught theoretical physics 'genius' who believed that his insights into physics were associated with his illness and that psychotropic medications blunted or indeed destroyed his inspiration and destroyed his true self. He had executed an advance directive, while competent, to say that he refused the administration of all psychotropic medications in the event he lost competence. Starson had been compulsorily detained under mental health legislation after threatening to kill two people. His psychiatrist sought leave from the courts to override his advance directive and current refusal to treat him with a variety of psychotropic medications. On appeal the majority of the Canadian Supreme Court, the highest Canadian court, agreed that Starson had the capacity or was competent to refuse medications, as under Ontario legislation it was clear that people may make decisions that are contrary to doctors' advice.

Beneficence and non-maleficence

One of the concerns about the scope of the principle of beneficence, as discussed in previous chapters, is that it can be used to justify paternalism. Paternalism is generally considered to be a negative in a society that values individual rights and responsibilities. However, the debates about providing care and treatment to people experiencing mental illness, particularly in its serious and acute forms, often approaches, if not encroaches on paternalism. When considering mental illness, the best interest analysis goes beyond what is in the best interests of the patient as an individual to also encompass what is in the best interests for the community. Now you might say that this is so for all forms of treatment, and indeed it is, but attaining the appropriate balance between individual and community interests is particularly acute in the mental health context. Those persons experiencing mental illness, particularly in its serious or acute form, are perceived as being vulnerable and in need of protection for their own good and for the good of society as a whole. This protective argument is characteristic of the traditional approach to managing the care and treatment needs of persons with a mental illness. But we need to raise the question as to whether this protective approach is appropriate or not. Could it undermine a person's well-being and their personhood to be considered to be in need of protection by reason of their having one or more of a relatively common set of illnesses? Rather than seeing persons experiencing mental illness as being in need of protection, should we perhaps be considering how we could shape our systems and environment to enable them to exercise their autonomy and personhood, despite their illness?

The beneficence analysis is strongly linked to the ethical principle of non-maleficence which focuses on harm and preventing needless harm, again both in respect of the individual and in respect of the community. The ethical principle of non-maleficence interacts with the principle of autonomy. As discussed in earlier chapters, John Stuart Mill suggested that the only justification for curbing the principle of autonomy was when its exercise threatened to harm others. Many people experiencing serious mental illness pose no direct threat of any kind to others. However, that appears not to be the case for everyone. In the *Starson* case (see the box on '*Starson v Swayze* 2003 SCCC 32'), Starson had threatened physical harm to others, causing those people a degree of anxiety and fear for their own well-being and that of family, friends and colleagues. The link between certain forms of serious and acute mental illness and actual violent offending is controversial – with previous research concluding the rates of violent offending among persons experiencing serious mental illness was no greater than the general population and recent research indicating that the rates are somewhat higher (Morgan et al. 2012). A primary justification for the detention, and treatment, of persons experiencing serious mental illnesses is that they pose a risk of causing serious harm to others, a risk best managed by detaining them, and, in Australia, treating them until that risk has passed. One of the significant challenges for health professionals working in the mental health area is how to judge and measure the level of risk posed by an individual to others.

The other justification that is recognised, albeit not by Mill, is when the individual poses a risk of harm to themselves. On the one hand suicide is not an unlawful act, although assisting a suicide currently is (however, note that in limited circumstances assisting a suicide will be lawful in Victoria from 2019; see Chapter 11), and an argument is made that competent adults should be able to, and in fact practically can, choose to end their lives as part of exercising their right to autonomy. On the other hand there is an arguable moral imperative on both health professionals and the state to prevent harm, in this case death – a death that might be preventable if treatment is provided. In this context, both ethics and law grapple with achieving an appropriate balance between respecting the rights and interests of individuals and promoting what are perceived to be the interests of the community.

Non-maleficence is also relevant in respect of the misuse of powers under mental health legislation and the abuse and exploitation of persons experiencing mental illness by health professionals. The powers conferred on designated people under mental health laws to control persons experiencing serious mental illness create a difficult and challenging environment that historically has seen a number of abuses of those powers. In addition, the nature of mental illness makes persons experiencing mental illness especially vulnerable to physical, psychological and emotional exploitation by others. The nature of certain forms of treatment for those experiencing mental illness creates a relationship where a health professional knows intimate details of that patient's life, relationships, thoughts, feelings and vulnerabilities. Two relevant concepts from psychotherapy are: transference – where a patient's feelings are redirected towards their therapist often in the form of attraction, dependence or ideation; and counter-transference – where a therapist's feelings can be redirected to towards their patient. If a health professional takes advantage of that knowledge and that clinical relationship, or is vulnerable to counter-transference, it can cause significant harm to the patient and is inherently exploitative of an individual with significant vulnerabilities. The case *Jacobsen v Nurses Tribunal & Anor* (see Chapter 4) illustrates that conduct that exploits the vulnerabilities of a person experiencing mental illness is considered an ethical and legal wrong and a violation of professional standards.

Justice

One of the faces of justice is distributive justice – the fair allocation of resources. Traditionally, services that support persons with mental illness have been under-resourced given the extent of mental illness within the community (Australian Medical Association 2018) and these services were generally the first to be cut during times of resource constraint. Critics suggest that the disproportionate gap in funding of mental health services was due to the stigmatisation and discrimination traditionally associated with mental illness. In 2011/2012 the Australian Commonwealth committed to remedying the traditional funding shortfall by targeting $1.5 billion towards the provision of mental health services.

The history of how we as a society relate to those experiencing serious mental illness has been one marked with discrimination and oppression. The coercive power of the state has been historically used or misused to:

➢ Forcibly detain individuals experiencing serious mental illness (and at times those with moderate or no mental illness)

➢ Incarcerate them, often indefinitely, often in poor conditions (the history of the treatment of mental illness in the West has seen people chained to walls and this is still a reality in some areas in countries like Afghanistan where there is no mental health infrastructure) with no rights of appeal

➢ Remove the power of the individual patient to make decisions, irrespective of whether they are competent or not

➢ Impose treatment on them, whether or not they refuse it

➢ Create conditions where patients are vulnerable to being abused or exploited by those who care for them and which leads to them not being treated with respect and accorded any recognition of their inherent dignity as a person

➢ Create conditions where patients have become institutionalised, marginalised and discriminated against.

There has been, and is still, much attention paid to enhancing the rights of patients experiencing serious mental illness. These measures include; creating rights for those persons to access legal assistance; rights to review and appeal any orders authorising detention or treatment; and institutional measures to ensure some independent oversight of mental health facilities, their policies and practices, and the practices of their staff. Much attention has also been paid to ensuring that patients have the right to be told of the above measures as they cannot effectively use such measures if they are unaware of them. Perhaps more fundamentally it is also recognised that the use of the powers of the state in this area has a profound impact on an individual's human rights: the right to freedom of movement (liberty); the right to autonomy or self-determination; and the rights to dignity and respect, among others. This is recognised at the international level with the passing of the *United Nations Principles for the Protection of People with Mental Illness*, and the *Convention of the Rights of Persons with Disabilities*. Article 17 of the Convention states that: 'Every person with disabilities has a right to respect for his or her physical and mental integrity on an equal basis with others.'

The nursing and midwifery codes

Discrimination

Discrimination directed towards persons experiencing mental illness by individuals and at the societal level is well-reported in Australia and internationally. The ICM Code of Ethics notes at II.d: 'Midwives respond to the psychological, physical, emotional and spiritual needs of women seeking health care, whatever their circumstances (non-discrimination).' The ICN Code of Ethics in its preamble notes: 'Nursing care is respectful of and unrestricted by considerations of age, colour, creed, culture, disability, race or social status.' Both also refer to respecting human rights which would include the right not to be discriminated against. The Codes of Conduct reinforce this at 3.2.d by stating nurses and midwives must 'adopt practices that respect diversity, avoid bias, discrimination and racism and challenge belief based on assumption (for example, based on gender, disability, race, ethnicity, religion, sexuality, age or political beliefs'.

Decision-making

There are a number of statements from the nursing and midwifery Codes of Conduct that discuss decision-making and these are extensively covered in Chapter 5. Especially relevant are that nurses and midwives must 'act according to the person's capacity for decision-making and consent ... based on their maturity and capacity to understand, and the nature of the proposed care' (2.3.c).

Power relationships

There are significant power-related issues between persons experiencing serious mental illness and health professionals who have the power to refer them for assessment, to section them under mental health legislation, to restrain or seclude them, and to decide when their compulsory detention and/or treatment ends. The Codes of Conduct recognise (2.2.h) that nurses and midwives should 'recognise that their context of practice can influence decision-making. This includes the type and location of practice setting.' It is recognised that institutional environments can impact their decision-making. If an institutional culture is similar to that described by C. Jones (2012) earlier in this chapter, then this can impact on their practice and may mean that they are more likely to act in certain ways towards their patients.

Exploitation

As discussed earlier, persons experiencing a mental illness may be vulnerable to exploitation. The Codes of Conduct (1.3.b) note nurses and midwives must 'remain alert to ... groups who may be vulnerable and at risk of physical harm and sexual exploitation and act on welfare concerns where appropriate'.

Confidentiality

Confidentiality is discussed in more detail in Chapter 7. However, both Codes of Ethics emphasise the importance of maintaining confidentiality and being aware of the conditions under which information may or may not be shared with others (element 1 ICN and III.a ICM). The Codes of Conduct also extensively discuss confidentiality at 3.5.

Law and mental health

Defining mental illness

Each jurisdiction defines mental illness slightly differently. The wording may vary slightly but the definition of mental illness in most jurisdictions generally relates to a condition that seriously affects a person's mental functioning often combined with a list of symptoms (for example, delusions, hallucinations, serious disorder of thought form, serious disturbance of mood, and sustained or repeated irrational behaviour indicating the presence of one of the aforementioned symptoms) (*Mental Health Act 2015* (ACT) s 10; *Mental Health Act 2007* (NSW) s 4; *Mental Health and Related Services Act* (NT) s 6; *Mental Health Act 2013* (Tas) s 3).

Queensland defines mental illness as a 'condition characterised by a clinically significant disturbance of thought, mood, perception or memory' (*Mental Health Act 2016* (Qld) s 10). A very similar definition is used in Victoria (*Mental Health Act 2014* (Vic) s 4(1)) and Western Australia (*Mental Health Act 2014* (WA) s 4). South Australia has a very generic definition: an 'illness or disorder of the mind' (*Mental Health Act 2009* (SA) s 3).

In a clear recognition of past history and the enduring potential of mental health law to be used as a tool of personal or state oppression, mental health legislation is clear that a person should not be considered to have a mental illness solely because they, for example:

➢ Express or fail to express a political, religious, legal or moral opinion

➢ Engage or do not engage in political, religious, illegal or immoral (including sexual activity and promiscuity) conduct or anti-social behaviour

➢ Take alcohol or drugs

➢ Have a particular economic or social status

➢ Are a member of a particular culture or racial group

➤ Have an intellectual disability

➤ Are involved in family conflict

(*Mental Health Act 2015* (ACT) s 1; *Mental Health Act 2007* (NSW) s 14(1); *Mental Health and Related Services Act* (NT) s 6; *Mental Health Act 2016* (Qld) s 10(2); *Mental Health Act 2009* (SA) sch. 1; *Mental Health Act 2013* (Tas) s 4(2); *Mental Health Act 2014* (Vic) s 4(2); *Mental Health Act 2014* (WA) s 6(2)).

Involuntary patients

The legal framework in Australia, in some circumstances, enables a person experiencing mental illness to be detained and treated without their consent and in the face of their express refusal (involuntary inpatients) or to be treated in the community without their consent under a community treatment order (CTO). These patients have been what is colloquially termed 'sectioned' under mental health legislation and lose several of their rights during the period of time that they fall under the legislation. Justice O'Brien of the Victorian Supreme Court noted in *Wilson v Mental Health Review Board* [2000] VSC 404 at [32]: 'The status of an involuntary patient … is a restriction upon the liberty of a person and an interference with their rights, dignity and self-respect.' Because of the draconian impact of mental health law and the history of misuse and abuse of its powers, there are a number of safeguards in place to try and ensure people are not arbitrarily detained and provided with unwarranted treatment.

The following sections present a summary of what are often complicated legislative frameworks. Nurses and midwives working in this area should familiarise themselves with the specifics of the legislation in the jurisdiction they practise in.

Australian Capital Territory

Mental Health Act 2015 (ACT)

A person experiencing a mental illness may voluntarily apply to be assessed if they believe that they are unable to make 'reasonable judgments' about their health or safety or unable to take care of their own health or safety or are likely to cause serious harm to others (s 33). Any person can apply for another person to be assessed:

➤ If the applicant reasonably believes that the other person's health or safety is, or is likely to be, 'substantially at risk' because they are unable, due to mental illness, to make 'reasonable judgments' about their health or safety or they cannot care for their health and safety.

> If the other person, because of mental illness, is doing, or is likely to do, serious harm to others.

After receiving an application the Australian Capital Territory Civil and Administrative Tribunal may issue an assessment order if:

> The person appears to have a mental illness; and

> Either the person's health or safety is or is likely to be substantially at risk or that person is doing or is likely to do serious harm to others (s 37).

An emergency assessment order can also be issued (s 37(2)).

The Tribunal must consider the assessment (s 53) and consult with people listed in section 54. It can then issue:

> A mental health order (ss 28, 29);

> A psychiatric treatment order (involuntary treatment) (s 58);

> A restriction order (s 60) (order that a person must live or be detained at a particular place); or

> A community care order (s 66).

The Tribunal may issue a psychiatric treatment order if it considers that the person has a mental illness and does not have decision-making capacity to provide consent and refuses the treatment, or the person has capacity but refuses to consent. It must also reasonably believe that the person is doing or is likely to do serious harm to self or to others, or is likely to experience a serious mental or physical deterioration which is of such a serious nature that it outweighs the person's right to refuse consent. The Tribunal must also be satisfied that psychiatric treatment is likely to reduce the harm or deterioration or result in an improvement in the person's condition. The Tribunal must also be satisfied that the treatment cannot be adequately provided in a way that would involve less restriction of the freedom of choice and movement of the person (s 58(2)). A restriction order can be issued if the Tribunal reasonably believes that it is in the interests of the person's health or safety or the safety of others to do so and the treatment to be provided under a psychiatric treatment order cannot be adequately provided to involve less restriction of the freedom of choice and movement of the person (s 60). The treatment must be explained to the person (s 63) after orders are issued.

Emergency apprehension by the police or ambulance paramedics is permitted under section 80(1) if they believe on reasonable grounds that the person has a mental illness and they have attempted or are likely to attempt suicide or to inflict serious harm on themselves or others. Similarly, a doctor or mental health officer may apprehend a person if that person has a mental illness and either the person requires immediate treatment or their condition will deteriorate within three days so that they would require immediate treatment (s 80(2)). They must have refused that treatment and detention is necessary for their health or safety, social or financial well-being or for the protection of others, and adequate treatment cannot be provided in a less restrictive environment.

New South Wales

Mental Health Act 2007 (NSW)

A person may be detained and admitted as a patient in a mental health facility:

➢ If a primary carer, relative or friend requests it in circumstances where it is not reasonably practicable to get a certificate from a doctor (i.e. long distance to travel and it is urgent in the circumstances) (s 26).

➢ If a doctor or 'accredited person' (including a qualified and experienced mental health nurse) examines a person and forms the opinion they are mentally ill or mentally disordered and completes a certificate to that effect (s 19).

➢ If an ambulance officer believes on reasonable grounds that a person appears mentally ill or mentally disordered and it would be beneficial to transport them to hospital (s 20) – they can request police assistance who can enter premises without a warrant and use reasonable force (ss 21, 81).

➢ If a police officer: (a) finds a person in a public place; (b) believes the person is mentally ill or mentally disordered; (c) believes the person has recently attempted to kill themselves or will try to or will attempt to cause serious bodily harm to themselves or has committed or is committing an offence; and (d) they believe it would be preferable to deal with the person under mental health law not the criminal law (s 22).

➢ If a magistrate orders a person undergoes examination by a doctor or accredited person (with the assistance of the police if required). Such an order can be made if they receive evidence under oath that the person may be mentally ill or disordered but could not be examined because of inaccessibility (s 23).

➤ If a magistrate believes a person appearing before them in a criminal matter is mentally ill they can issue an order requiring detention and assessment (s 24).

➤ If a doctor working in a facility believes the person should be transferred to a mental health facility and detained there because they are mentally ill (ss 19, 25).

The first examination by a doctor must occur as soon as practicable, no later than 12 hours after admission. If the doctor deems them mentally ill (has a mental illness and needs treatment to protect them from serious harm or to protect others from serious harm) or mentally disordered (a mental illness is not required but they must be irrational such that treatment is required to protect the person from serious physical harm or to protect others from serious harm) then they must be examined by a psychiatrist, otherwise they are released (s 27). The second examination must occur as soon as practicable and if the second doctor concludes the person is mentally ill or disordered the person may be detained for a maximum of three days and must be reviewed by the Tribunal. If the doctor does not agree then a third examination is required (s 27(b)), and while this is being organised the patient may be admitted voluntarily or discharged if appropriate. A mentally disordered person may only be detained for no more than three working days and must be examined every 24 hours by a doctor and must not be detained if less restrictive care is available and appropriate (s 31). If a person is deemed mentally ill on admission then this must be reviewed by the Tribunal as soon as practicable to determine they are, in fact, mentally ill within the meaning of the Act, how long they should be detained and what care should be provided. The patient is highly engaged in this process. If the Tribunal determines the person is mentally ill within the meaning of the Act it may:

➤ discharge the person;

➤ place the person on a CTO for a maximum of 12 months; or

➤ make an involuntary patient order directing detention for a maximum of three months.

Northern Territory

Mental Health and Related Services Act (NT)

A person may request a doctor, psychiatrist or designated mental health practitioner (a person appointed under the Act who might be a registered nurse with at least two years' experience and with approved training) to make an assessment to determine whether they need treatment under the Act or another concerned person may make the request (s 32). A police officer may also bring a person to a doctor, psychiatrist or designated mental health practitioner for assessment if he or she believes the person may need treatment under the Act and is likely to cause harm to themselves or others (s 32A).

An assessment must occur as soon as practicable (s 33) and the assessor can recommend an examination if they are satisfied the person meets the criteria for involuntary admission because of mental illness or mental disturbance (irrational such that without treatment they may cause harm to self or others, may be a danger to the community or likely to seriously deteriorate) (s 34). Once a recommendation is made the practitioner, an ambulance officer or another specified person may transfer the person to a facility, with the assistance of police if required. Police may use reasonable force (s 32A). Once at the facility they may be detained for a maximum of 24 hours for examination by a psychiatrist or 72 hours if they are detained on the basis of mental disturbance. If, after examination, the psychiatrist believes the person meets the criteria for involuntary admission (mental illness, needs treatment, without treatment they might harm self or others or seriously deteriorate, cannot give consent or have unreasonably refused and there is no less restrictive treatment) they may be detained for 14 days if they are detained on the basis on mental illness (s 39), although this may be extended, or they may be placed on a CTO (s 38). Once admitted as an involuntary patient they must be examined by a psychiatrist every 72 hours.

Queensland

Mental Health Act 2016 (Qld)

A doctor or authorised mental health practitioner (AMHP) may examine a person to decide whether to recommend that that person be assessed, if the person asks for, or consents to, the examination under the Act (s 31) and can detain that person for an hour to examine them (s 36(2)). After the examination if they are satisfied the treatment criteria may apply to the person the doctor or AMHP may recommend that the person be assessed, as long as there appears to be no less restrictive way for the person to be treated for their mental illness (s 39(1)).

An authorised doctor assesses whether the treatment criteria apply to the person and whether there is a less restrictive way for the person to receive treatment for their mental illness (s 43(1)). The person can be held for assessment for 24 hours (s 45(1)). After the assessment, the doctor may make a treatment authority for the person as either an inpatient or in the community (s 51). The treatment criteria are:

a) the person has a mental illness;
b) the person lacks capacity to consent to treatment;
c) due to their mental illness the lack of involuntary treatment or its continuance is likely to result in imminent serious harm to self or others or the person suffering serious mental or physical deterioration (s 12(1)).

South Australia

Mental Health Act 2009 (SA)

The police and authorised officers (ambulance officer, medical officer or flight nurse employed by the Flying Doctors or a mental health clinician – a person engaged in care and treatment of patients and designated by the Chief Psychiatrist) can apprehend persons who appear to be suffering from a mental illness (ss 56, 57). If they have reasonable cause to suspect that the person has a mental illness and has caused harm they may enter any place and apprehend the person using reasonable force to transfer them to a mental health facility.

A person may receive treatment pursuant to a CTO or a detention and treatment order (DTO).

There are two levels of CTOs. A Level 1 CTO may be issued in writing by a doctor or authorised health professional (as authorised by the Minister so registered nurses may fall into this category) if it appears:

➤ the person has a mental illness;

➤ the person requires treatment for their protection or to protect others;

➤ there are facilities and services available; and

➤ there is no less restrictive means than a CTO to manage the person's illness (s 10).

It lasts 28 days and if not made by a doctor must be reviewed by a doctor within 24 hours.

A Level 2 CTO is issued by the Guardianship Board pursuant to the criteria used in relation to Level 1 CTOs after application by the public advocate, a doctor, a mental health clinician, guardian, carer, relative or friend of the person or any other person with an interest in the patient's welfare. A Level 2 CTO lasts 6 months for children and 12 months for adults.

There are three levels of CTOs and the criterion for each is:

➢ the person has a mental illness;

➢ the person requires treatment for their protection or to protect others from harm; and

➢ there is no less restrictive means other than detention and treatment in a mental health facility.

A Level 1 CTO may be made by a doctor or authorised health professional who, after examination, is satisfied the person meets the criteria. It is valid for 7 days. The patient must be examined by a psychiatrist or authorised doctor (although not the one who made the first assessment) within 24 hours or as soon as practicable to confirm it. They may then issue a Level 2 CTO which lasts 42 days. A Level 3 CTO is made by the Guardianship Board and expires after 6 months for a child and 12 months for an adult (s 29).

Tasmania

Mental Health Act 2013 (Tas)

Any medical practitioner may issue an assessment order (s 22) if they have examined the person within the 24 hours immediately before the assessment order is made. As a result of that examination, the doctor needs to be satisfied that the person needs to be assessed against the assessment criteria. The criteria is defined in section 25 as:

➢ the person has, or appears to have, a mental illness that requires or is likely to require treatment for:

the person's health or safety; or

the safety of other persons; and

➢ the person cannot be properly assessed except under the authority of the assessment order; and

➢ the person does not have decision-making capacity.

A reasonable attempt to have the person assessed, with their informed consent, needs to have failed or it needs to be considered futile or inappropriate to make an attempt (s 24(1)). A medical practitioner may make an assessment order authorising a patient's admission to, and, if necessary, detention in, an approved hospital (s 24(2)). An assessment order gives authority for that person to be assessed without their consent by an approved medical practitioner to confirm whether the patient meets the assessment and treatment criterion (s 27(1)). After an assessment order is issued an assessment needs to be undertaken by an independent medical practitioner within 24 hours (s 30).

A treatment order can only be issued by the Tribunal (s 36) on application by a medical practitioner. A treatment order can only be issued if it is satisfied that an approved medical practitioner has validly applied for a treatment order in respect of the person, the person meets the treatment criteria and a treatment plan has been prepared in consultation with the patient (s 39). A treatment order may include a requirements in respect of the treatment setting and that the person may be detained in a specific setting (s 39). The treatment criteria are that the person has a mental illness and without treatment the mental illness will or is likely to seriously harm the person's health or safety or the safety of others. The proposed treatment needs to be considered appropriate and effective, cannot be adequately given except under a treatment order and the person does not have decision-making capacity (s 40). If the person does not comply with a treatment order, despite reasonable steps being taken to obtain the patient's 'compliance' with the order, and this has seriously harmed, or is likely to seriously harm the patient's health or safety or the safety of others and the harm cannot be addressed other than way of alternative treatment, a medical practitioner may apply to the Tribunal for an order (s 47(1)). The Tribunal may vary the order, provide authorisation to admit or detain the person, or authorise immediate treatment (s 47(2)). Section 55(1) and(2) states that a person may be given treatment without informed consent or Tribunal authorisation if an approved medical practitioner authorises the treatment as being urgently needed in the patient's best interests and the necessary treatment outcome would be compromised by waiting for Tribunal authorisation. The criteria for a medical practitioner to determine this is the patient has a mental illness that needs treatment and urgent treatment is necessary for the patient's health or safety or the safety of others and it is likely to be effective and appropriate.

Victoria

Mental Health Act 2014 (Vic)

An assessment order may be issued by a medical practitioner to assess whether a person meets the treatment criteria. After an order is issued a person may compulsorily be examined or examined and detained (s 28). Section 29 sets out the criteria requiring the person to appear to have a mental illness and needs immediate treatment to prevent a serious deterioration in the person's mental or physical health or serious harm to the person or to others and there is no less restrictive means reasonably available to enable the person to be assessed. The assessment needs to occur between 24 and 72 hours of the order being issued (depending on the circumstances) (s 34). Section 52 states that after an assessment a Tribunal may issue a treatment order for that person to be treated in the community (CTO) or in a mental health facility (inpatient treatment order). The Tribunal must decide whether the person meets the criteria and have regard to the views of a number of people, including the person (s 55). The treatment criteria are set out in section 5 and include that the person has a mental illness and needs immediate treatment to prevent either a serious deterioration in their mental or physical health or serious harm to the person or to another person which can be immediately provided. There needs to be no less restrictive means reasonably available to enable the person to receive immediate treatment.

Western Australia

Mental Health Act 2014 (WA)

A medical practitioner may refer a person for examination by a psychiatrist if the practitioner reasonably suspects that the person needs involuntary treatment (s 26). A person who is referred for examination may be detained for up to 24 hours. Only a psychiatrist may make an involuntary treatment order. Before deciding whether or not to make an inpatient treatment order, a psychiatrist must consider whether the objects of the Act would be better achieved by making a CTO (s 24). Two types of involuntary treatment orders may be issued: an inpatient treatment order (admission and detention to a hospital to enable treatment without informed consent (s 22)); or a CTO, which enables the provision of treatment in the community without informed consent (s 23). The criteria for an inpatient treatment order is set out in section 25(1). The person must have a mental illness needing treatment and the mental illness results in a significant risk to the health or safety of the person or to the safety of others or a significant risk of serious harm to the person or to another person. The person must also not demonstrate the required capacity to make a treatment decision about their treatment, treatment in the community cannot reasonably be provided and the person cannot be adequately provided with treatment in a way that is less restrictive to the person's freedom of choice and movement than an inpatient order. The criteria for a community treatment is similar. However, unlike for the inpatient treatment order, a CTO may be issued if there is a significant risk of the person suffering serious physical or mental deterioration.

Also it needs to be considered whether treatment in the community can reasonably be provided to the person and the person cannot be adequately provided with treatment in a way that would involve less restriction on the person's freedom of choice and movement than making a CTO (s 25(2)).

Safeguards against abuse of process

Review Tribunals/Boards

An important element of the framework to limit the possibilities of abuse of mental health legislation is the role of independent Tribunals or Boards that review involuntary treatment orders or CTOs. These Boards or Tribunals have the power to confirm, vary or to revoke such orders. The specifics vary between jurisdictions, but a review may occur after it receives an application from the person or their representative, on its own initiative, or immediately after an order is imposed and at specific intervals after the order is imposed (*Mental Health Act 2015* (ACT) s 79; *Mental Health and Related Services Act* (NT) ss 122–127; *Mental Health Act 2016* (Qld) s 28 and Ch 5; *Mental Health Act 2009* (SA) ss 81–82; *Mental Health Act 2013* (Tas) Ch 3, Pt 3; *Mental Health Act 2014* (Vic) Pt 8; *Mental Health Act 2014* (WA) Pt 21).

Official visitors

Another important safeguard against the misuse or abuse of mental health legislation is the role of the 'official visitors' or 'authorised officers' or 'community visitors' (official visitors). While the Mental Health Tribunals/Boards can review matters on paper, they cannot assess the day-to-day conditions or treatment experienced by patients receiving mental health services within institutions. Official visitors are government-appointed officers charged with the oversight of the care and treatment provided within facilities to patients. The responsibilities of official visitors vary slightly between jurisdictions, but in general they are required to regularly visit facilities, with or without notice, to, among other things, inspect, enquire into and assess facilities and services, enquire into complaints and make sure patients are aware of their rights and that these are respected. They have the power to access any areas of the facility, see any patient, make any enquiries and inspect documentation without obstruction by staff (*Mental Health Act 2015* (ACT) Pt 12.3; *Mental Health and Related Services Act* (NT) s 104; *Mental Health Act 2009* (SA) Pt 8, div 2; *Mental Health Act 2013* (Tas) Ch 3, Pt 2 and sch. 5; *Mental Health Act 2014* (Vic) Pt 9). In New South Wales these responsibilities are split between authorised officers and official visitors (*Mental Health Act 2007* (NSW) ss 128–139). In Western Australia they are termed mental health advocates (*Mental Health Act 2014* (WA) Pt 20, div. 2).

Rights

Historically, patients receiving mental health services within institutions have not always been aware of their rights, especially involuntary patients who were not always aware that they had rights to appear before the Tribunal to seek a review of their status. Most jurisdictions require the provision of information to all patients admitted to receive mental health services about their rights and entitlements (*Mental Health Act 2015* (ACT) Pt 3.1; *Mental Health Act 2007* (NSW) s 74; *Mental Health and Related Services Act* (NT) s 87; *Mental Health Act 2016* (Qld) Ch 9; *Mental Health Act 2009* (SA) ss 9, 12, 23, 27; *Mental Health Act 2013* (Tas) s 129; *Mental Health Act 2014* (Vic) Pt 3; *Mental Health Act 2014* (WA) Pt 16).

Restraint and seclusion

The techniques of restraint and seclusion (see Figure 9.1) may be used in a mental health context. Seclusion and restraint raise significant human rights-related questions as by definition they involve limiting or removing a person's freedom of movement – their liberty – to an extent greater than detaining them in hospital and may also involve the use of reasonable force. The justification for using these techniques is to protect the individual from self-harm (for example, suicide or cutting) and to protect others from harm (in this context other patients or staff). These techniques are not without risk – some patients have died from suffocation while restrained – and long periods of seclusion have been shown to cause mental illness. There is also a risk that restraint or seclusion may be used for the convenience of staff, or to coerce patients to be compliant, or as a tool to punish an individual for non-compliance. Accordingly, there are legislative protections in place in all Australian jurisdictions to limit the circumstances in which restraints or seclusion can be used and to reduce the risks to those who are being restrained or secluded. These restrictions differ from jurisdiction to jurisdiction ranging from minimal to comprehensive. Some jurisdictions confer specific responsibilities on registered nurses.

Restraint and seclusion	Mechanical restraint - the application of devices (straps, manacles, harnesses, bed rails, chairs that are difficult to get out of etc) to a person's body to restrict movement.
	Physical restraint - the application of physical force to a person's body to restrict movement.
	Chemical restraint - the use of pharmaceuticals to restrict movement.
	Seclusion - the confinement of a person in a locked room.

Figure 9.1 Definitions of restraint and seclusion

Australian Capital Territory

An involuntary patient may be restrained if the Chief Psychiatrist considers it 'necessary' and 'reasonable' to 'prevent the person from causing harm to themselves or someone else' and may place a patient in seclusion if 'it is the only way in the circumstances to prevent the person from causing harm to themself or someone else' under section 65(2) of the *Mental Health Act 2015* (ACT). If the person is placed in seclusion they need to be checked by a doctor at least once every four hours (s 65(3)). The Chief Psychiatrist must enter into the patient's record and a register of involuntary restraint and seclusion that they were restrained or secluded and for what reason, and must inform the Public Advocate (s 65(5)).

New South Wales

There is limited legislative regulation of restraint and seclusion in New South Wales with section 68(f) of the *Mental Health Act 2007* (NSW) saying that 'any restriction on the liberty of patients and other people with a mental illness or a mental disorder and any interference with their rights, dignity and self-respect is to be kept to the minimum necessary in the circumstances'.

Northern Territory

It is a criminal offence to apply mechanical restraint to a person being assessed or treated under the *Mental Health and Related Services Act* (NT) (s 61(2)) unless the procedures set out in section 61 are followed.

Mechanical restraint or seclusion can only be applied without consent if it is necessary:

➤ For the purpose of medical treatment; or

➤ To prevent the person from harming themselves or any other person; or

➤ To prevent the person from persistently damaging property; or

➤ To prevent the person from absconding from the facility; and

➤ There must be no other less restrictive alternative (ss 61(3), 62(3)).

Restraint or seclusion must be approved by an authorised psychiatric practitioner or, in an emergency, by the senior registered nurse on duty (ss 61(4), 62(4)). If the senior registered nurse authorises the restraint they must notify the person in charge of the facility and the authorised psychiatrist as soon as practicable.

There are a number of restrictions on the use of restraint or seclusion:

➤ A registered nurse or doctor must keep a patient under continuous observation if they are mechanically restrained.

➤ A registered nurse must review the patient at intervals of no longer than 15 minutes.

➤ A registered medical practitioner must examine mechanically restrained patients every 4 hours or at specified intervals in relation to seclusion.

➤ The patient must be provided with appropriate bedding and clothing.

➤ The patient must be provided with food and drink at appropriate times.

➤ The patient must have access to appropriate toilet facilities.

➤ The patient must be provided with physical and psychological care appropriate to their needs (ss 61(8), 62(8)).

If the senior registered nurse on duty, a doctor or an authorised psychiatric practitioner is satisfied that the continued use of restraint or seclusion is not necessary, having regard to the reasons why restraint or seclusion may be used set out in sections 61(3) and 62(3), they must without delay release the patient (ss 61(11), 62(11)). There are also requirements that as soon as practicable after the restraint or seclusion has ceased that records be made, including the form of restraint, the reasons, the name of the approver, the name of the person who applied the restraints and the period of time the restraint/seclusion was imposed (s 61(12)). The adult guardian (a public official) must also be notified about the use of restraint.

Queensland

Chapter 8 of the *Mental Health Act 2016* (Qld) regulates mechanical restraint, seclusion and physical restraint. Section 270 states that an authorised doctor or a health practitioner in charge of an inpatient unit may authorise the use of physical restraints if there is no other reasonably practicable way to protect the patient or others from physical harm, to provide treatment and care to the patient, prevent the patient from causing serious damage to property, or to stop an involuntary patient from leaving.

An authorised doctor, or a health practitioner authorised by that doctor, may keep a patient in seclusion if the seclusion is authorised by an authorised doctor, if a written direction is given the seclusion complies with it, it complies with the restraint and seclusion policy and with any reduction and elimination plan if there is one, no more force than necessary and reasonable is used and the person is observed continuously or at no less than 15 minute intervals (s 256). Authorisation by an authorised doctor can be provided if there is no other reasonably practicable way to protect the patient or others from physical harm and the seclusion complies with the restraint and seclusion policy and with any reduction and elimination plan if there is one. It must be in writing and specify the start and end time, the time period of no more than three hours, the measures that must be taken to ensure the health, safety and comfort of the patient, the frequency of observation and whether a health practitioner can remove the person from seclusion before the end of the period (s 258). The health practitioner in charge of an inpatient unit has responsibilities to ensure that the seclusion complies with the authorisation and the patient's reasonable needs are met, including being given bedding and clothing, sufficient food and drink, and access to toilet facilities, and they must record information about the seclusion (s 260). The authorised doctor or the health practitioner in charge of the inpatient unit (if authorised to do so) must stop the seclusion if they are satisfied it is no longer necessary to protect the patient or others from harm (s 261).

Mechanical restraint is also permitted only if authorised by both the chief psychiatrist and an authorised doctor under similar conditions to that required to authorise seclusion. However, a patient must be continuously observed and cannot be mechanically restrained for more than three hours at a time and for no more than nine hours in a day (Div. 2).

South Australia

South Australia also has limited legislative regulation, with section 7(1) (f) of the *Mental Health Act 2009* (SA) stating: 'mechanical body restraints and seclusion should be used only as a last resort for safety reasons and not as a punishment or for the convenience of others'.

Tasmania

In Tasmania section 57 of the *Mental Health Act 2013* (Tas) states that an involuntary patient in an approved hospital may be restrained to prevent the person from harming themselves or others or to prevent: the patient from damaging property or equipment in a facility; to break up a dispute involving the patient; or to ensure the patient's movement for a lawful purpose if they are uncooperative. Seclusion is also permitted to facilitate the patient's treatment; ensure the person's health and safety; ensure the safety of the other persons; or provide for the management, good order or security of the hospital (s 56(5)). They must be monitored at no more than 15-minute intervals or as specified in a standing order. Whether a patient is restrained or in seclusion, the patient must be provided with suitable clothing and bedding, food and fluids, toilet and sanitary arrangements, adequate ventilation and light and a means of summoning aid (ss 56, 57).

Victoria

The *Mental Health Act 2014* (Vic) speaks of restrictive interventions, which include seclusion or bodily restraint. These can only be employed after all reasonable and less intrusive options have been tried or considered and found to be unsuitable. A person can only be kept in seclusion if necessary to prevent imminent and serious harm to the person or another person or to enable treatment (s 105). A person who authorises the restrictive intervention must ensure that the person's needs are met and their dignity protected (s 106). A person who is subject to seclusion or bodily restraint must be monitored by a registered nurse or doctor either continuously or at no less than 15-minute intervals (Pt 6 div. 2 and 3).

Western Australia

Bodily or mechanical restraint can be used. There are principles for bodily restraint, which include that:

> The degree of force must be the minimum required in the circumstances.

> There must be the least possible restriction on the person's freedom of movement consistent with the restraint.

> The person must be treated with dignity and respect (*Mental Health Act 2014* (WA) s 228).

The person in charge of the ward where the person is restrained must ensure the requirements around monitoring are complied with. A mental health practitioner or a nurse must be in physical attendance on the person at all times and, as soon as practicable, must record any observations they make about the person. A medical practitioner must examine the person at least every 30 minutes and, as soon as possible record their name and qualifications, the date and time of the examination, the results of the examination, including whether or not the medical practitioner considers that person should continue to be restrained. If the person remains restrained for more than 6 hours, a psychiatrist must review them. The person must be provided with appropriate bedding and clothing, sufficient food and drink, access to toilet facilities and any other care appropriate to the person's needs (s 238).

Limitations on use of certain treatments

Three jurisdictions also ban and/or criminalise coma therapy (*Mental Health and Related Services Act* (NT) s 59; *Mental Health Act 2016* (Qld) s 240; *Mental Health Act 2007* (NSW) s 83)).

Two treatments attract very specific restrictive regulation because of their past history, side effects, and/or long-term implications. Electro-convulsive treatment (ECT) is used to treat mood disorders, especially severe depression, and induces a convulsion or fit through the application of electricity. It can cause serious physical harm if used without appropriate anaesthesia, as well as short- or long-term memory loss but can be effective in treating depression. The use of psychosurgery, such as lobotomy which removes brain tissue, is also limited by legislation and is very rarely performed.

Australian Capital Territory

ECT can be provided by a doctor to a voluntary patient if they give informed consent, have not had ECT administered on nine or more occasions since giving consent and have not withdrawn their consent (*Mental*

Health Act 2015 (ACT) s 148). For patients who do not have decision-making capacity it may be administered if they have given an advance consent direction consenting to ECT and they do not refuse or resist or if it is administered by an ECT order or an emergency ECT order. The ACT Civil and Administrative Tribunal may make an ECT order if it is satisfied (*Mental Health Act 2015* (ACT) s 157(1)):

➢ the patient has a mental illness;

➢ the person lacks capacity to consent to ECT;

➢ the person does not have an advance consent direction refusing consent to ECT;

➢ the therapy is likely to result in a substantial benefits to the person; and

➢ either:

  – it is the most appropriate form of available treatment reasonably available; or

  – all other forms of treatment have been tried and were not successful.

It can also be provided if the Tribunal issues an emergency ECT order. Such an order may only be made by the Tribunal if:

➢ the person has a mental illness;

➢ the person does not have decision-making capacity to consent to ECT;

➢ the person does not have an advance consent direction refusing ECT;

➢ the administration is necessary to save the person's life or prevent the likely onset of a risk to the person's life within three days; and

➢ either:

  – it is the most appropriate form of available treatment reasonably available; or

  – all other forms of treatment have been tried and are not successful.

Psychosurgery can only be performed with the approval of the Chief Psychiatrist (*Mental Health Act 2015* (ACT) s 168). The Chief Psychiatrist must convene a multidisciplinary committee for its recommendation and act according to that recommendation. The Committee may only recommend surgery if it is satisfied:

➤ there are reasonable grounds to believe that surgery will result in substantial benefit to the patient;

➤ all available alternative forms of treatment have failed or a likely to fail to benefit the person; and

➤ the recommendation must be supported by the psychiatrist and the neurosurgeon that sit on the committee (s 170(4)(a)–(b)).

Similarly, the Supreme Court must be satisfied:

➤ the patient has a mental illness;

➤ the patient does not have decision-making capacity to consent;

➤ the person has not consented or refused consent to the surgery;

➤ that the surgery will substantially benefit the patient; and

➤ all forms of treatment reasonably available have failed or are likely to fail to benefit them (s 173).

Surgery cannot be provided if the person refuses it, even with a court order (s 174).

New South Wales

In New South Wales ECT may be administered to a voluntary patient who has given informed consent. It may be administered to an involuntary patient after the Mental Health Tribunal has determined that the patient has the capacity to give consent and has given informed consent. If they are unable to consent or have refused the Tribunal can intervene and authorise the treatment if it is satisfied that it is 'reasonable and proper' and 'necessary and desirable' (*Mental Health Act 2007* (NSW) s 96). Psychosurgery is generally prohibited (s 83).

Northern Territory

ECT may not be used unless informed consent is obtained from the patient or the patient's adult guardian or if it is performed in accordance with the *Mental Health and Related Services Act 1998* (NT) (s 66(1)). Where a person is unable to give consent or there is no adult guardian the Tribunal may authorise it when two psychiatrists report that ECT is reasonable and proper treatment for the patient's condition (s 66(2)). ECT may be performed on an involuntary patient if two psychiatrists state it is necessary to save the person's life, to prevent the person suffering serious physical or mental harm, or to relieve severe distress (s 66(3)). All psychosurgery is prohibited (s 58(2)).

Queensland

ECT may be provided if the person has given informed consent or with the authorisation of the Mental Health Review Tribunal or in an emergency if it is considered necessary to save the person's life or prevent them suffering irreparable harm (*Mental Health Act 2016* (Qld) ss 236–237). The Mental Health Review Tribunal must consider (s 509(3)):

➢ Any views or preferences expressed by an adult in an advance directive

➢ The views of a child's parents and the views and preferences of the child

➢ Whether ECT is in the person's best interests

➢ Whether evidence supports the effectiveness of the therapy for the patient's form of mental illness (or age if the person is a minor)

➢ If it has been previously performed on the person, its past effectiveness.

Psychosurgery is prohibited (s 241). Non-ablative neurosurgical procedures are not permitted unless the patient has given informed consent and the Mental Health Review Tribunal has approved it (ss 238–239).

South Australia

ECT can only be administered to a patient if:

➢ they have a mental illness;

➢ it has been authorised by a psychiatrist; and

➢ written consent has been provided by the patient, or on behalf of the patient if they are under 18 years of age, or by the Guardianship Board if they are not competent (*Mental Health Act 2009* (SA) s 42(1)).

Surgery may only be undertaken:

➢ if the patient has a mental illness;

➢ if it has been authorised by the person who is to carry it out supported by two psychiatrists (one who must be senior) after separately examining the patient; and

> if the patient is over 16 years of age and has provided written consent or, if the patient is not able to give consent, it has been given by the Guardianship Board (s 43).

Tasmania

ECT is not dealt with as a special treatment under the *Mental Health Act 2013* (Tas). Psychosurgery is illegal in Tasmania unless the patient has provided informed consent and the Mental Health Tribunal gives approval in writing. It can only give approval if an approved medical practitioner has examined the person within the previous seven days and concluded that the patient has a mental illness which needs treatment and is amendable to psychosurgery, the surgery is a reasonable and appropriate treatment for the patient and necessary for that person's health and safety or the health and safety of others (*Mental Health Act 2013* (Tas) s 124).

Victoria

ECT may be performed on an adult patient with written patient consent or with the permission of the Tribunal if the patient lacks capacity to consent. The Tribunal must have regard to:

> The views and preferences of the patient about ECT and any alternative treatments that are reasonably available and the reasons for those views, including any recovery outcomes the patient has

> The views and preferences of the patient as expressed in an advance directive

> The views of the patient's nominated person

> The views of a guardian of a patient

> The views of a carer – if the ECT will directly affect the carer and the care relationship

> The likely consequences for the patient if the treatment is not performed

> Any second opinion (*Mental Health Act 2014* (Vic) s 93).

It is a criminal act to perform psychosurgery on a person unless the Mental Health Tribunal is satisfied that the person concerned has given informed consent and that it is satisfied that the surgery will benefit the person. In making the determination of benefit it must consider whether the surgery would remedy or alleviate symptoms and reduce ill effects;

the likely consequences on the person; any beneficial alternative treatments that are readily available and the person's views about them; and the nature and degree of any discomfort, risks and common side effects associated with surgery, including the person's views about this (*Mental Health Act 2014* (Vic) s 102).

Western Australia

ECT may not be provided to an involuntary patient unless the Mental Health Tribunal approves it. The Tribunal must consider a number of factors, including:

➢ The patient's wishes if practicable to ascertain them

➢ The views of relevant people, including the substitute decision-maker, a child's parent or guardian, a nominated person, a carer if they have one, a close family member

➢ The reasons why the treatment is recommended

➢ The consequences of not performing it

➢ The nature and degree of the risk of performing it

➢ Whether the ECT is likely to maintain the health and well-being of the patient

➢ Whether any alternatives are available

➢ The nature and degree of risk associated with any alternatives

➢ Any other relevant information (*Mental Health Act 2014* (WA) s 414).

Psychosurgery is a criminal offence unless the patient has given informed consent and the procedure has been approved by the Mental Health Tribunal (s 208(2)(a)–(b)). The Mental Health Tribunal must consider whether the surgery has clinical merit, whether it is appropriate, and whether all reasonably available alternatives have been trialled and not resulted in lasting benefit to the patient (s 419).

Voluntary patients

Most patients experiencing mental illness admit themselves into hospital voluntarily and consent to treatment. Mental health legislation in Australia is increasingly addressing this group of patients, albeit minimally. Most just define the term, that is, 'voluntarily' (*Mental Health Act 2009* (SA)

s 8; *Mental Health Act 2013* (Tas) ss 4–5; *Mental Health Act 2014* (WA) s 4). They are a vulnerable group in several ways. Only the Northern Territory has more extensive treatment of this group, which requires patients to be informed of their right to leave and that the psychiatric practitioner must discharge a person if it is in that person's best interest or the person will not benefit from a longer admission (*Mental Health and Related Services Act* (NT) s 29(2)–(3)). Health professionals may not use the threat of sectioning a person under the mental health legislation to induce compliance. For example, 'If you don't take your meds we'll section you.' This is clearly intended to be coercive and to exploit the vulnerabilities of the patient.

Voluntary patients are also vulnerable to a slippage in status in that, although they may be technically a voluntary patient, they may be treated as though they were an involuntary patient. As an example, in the United Kingdom a patient with autism and significant behavioural problems became agitated when attending a day centre. He was taken to an emergency department and admitted to hospital as a voluntary inpatient. However, the European Court of Human Rights determined that during his stay he had not been free to leave the hospital so while technically a voluntary patient he was in fact being treated as an involuntary patient. The Court concluded his treatment amounted to an unlawful deprivation of his liberty (*HL v United Kingdom* (2005) 40ERR 32). In New South Wales the *Mental Health Act 2007* (NSW), sections 5–8, regulates voluntary patients, especially it requires the Mental Health Tribunal to review voluntary patients who have been in a mental health facility for more than a continuous 12-month period.

Overview

The care and treatment provided to persons experiencing mental illness have historically been problematic, with patients experiencing discrimination, oppression, exploitation, misuse and abuse. The potential for misuse and abuse still remains. Nurses and midwives have ethical obligations to treat persons experiencing mental illness with dignity and respect, to maximise their autonomy and to ensure that patients are treated fairly and humanely. Because the state has chosen to create legal powers to detain and treat patients experiencing mental illness without their consent, nurses and midwives involved in the care of patients who have had certain human rights curtailed must carefully balance their ethical obligations, in respect of promoting autonomy and providing care and treatment that are in the best interests of the patient and do not needlessly harm them, with their legal responsibilities to provide care and treatment to the patient. This is a complex area of practice but an important one in

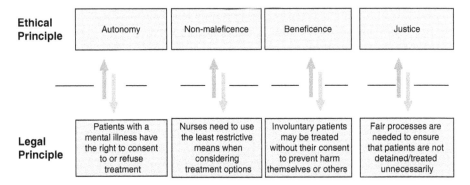

Figure 9.2 Ethical and legal principles relevant to the care and treatment of patients experiencing mental illness

terms of a nurse's or midwife's role in promoting and protecting human rights, practising in a moral and ethical way and recognising the inherent vulnerability of those they care for by respecting their patients' inherent human dignity.

Further reading

Jones, C. 2012, 'Life in a public mental ward: Enough to drive you insane', *Sydney Morning Herald*, 15 March 2012.
Nolan, P. 1993, *A History of Mental Health Nursing*. Chapman Hall: London.
Smith, S. 2017, 'Ethical issues in mental health nursing' in P. Scott (ed.) *Concepts and Issues in Nursing Ethics*. Springer: Basel, 145–157.

Questions

While compulsory detention and treatment for persons experiencing significant mental illness is lawful in Australia, only compulsory detention is lawful in Canada. Discuss the practical, professional, ethical and legal issues associated with each position.

Analyse the concept of 'authentic' autonomy with reference to the Canadian *Starson* case.

Scenarios

1. Casey James, a 21-year-old woman with anorexia nervosa, has been admitted as a voluntary patient to a psychiatric unit. Casey has been an inpatient at the facility on two previous occasions and has had multiple

treatment failures. During her previous admission, there had been a serious breakdown in Casey's confidence in the therapeutic relationship due to an issue involving breach of privacy during clinical monitoring of her weight and condition. Toshie Kikuchi is a registered nurse in charge of Casey's care and has worked closely with Casey over the past two years. Toshie is familiar with Casey's history of childhood abuse, her difficulties with trust and the circumstances which led to Casey's loss of confidence in medical staff during her previous admission. Casey stated on admission: 'I've come back because Toshie is the only person I can trust and she promised I can go at my own pace.' Toshie has worked extensively in the area of mental health and is familiar with the success of both coercive and non-coercive treatments in relation to eating disorders. Dr Ed Jensen has evaluated Casey's condition and has determined that her body weight is approaching a critical level and has concluded that Casey should be force fed through a nasogastric tube. Toshie is aware that Casey will refuse nasogastric feeding.

Apply the decision-making framework to this problem.

2. Mariam was the registered nurse in charge of a ward in an acute mental health unit for a night shift. She was supported by one other newly graduated registered nurse who had been practising for one week. There were nine patients in six rooms. Mariam had responsibility to carry out observations. She chose not to ask the new nurse to assist with the observations as she thought she needed more experience. Psychiatrists had ordered that four patients required observations at 10-minute intervals, four other patients for 30-minute intervals and for the remaining patient, 120-minute intervals. Mariam did not ensure the observations occurred as required and those that were undertaken were not taken in accordance with the standard required, that is, passive rather than active checking. Between 3 a.m. and 4 a.m. one patient killed another patient in their shared room. Mariam recorded observations of those patients at 4.35 a.m. and 6.26 a.m.; she did not notice that one of the patients had been killed. The patient's death was not discovered until shortly after Mariam had finished her shift. She subsequently admitted that she had reduced the frequency of the checks on her own initiative as patients disliked the disruption, she had been verbally and physically abused doing observations at night, and in her opinion it was better for patients to sleep. She had been doing this for a year with no harm to patients.

Apply the decision-making framework to this problem.

10

Ethics, law and the elderly

Introduction

An eminent gerontologist has commented 'it is still clear that many healthcare workers have a troubling moral and professional blindness to the humanity and complex care needs of older people' (O'Neill 2011, p. 3395). This view is confirmed by empirical research. For example, a study of health professionals working in the oncology area found they held consistently negative attitudes towards the elderly (Kearney et al. 2000) as did an Australian study of nurses in the acute care setting (Higgins et al. 2007). The Australian study reported that some nurses regarded older people as having a lower status in the health system, that some nurses perceived they did not have time to deal with 'the oldies in the corner' and that older patients were characterised as a 'burden' to some nurses and as being 'difficult'. There is a body of evidence that negative attitudes towards the aged are held by some health professionals (Wyman et al. 2018). These types of views are immensely disturbing and concerning as 'Ageist stereotypes, prejudice, and discrimination are potential barriers for health equality, in terms of the quantity and quality of care provided to older patients and their health-related outcomes' (Wyman et al. 2018, p. 194). Butler (1975) developed the term ageism and notes it results in older persons being 'categorized as senile, rigid, and old-fashioned in morality and skills. Ageism allows those of us who are younger to see old people as "different." We subtly cease to identify with them as human beings, which enables us to feel more comfortable about our neglect and dislike of them' (p. 894).

Ageing is, after all, an inevitable consequence of being a living human being. We will all age, although we might not all live to grow old. So let us ask the question how would we, as individuals, want to be treated as we age? As a nurse are you treating patients as you would like to be treated yourself? However, it is important to emphasise that this is not just an issue for individual health professionals but is also a societal issue.

How do we as a society value the elderly as groups, communities and societies? How do these values affect the way in which we all relate to the elderly and provide services to them?

O'Neill (2011) went on to suggest that there was a twofold reason to explain the moral blindness of some health professionals in developed nations to the elderly. He argues that it might partly be a function of the complexity of health care, which leads some health professionals to become focused on particular tasks or organs (e.g. hip). Primarily, he suggests that many of us living in developed western societies have difficulties in appreciating the value of the existence of life at an advanced age. He notes that the metaphor of a 'good innings' is pervasive and unhelpful in valuing life as an older person, as is the conceptualisation of dementia as a 'marker of dehumanisation', rather than being characterised as a series of impairments that can be engaged with (O'Neill 2011, p. 3395).

In addition to the factors identified by O'Neill, we are surrounded by rhetoric that urges us to defy age – think of advertisements for the latest miracle face cream, for cosmetic surgery and for various supplements and foods. In a sense the effects of ageing seem to be increasingly considered to be the fault of the individual for not eating the right foods (or too many of the wrong ones), not exercising correctly or sufficiently, or for failing in some way to do the 'right' thing – whatever that might be. If the impacts of ageing are seen as something to be avoided then a logical consequence of that view is to devalue those who are not ageing 'well' or indeed who are just ageing. Another significant factor is that the elderly are also sometimes portrayed or sometimes perceive themselves as being a 'useless drain on the energies of the young' (McCallum 1997), not to mention a drain on the economy due to the high cost of care.

Lastly, it is important to acknowledge the structural factors that contribute to some persons having a negative view of the aged in the context of providing health services. It is well known that those who work in the aged care sector of the health system, whether they be nurses or care assistants, are not paid as well as those who work in other parts of the health system (Commonwealth of Australia 2017b). The aged care sector is also a sector where care is often provided by a number of for-profit companies where cost control is a critical part of achieving a profit. As such, there may be issues in respect of staffing levels and mix (i.e. the ratio of registered nurses to enrolled nurses and care attendants), the availability of training and the adequacy of supervision. These structural factors may contribute to some staff being unable or unwilling to provide appropriate care or treatment to the elderly.

But this view of ageing is not universal. Many cultures deeply respect the aged members of their population believing that age confers wisdom, knowledge, understanding and dignity. The Aunties and Uncles in Aboriginal and Torres Strait Islander cultures and the elders in Polynesian and Melanesian cultures in the South Pacific have special places in their communities as teachers, guides and leaders. In many cultures it is unimaginable to place an elder in a care facility, as it is strongly believed that a family has obligations to care for the elderly in the home and also that it is important for that elderly person to continue to share their wisdom with their family and/or their community. That sense of caring for and valuing the elderly is not limited to indigenous or non-western cultures. It is also present in individualised western cultures, as can be seen by the public outrage relating to cases where elderly members of society have died alone and unnoticed, have been abused, exploited or neglected by family or by caregivers, including health professionals, or have been discriminated against by individuals, groups or society.

In addition to the moral dimension, how we treat the elderly also has significant implications for policy and practice. The population of the world is ageing. The United Nations estimated that there were approximately 962 million people aged 60 or over in the world, accounting for 13 per cent of the world's population (United Nations n.d.). It estimates that this figure will rise to more than 2.1 billion by 2050 (United Nations 2018). In Australia the numbers of people aged 65 and over is expected to rise from 15 per cent of the population in 2016 (3.7 million people) to between 22 per cent of the population in 2056 (8.7 million) (Australian Institute of Health and Welfare 2017). With an increasing population of ageing persons how societies treat the aged becomes a significant issue, so significant that at the international level the General Assembly of the United Nations has issued the *United Nations Principles for Older Persons* (1991). The principles emphasise the importance of providing opportunities for older persons to realise their potential to participate fully in all aspects of life, to eliminate discrimination, abuse, neglect and violence, and for the elderly to be treated with dignity and respect.

Many who practise gerontological medicine and nursing note the remarkable nature of elder life, the possibilities of adaption to loss and/or age-related conditions, and that providing care to the elderly can be both rewarding and fulfilling with the right 'attitudes, skills and approaches' (O'Neill 2011). This chapter focuses on the ethical and legal obligations nurses have to older patients in their care.

Ethics and nursing practice

The principles approach

Justice

One of the faces of the ethical principle of justice is distributive justice – ensuring the fair distribution of benefits and burdens. This has been a contentious issue in respect of providing life-prolonging interventions to the elderly – certainly at the theoretical level (see also the discussion in Chapter 2). New medical technologies have made it possible for an individual's life to be extended, but the high costs of new technology raise questions about the sustainability of funding these technologies in the long term. The economic question is also accompanied with a moral question about the costs (in a non-financial sense) and consequences for the individual of prolonging life, or deferring death depending on how you look at it. Daniel Callahan, a respected American bioethicist, has proposed that government should not pay for life-extending medical care for adults aged over a certain age (1995, 1996). Government should only pay for routine care for the elderly aimed at relieving pain. He suggests governments have a duty to help people live a normal life span but not to promote extension of life through the use of technology. Callahan's argument is based on the following premises:

> ➤ It is possible to live a meaningful old age that is limited in time but does not require compulsive efforts to extend life.

> ➤ Society needs a more supportive context for ageing and death that cherishes and respects the elderly, while recognising that their primary orientation should be to the young and to future generations.

A utilitarian argument has also been advanced that the costs of treating one elderly person may fund the care and treatment of a number of younger persons (Callahan 1995, 1996; see also Daniels 1988). It is argued that this may be better for the economy in terms of young peoples' social productivity compared with the social productivity of the elderly. An equity argument has also been made that spending much more on health care for the elderly is unequitable (Veatch 1988). Unsurprisingly, these arguments have been extensively critiqued (see, for example, Brock 1989). Some argue that these approaches treat the elderly as a means to an economic end rather than respecting their inherent dignity. It also assumes that the elderly are less valuable than the young, not taking into account the wisdom and experience of the elderly and undervaluing the unpaid contributions they make to society as caregivers, volunteers and citizens. Additionally, it is suggested that a proposal that government no longer pay for certain types of care may add to the societal fear of ageing and take away hope from elderly persons. Lastly, it is suggested that an elderly person should be able to make a choice about whether they want to prolong their life, aware of the costs and consequences of that choice, rather than the government making that choice for them. The cases set out below discuss some of the challenges involved in allocating resources.

James McKeown and Rau Williams (*Shortland v Northland Health* [1998] 1 NZLR 433)

In New Zealand two men were denied access to renal dialysis within a short time of each other. James McKeown, a 76-year-old man, was denied access to renal dialysis on the basis of guidelines that said it should not be available to persons over 75 years of age. His family alleged age discrimination. South Auckland Health ordered a reassessment and he was subsequently provided with dialysis.

Shortly afterwards Rau Williams, a 63-year-old Maori man with renal failure, diabetes and dementia, was denied access to renal dialysis. Mr Williams' family were strongly of the view that he should be able to access dialysis as his life still had value and meaning to him, to his family and to his community, as he was a respected elder. The family challenged the decision in the courts and the refusal was upheld. Mr Williams died shortly afterwards. The court concluded that the decision to deny access to dialysis was not based on resources (or age) but was a clinical decision made after an extensive multidisciplinary evaluation, a trial period of dialysis and application of guidelines about who was eligible for dialysis. As a result of the assessment a determination was made that Mr Williams was unsuitable for long-term dialysis as his dementia made him unable to manage the treatment at home (no consideration was given as to whether it could or should be available in hospital).

Beneficence

Beneficence – the concept of acting in the best interests of the patient – is an important principle in this context. The question that constantly needs to be asked is whether it is the nurse's conception of what the patient's best interest is or whether it is the patient's understanding of what they believe to be in their best interest that is at the forefront. As discussed in Chapter 2, one of the concerns about the principle of beneficence is that it can become paternalistic – something that undermines the important ethical principle of autonomy. It is also important to emphasise that perceptions of what is in the best interests of patients may be culturally specific. Two examples of this may be where the elderly person or elderly persons more generally play a significant role in a community and decisions about what is in that person's or those persons' best interests may be mediated through what is in the best interests of their community, or where there is a generally understood and accepted cultural norm about what an individual can and ought to be told about their health. In Japan, for example, there has been a traditional norm that people should not be told of a cancer diagnosis as it would remove hope – however, it is possible that this norm is no longer as universal as it once was, especially for younger generations (Ells and Caniano 2002).

The ways in which paternalism may manifest itself in the context of providing care to the elderly is twofold. First, as discussed in the introduction to the chapter, is through what might be described as ageism – a systematic stereotyping and discrimination against people because they are old – this may be seen through presumptions that an elderly person's life is not worth living, or has no value, with consequences for the way in which care is provided and/or what treatment is provided (see discussion of the McKeown and Williams cases).

Second, it may be seen through a desire to 'protect' elderly persons – even if that 'protection' constrains an elderly person's ability to exercise their autonomy. This is sometimes referred to as the 'dignity of risk': the ability to take risks is essential for the dignity and self-respect of individuals (Ibrahim and Davis 2013). This protectionism can be seen when individuals or institutions attempt to stop elderly persons from having sexual relationships, for example (Bauer and Fetherstonhaugh 2016). It may also be seen where an individual's free movement is constrained by those caring for that person on the basis that such constraints protect them from wandering off and becoming lost and distressed or from falling and sustaining harm. This is not to understate the complexity of the issues around managing the risks of falling and wandering, but it is to say that careful consideration has to be given to the protection versus autonomy question. If restraint or seclusion is used for the convenience of staff or as a threat to induce compliance with institutional norms this would not be in the individual's best interest.

Non-maleficence

One issue that is particularly important to highlight in context of the ethical principle of non-maleficence (avoiding needless harm) is elder abuse. What is elder abuse? Elder abuse can be defined in various ways but a widely used definition comes from the World Health Organization (WHO 2002). It defines elder abuse as: 'a single, or repeated act, or lack of appropriate action, occurring within any relationship where there is an expectation of trust which causes harm or distress to an older person'. Elder abuse includes several forms of abuse including physical, sexual, financial, psychological abuse and neglect.

A relationship with an implication of trust refers to familial relationships or caregiving relationships – whether volunteer (for example, meals on wheels volunteers) or professional (enrolled or registered nurses, personal care attendants, home care workers). Elder abuse may occur within the elderly person's private residence or in some form of residential care, including aged care facilities and hospitals.

Little research has been done to establish the incidence of elder abuse in Australia or indeed internationally and the research that has been done is variable as different definitions of abuse have been used. However, Kaspiew, Carson and Rhoades (2016) suggested that the little evidence around elder abuse in Australia suggests incidence varies across abuse types, with psychological and financial abuse being the most common types reported.

A recent report of the Australian Law Reform Commission (2017) noted that elder abuse is a significant public health and social problem. Obviously there is an ethical imperative for all health professionals, including nurses, not to abuse their elderly patients. Elder abuse committed by family members or other health professionals raises issues for nurses to identify any concerns and respond appropriately in order to protect the elderly person.

Autonomy

The basic rule of autonomy is that a competent adult has a right to consent or refuse consent to treatment, irrespective of whether the health professional considers a refusal to be rational or not (see Chapter 5). Illnesses, such as dementia, may have an impact on an individual's competence to make decisions. However, just because a person has dementia, or indeed other age-related cognitive conditions, does not mean they are not competent. Persons with dementia, and similar illnesses, may be competent, may have variable competency (at times being quite lucid and other times being confused or being able to make some types of decisions but not particularly complex ones) or may lack competency (see Chapter 5). A nurse's ethical responsibility could therefore be seen to be to assist individuals to maximise their capacity to make autonomous decisions and to maximise their independence. In part nurses can do this by not making assumptions about a person's capacity based on that person's age or medical condition, by seeking or conducting comprehensive competency assessments, and by providing appropriate information to that person to support their autonomy. If an individual is found to lack decision-making capacity, their wishes can be respected if they have an advance directive or through their substitute decision-makers being provided with the information necessary to support informed decision-making (see discussion in Chapter 5). If a person does not have capacity, that person should still be encouraged by nurses to participate in decision-making about their care to the greatest extent possible.

It is also important to emphasise that the decisions made by elderly people may be quite relational, rather than individualistic, in their orientation. It may be that some elderly persons make health care decisions based on their concerns about being or becoming a 'burden' to their families. They may choose to make decisions because they think it is in everyone's best interests but it may or may not reflect their inclination if they did not have family to think about and care for.

A constraint on autonomy that we must acknowledge is the institutionalisation of many elderly persons. While some aged care facilities focus on the needs of the individual and maximise the autonomy of residents, others are much more focused on the needs of the institution, and its staff, at the expense of the individual. In an aged care facility individuals may not have much control or choice in respect of when they get up, when they shower, when they eat, what they eat and what they do as their autonomy may be constrained, to a greater or lesser extent, by the norms of that institution and by the goodwill or otherwise of their caregivers. This vulnerability may affect their decision-making. For example, it may be less likely that residents of aged care facilities will complain about anything that occurs in a residential facility for fear of repercussions.

Institutionalisation does not just relate to residents of aged care facilities. It may also create assumptions by health professionals, working in this context, that residents/patients will be compliant with institutional norms. Patients/residents on the other hand may want to maintain as much independence of mind and conduct as possible, even if they cannot maintain physical independence. This may be characterised by what may be perceived by health professionals as 'unreasonable', 'exasperating' and 'disruptive' behaviour, when in fact an important component of autonomy is not just the ability to control what happens to one's own body but to control what and how one lives one's life and relates to others. A legitimate constraint on autonomy is that it can only be exercised in such a way that does not harm others. But what does harm mean? The challenge in an institutional context particularly is that it is easy to reframe behaviour as disrupting the peace of others and therefore requiring interference (i.e. a noisy person being placed in seclusion). It is also easy to suggest that a person who resists personal cares, like having one's clothing removed, is being unreasonable and difficult and so should be forced to comply, when in fact that refusal may be based on their past experience. A person who was physically and sexually abused as a child by a carer would, not unreasonably, resist when someone in a position of power over them attempts to remove their clothing. Autonomy should not only be respected in patients or residents who are perceived as compliant – autonomy should be respected for all of those persons who are able to fully or partially exercise it. Even when a person is not capable of exercising their autonomy in any meaningful way, it does not mean that there should be any less respect for their innate humanity and their inherent dignity.

Another way in which elderly persons may have their autonomy limited and may be harmed is through the use of restraint and seclusion techniques. Restraint or seclusion (see definitions in Figure 9.1) are controversial techniques as they involve measures aimed at limiting the liberty of individuals. These measures are usually justified on the basis of protecting the individual, or of protecting others, such as health professionals, staff and other residents, from harm. In Chapter 1, we discussed John Stuart Mill's perspective that the only justification for limiting autonomy was to protect others – but to protect others from what? There appears to be a justification for the use of restraint or seclusion if the person is physically violent towards others, creating an immediate risk of physical harm, but what if the 'violence' is verbal? What if the person is creating a disturbance – does that justify restraining or secluding them? The self-protection of individuals is also accepted as a limited justification for some forms of intervention. Thus the justification for restraint and seclusion also draws on the principle of beneficence to suggest it is in the person's best interests to protect them from harm, for example from falling. This raises some complex issues. On the one hand a claim can be made that restraining a person may protect them from harm, for example from wandering or falling. However, taken too far claims to protect can constitute paternalism, as McDonald (2003 at 23) notes: 'risks are a part of life and to deny the [competent] elderly the chance to take risks can be to deny their autonomy.'

If a justification for the use of restraints is that their use may prevent harm to self or others we must also consider whether the techniques used to restrain people, especially those who are older, may actually be harmful. The physical harms that can result from restraint can be illustrated with reference to a 1998 incident. In 1998 Harry Robertson died from asphyxia at the Begonia Nursing Home in Ballarat. He was blind and experienced florid dementia. He had been left on a commode next to his bed, with a rug wrapped around his abdomen and tied to the bed rail. He was left unobserved for 20 minutes and was subsequently found dead on the floor with the rug caught around his neck (*Plover v McIndoe* (2000) VR 385). The decision whether or not to use restraint or seclusion therefore must involve a careful consideration of the risks versus the benefits of its use, other less restrictive interventions, and the development of a management plan to monitor the patient to ensure his or her wellbeing.

However, it is also important to note that there has been a history of health professionals threatening to use and/or using restraints and/or seclusion punitively or coercively (i.e. 'If you don't behave I'll tie you to your chair') or for the convenience of staff who are overworked, short-staffed or, sadly, who just cannot be bothered. This reason for the use of restraints is contrary to the ethical principles of beneficence and non-maleficence.

The nursing codes

Many of the value statements and conduct statements in the ICN Code of Ethics for Nurses and the Code of Conduct for Nurses are relevant to caring for elderly patients but the most directly relevant are discussed below.

Consent

As discussed in more detail in Chapter 5, the ICN Code of Ethics, at 1, states: 'The nurse ensures that the individual receives accurate, sufficient and timely information in a culturally appropriate manner on which to base consent for care and related treatment.' The Nursing Code of Conduct in 2.2 notes that making decisions is a shared responsibility of the patient and the nurse and other health professionals and they should 'take a person centred approach to managing a person's care and concerns, supporting the person in a manner consistent with that person's values and preferences' (2.2.a). Principle 2.2.b also notes that nurses should 'advocate on behalf of the person where necessary, and recognise when substitute decision-makers are needed (including legal guardians or holders of power of attorney)'. Principle 2.3.c notes that nurses should 'act according to the person's capacity for decision-making and consent'.

Discrimination

There is concern that ageism is a significant barrier to the ethical provision of health care. Ageism can be manifest in the day-to-day environment or in the health system and society more generally. In the ICN Code of Ethics, Element 1 notes: 'In providing care, the nurse promotes an environment in which the human rights, values, customs and spiritual beliefs of the individual, family and community are respected.' A recognised human right in Australia is the right not to be discriminated against on the basis of age. The Code of Conduct, at Principle 3.2.d, notes that nurses should 'adopt practices that respect diversity, avoid bias, discrimination and racism, and challenge belief based on assumption (for example, based on gender, disability, race, ethnicity, religion, sexuality, age or political beliefs)'.

This speaks of a broader obligation, not only to individual patients but also to the community to combat ageism. What these statements imply is that individual nurses must take responsibility for their own attitudes but also that individually, and as a profession, nurses need to work towards the elimination of discriminatory and prejudicial attitudes, especially in this context – ageism. This may include acting as an advocate for the patient and for the values of the profession by questioning colleagues who display such attitudes. Principle 2.1.c of the Code of Conduct also implies that if nurses are concerned that structural factors, such as staffing levels or staff mix, are impacting negatively on the ability to provide quality nursing and health care then they should be acting as an advocate for patients in this respect also by documenting concerns.

Abuse

Elder abuse is a significant issue for health professionals and is more explicitly recognised in the Nursing Code of Conduct. This is also reflected in the ICN Code of Ethics, which notes, at 1, that a nurse 'shares with society the responsibility for initiating and supporting action to meet the health and social needs of the public, in particular those of vulnerable populations'. Nurses, along with other health professionals, are often in a unique trusted position when they come into contact with older patients. This raises particular ethical obligations to consider the welfare of this potentially vulnerable group. Principle 1.3.a notes that nurses must 'abide by the relevant mandatory reporting legislation that is imposed to protect groups that are particularly at risk, including reporting obligations about the aged'. Principle 2.1.b also notes that nurses must 'provide leadership to ensure the delivery of safe and quality care and understand their professional responsibility to protect people, ensuring that employees comply with their obligations'. The statement recognises that some people will need protection due to their health condition or their vulnerability due to their power imbalance in respect of the systems that provide health care, which, as discussed, is a particular issue for elderly persons residing in residential care facilities. More generally, at 1.1 and 1.2, the Code of Conduct recognises the need for nurses and midwives to act in accordance with the law. In this context, this relates to the laws regarding mandatory reporting of reportable assaults (discussed further in the 'Reporting abuse' section below).

Restraints

The nursing code of conduct notes (4.1.j) that nurses and midwives should 'not participate in physical assault such as striking, unauthorised restraining and/or applying unnecessary force'.

Elder law

There are a number of areas of law that relate to providing care to the elderly, some of which are covered in this chapter. Other particularly relevant aspects of law are covered in Chapters 5 and 11 (in the discussions on consent and end-of-life issues, respectively).

Civil liability

Negligence is discussed extensively in Chapter 8. But there are other grounds on which compensation can be sought for wrongful acts, some of which are particularly relevant to the care of the elderly.

Battery (unlawful and unpermitted touching of another) and assault (where a person has received or perceives a threat of violence) are two grounds for a person to bring a civil action under the common law seeking compensation for harm (battery and assault are also potentially criminal acts) (see discussion in Chapter 8). A defence to civil claims of assault and battery is the voluntary consent of the individual, although there are some things to which consent is not a defence, for example assisting someone to die in Australian jurisdictions (except Victoria from 2019; see Chapter 11). Another available defence is self-defence. If seriously threatened people are permitted to use *reasonable* force to defend themselves or others. Any excessive force could see a nurse faced with criminal or civil charges of assault and/or battery and also disciplinary proceedings.

Nursing and Midwifery Board of Australia v Hughes-Fischer
[2011] QCAT 627.

An 85-year-old resident of a long-term facility, who had dementia, a hearing impairment and was using a nebuliser, placed his hands around a registered nurse's throat after apparently being startled when the nurse bent to check him. The nurse's response was to push against the patient's jaw, fracturing it in two places. The Tribunal found the nurse could have stepped away from the patient, breaking the patient's hold, or pushed his hands away without injuring the patient. The Tribunal also found that the nurse did not report the incident and/or follow up the patient's injuries appropriately. The Tribunal reprimanded and suspended the nurse. Conditions were placed on the nurse's practice (training and mentoring requirements).

False imprisonment, or unlawful restraint on the liberty of a person, can also be a ground for a person to bring a civil action. To establish a person has been falsely imprisoned the person bringing the action must establish the following (*Myer Stores Ltd v Soo* [1991] 2 VR 597; *Ruddock v Taylor* [2003] NSWCA 262):

➤ That there was no practical or reasonable means of escape

➤ There was a total restriction on that person's freedom of movement

➤ There was no lawful authority for that restraint.

False imprisonment does not require physical detention (i.e. being physically restrained or locked in a room). Being detained by the use of authority (i.e. 'I require you to stay here') is sufficient. Damage, or physical or serious psychological harm to the person, is not required if the imprisonment is intentional but is required if the false imprisonment is due to negligence (i.e. accidently locking someone in) (*Myer Stores Ltd v Soo* [1991] 2 VR 597; *Ruddock v Taylor* [2003] NSWCA 262).

Chief Justice Spigelman in *Ruddock v Taylor* [2003] NSWCA 262 at 3 noted:

> The protection of the personal liberty of individuals has been a fundamental purpose of the common law for centuries. The tort of trespass in the form of false imprisonment has been one of the ways in which that protection has been provided throughout the period.

The relevance of false imprisonment to the care of elderly persons is apparent when considering the techniques of restraint and seclusion (see definitions in Figure 9.1) as these are designed to limit the liberty of a person. Limitations on liberty are justified on the basis of protecting the patient or protecting others from serious harm (for example, health professionals, other staff and other residents). However, restraint and seclusion limit personal liberty and there must be lawful authority to justify usage of these techniques – needless to say the convenience of health professionals does not constitute lawful authority. In general, consent by a competent adult is a defence to false imprisonment, as it is for assault and battery.

What if the person lacks capacity to give consent? Does this mean that every time a nurse touches an older person that nurse commits a battery? That every use of restraint or seclusion constitutes false imprisonment? As discussed in Chapter 5, substitute decision-makers can consent to most health care and treatment on behalf of those who do not have decision-making capacity, as long as it is in the best interests of that person, but it is not clear whether this includes restraint or seclusion. The courts appear to have the power to authorise the use of restraint and seclusion techniques in respect of adult patients who lack decision-making capacity. In relation to seclusion, in *Re WMC* [2005] QGAAT 26 the patient was a 45-year-old intellectually disabled man with a history of yelling, pounding walls and doors, and punching and breaking windows. Seclusion was used to settle him down. The Tribunal accepted that the use of seclusion could be permissible for this patient but only if it promoted the patient's health and wellbeing and was in his overall best interest. In relation to restraint, in *Re HAB* [2007] QGAAT 13 the Tribunal did not object to the use of a lap band to restrain an 88-year-old woman with dementia and impaired mobility who had sustained a number of serious falls when trying to rise, including a fall that broke her hip.

Some states have also enacted legislation to address these issues. In both Queensland and South Australia legislation permits a health professional to use minimum force to provide treatment authorised under the Act (*Guardianship and Administration Act 1993* (SA) s 32(1)(c); *Guardianship and Administration Act 2000* (Qld) s 75).

In general, the following principles apply to the use of restraint and seclusion:

➤ It should be the least restrictive option or involve minimal force

➤ There needs to be a serious risk of harm to the person who is to be restrained or secluded or to other persons

➤ It should be in the person's best interests

➤ It should be acknowledged that restraint, seclusion and the use of force create a risk of harm and that risk should be managed – that is, through regular checks and reviews while restraint or seclusion is being used to ensure the welfare of the patient

➤ Chemical restraints should only be used if prescribed by a doctor and administered according to the doctor's instructions

➤ Restraint or seclusion should not be indefinite (it must have a beginning point and an end point).

The Australian Law Reform Commission (2017) has recently recommended regulating the use of restraint and seclusion in aged care.

Disciplinary proceedings

Disciplinary proceedings are extensively discussed in Chapter 4. Disciplinary proceedings are also important accountability mechanisms in respect of the care and treatment provided to the elderly by registered nurses. Four examples are set out below.

Abuse: Verbal and physical

In *Tasmanian Board of the Nursing and Midwifery Board of Australia v Wiggins* [2011] TASHPT 4 a registered nurse faced disciplinary proceedings in respect of allegations she had verbally abused and humiliated residents and swore at them, for example by calling down a passage 'the fucking old dickhead is out of his bed again'. She was also said to have instructed Extended Care Assistants to leave a resident with dementia on the floor after he had fallen out of bed for the second time and subsequently dragged him to a mattress on the floor. She was suspended from practice when the allegations were made. The Tribunal lifted the suspension and imposed conditions on her practice. It noted (at 6):

> The respondent misused her authority as a Registered Nurse and also the trust imposed upon her to oversee the care of these patients (residents) in a professional and ethical manner consistent with the standard of care expected by her profession. On the subject nights she fell well short of those expectations and the Tribunal infers she allowed her temper or the challenging behaviour of the patients (residents) to override her professional duty.

In *Nursing and Midwifery Board of Australia v Csepregi* [2016] SAHPT 5 an enrolled registered nurse put her hand over the mouth of a 98-year-old agitated patient in a hospital, causing a bruise. The nurse then made a false report alleging the bruise was caused by the patient making contact with the bed rail. The nurse tried to get another enrolled nurse to back up her story. The Tribunal noted (at 25–26):

> It is admitted the conduct involves a breach of trust. It involved an exploitation of the power imbalance between the respondent and a vulnerable patient. It involved the unnecessary application of force. Whatever force the respondent did apply was sufficient to generate a bruise. Irrespective of the degree of force the fact of physical contact is what is significant. It is not just about the physical contact between the respondent and patient but also what the respondent did thereafter namely the falsification of the SLS [safety learning system] Report and her approaches to a fellow nurse with a view to having her corroborate her story. It is a combination of these matters that the complainant relies on as sustaining professional misconduct and the need for a proper sanction to be imposed.

Exploitation

In *HCCC v Belkadi* (No 2) [2012] NSWNMT 14 a registered nurse faced disciplinary proceedings for not disclosing three convictions for theft, larceny and shoplifting and for obtaining substantial loans from patients or their family members. The nurse claimed to be in financial difficulties at the time. In respect of the first patient, the nurse provided care to the female patient in the palliative care ward at the hospital in which she worked. After the patient's death the nurse inappropriately accessed confidential information which she used to visit the patient's husband and asked to borrow $25,000. A few weeks later she asked to borrow an additional $19,000. A court subsequently ordered her to repay the $44,000 that she had borrowed which she failed to do. She also inappropriately accessed the personal information of an elderly patient who had been admitted to the hospital for just over four weeks and visited her asking for a loan of $2,500. She afterwards tried to borrow more over the phone. The nurse then returned to the patient's house asking for more money and wrote to the patient and wrote and visited the patient's daughter asking for money. She did not repay the $2,500. The nurse was de-registered.

In *Nursing and Midwifery Board Australia v Montero* [2015] QCAT 316 an enrolled registered nurse was disciplined in respect of her conduct towards a 90-year-old male patient with dementia and a mild intellectual disability. She accepted an appointment as his enduring power of attorney, redirected his mail to her address and made false statements to the assessment agency that the patient lived with her and was related to either her or her husband and made a further false statement to the Office of the Adult Guardian.

Restraint

In *Nursing & Midwifery Board of Australia v Kiroff & Nyhan* [2016] SAHPT 9 an elderly male patient with dementia was restrained to a chair with a pelvic restraint for two hours in the lounge of the aged care facility. Then his chair was moved closer to the nurses station and a second pelvic posey was used to attach the chair to the railing. He remained restrained in that position for a further nine hours. He was in a state of complete or partial undress for most of that time, including being naked from the waist down, and was sitting in a pool of urine. He was not released or toileted during this period and no attempt was made to seek a review by a doctor or the managing nurse. The registered nurse and the enrolled nurse were found to have committed professional misconduct and were reprimanded; their registration was suspended for nine months and conditions were imposed on their practice. A third nurse voluntarily de-registered himself.

Timely treatment

In *Kahler v Nurses Registration Board* (unreported, 21 February 1995, SCNSW) Kahler, a registered nurse, was the administrator of a complex providing various levels of care to veterans. A resident in its hostel had worsening dementia and his care needs were growing more complex, necessitating a transfer to the nursing home within the complex. Kahler failed to organise the transfer for several months and did not organise appropriate care. When the patient was finally transferred to the nursing home he was in a serious condition with severe dehydration and multiple bed sores and lesions. Kahler was de-registered.

Criminal law

Some aspects of the criminal law in relation to the end-of-life are described more extensively in Chapter 11 and in respect of health care more generally in Chapter 8.

Under the common law, criminal charges can be laid for failing to provide the necessaries of life. These cases arise where someone in a position of responsibility neglects the person in their care, for example by not providing food or medical assistance, and that neglect results in that person's death or serious injury. In states and territories in Australia with a codified or partially codified criminal law there is a specific offence of failing to provide the necessaries of life (see Table 10.1).

Table 10.1 Failing to provide the necessaries of life

Jurisdiction	Act	Content
New South Wales	Crimes Act 1900, s 44(1)	A person (a) who is under a legal duty to provide another person with the necessaries of life, and (b) who, without reasonable excuse, intentionally or recklessly fails to provide that person with the necessaries of life, is guilty of an offence if the failure causes a danger of death or causes serious injury, or the likelihood of serious injury, to that person.
Northern Territory	Criminal Code Act, s 183	Any person who, being charged with the duty of providing for another the necessaries of life, unlawfully fails to do so whereby the life of that person is or is likely to be endangered or his health is or is likely to be permanently injured, is guilty of a crime and is liable to imprisonment for 7 years.
Queensland	Criminal Code, s 285	It is the duty of every person having charge of another who is unable by reason of age, sickness, unsoundness of mind, detention, or any other cause, to withdraw himself or herself from such charge, and who is unable to provide himself or herself with the necessaries of life … to provide for that person the necessaries of life; and the person is held to have caused any consequences which result to the life or health of the other person by reason of any omission to perform the duty.
South Australia	Criminal Law Consolidation Act 1935, s 30	Where (a) a person is liable to provide necessary food, clothing or accommodation to another person who is (i) a minor; or (ii) suffering from an illness; or (iii) disabled; and (b) the person without lawful excuse, fails to provide that food, clothing or accommodation, that person shall be guilty of an indictable offence and liable to be imprisoned for a term not exceeding 3 years.

Jurisdiction	Act	Content
Tasmania	*Criminal Code Act 1924*, s 144	It is the duty of every person having charge of another, who is unable by reason of age, sickness, unsoundness of mind, detention, or any other cause to withdraw himself from such charge, and who is unable to provide himself with the necessaries of life, to provide such necessaries for the other person.
Western Australia	*Criminal Code*, s 262	It is the duty of every person having charge of another who is unable by reason of age, sickness, mental impairment, detention, or any other cause, to withdraw himself from such a charge, and who is unable to provide himself with the necessaries of life, whether the charge is undertaken under a contract, or is imposed by law, or arises by reason of any act, whether the lawful or unlawful, of the person who has such charge, to provide for that other person the necessaries of life; and he is held to have caused any consequences which result to the life or health of the other person by reason of any omission to perform that duty.

Failure to provide the necessaries of life

In 2006 a Canadian registered nurse, Janet Longford, was found guilty of failing to provide the necessaries of life to a female patient in her 80s, placing that patient's life in danger. The patient had been admitted to an aged care facility run by the nurse. She had mobility difficulties and dementia and was entirely reliant on her caregivers. When she was admitted in November she weighed approximately 86 kilos and when she left in April she weighed approximately 50 kilos and had developed pressure sores on both hips, both heels and her tail bone that required surgery. The nurse did not seek medical attention for this patient at any point during her residence at the facility. The nurse was convicted of failing to provide the necessaries of life and sentenced to six months' home detention. She was also de-registered (*College of Nurses of Ontario v Janet Longford*, 30 April 2007).

Reporting abuse

Concerns about the abuse of residents in aged care facilities, highlighted by the criminal prosecution of a personal care assistant, Alexander (see the box 'R v Alexander [2008] VSCA 191'), led the Commonwealth government in 2007 to amend the *Aged Care Act 1997* to require the reporting of certain types of conduct.

R v Alexander [2008] VSCA 191

Alexander was a personal care assistant in an aged care facility in Victoria. He was convicted of one count of rape. The victim, M, was an 85-year-old female resident of that facility who had dementia and was incontinent. Alexander and another care assistant were cleaning the patient after an episode of incontinence when Alexander digitally penetrated her. There was some delay in the other care assistant reporting what had occurred. The appeal court noted:

> Neither the extreme vulnerability of M nor the flagrant disregard of her humanity and dignity inherent in the respondent's conduct requires emphasis. ... It is no easy thing for members of a family, who for one reason or another find it impossible to care for an elderly relative, to entrust their care to strangers in a nursing home. At minimum they must be able to have confidence that the elderly will not be abused in such settings.'

Section 63–1AA of the *Aged Care Act 1997* makes it mandatory for approved providers of aged care services and their staff to report allegations or reasonable suspicions about what is termed 'reportable assaults' made against persons in aged care. A reportable assault is in turn defined in section 63–1AA(9) as 'unlawful sexual contact, unreasonable use of force or assault ... constituting an offence against the law of the Commonwealth or a State or Territory'. Approved providers must make reports as soon as is reasonably practicable or within 24 hours (s 63–1AA(2)) to either the police or the Department of Health and Aging. Staff members must report to one or more of the following: (1) the approved provider (i.e. the institution); (2) key personnel within that institution; (3) a person authorised by the provider to receive such reports; (4) a police officer; or (5) the Department of Health and Aging (s 63–1AA(5)). A central responsibility of residential aged care facilities is therefore to actively require staff to make such reports. Providers can choose whether to report an alleged reportable assault committed by a resident with an assessed cognitive or mental impairment. Individual staff members who report allegations in a way that is consistent with the process set out in the Act and in good faith may be protected under section 98–8 from civil or criminal liability for making the disclosure (unless they are disclosing their own abuse of a resident), from employment-related proceedings for breaching any confidentiality requirements in their employment contract and from victimisation. Residential care facilities may face sanctions if they do not comply with the requirements of the *Aged Care Act 1997* (s 66–1).

On the face of it this appears to be a useful mechanism to detect abuse of the elderly in residential facilities. However, it has been criticised as it only applies to approved residential care facilities and subsidised in home services – it does not apply to privately owned residential care facilities. Another limitation is that it does not cover financial abuse or neglect. The Australian Law Reform Commission (2017) has recommended the institution of a serious incident report scheme to replace section 63–1AA and the development of an independent oversight body to oversee the scheme and investigate incidents.

Overview

This chapter highlights that the ethical principles, professional ethics and legal rules relating to the profession of nursing emphasise that they have responsibilities to individuals and to society to act with care and compassion towards older patients in the course of their professional practice. The legal framework emphasises professional obligations to not cause harm to elderly patients and to actively protect them from harm through mandatory reporting requirements. The ethical frameworks and the legal frameworks also emphasise that nurses must be accountable to their profession and through that profession to the public for their actions.

Figure 10.1 highlights the interactions between the ethical principles and the legal principles relevant to care of the elderly.

Further reading

Brock, D. 1989, 'Justice, health care and the elderly', *Philosophy and Public Affairs*, 18: 3, 297–312.
Rees, J., King, L. & Schmitz, K. 2009, 'Nurses perceptions of ethical issues in the care of older people', *Nursing Ethics*, 16, 436–452.

Questions

Should governments stop funding life-prolonging treatment for persons over the age of 75 years in Australia? Discuss the ethical and legal implications with reference to the cases of James McKeown and Rau Williams.

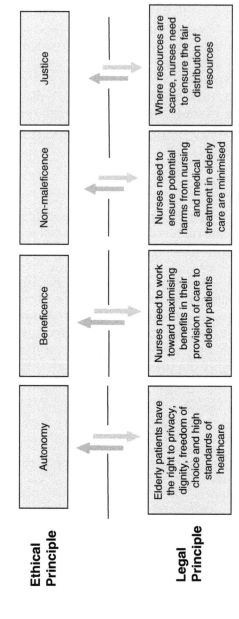

Ethical Principle

Autonomy | Beneficence | Non-maleficence | Justice

Legal Principle

Elderly patients have the right to privacy, dignity, freedom of choice and high standards of healthcare

Nurses need to work toward maximising benefits in their provision of care to elderly patients

Nurses need to ensure potential harms from nursing and medical treatment in elderly care are minimised

Where resources are scarce, nurses need to ensure the fair distribution of resources

Figure 10.1 Ethical and legal principles relevant to care of the elderly

If you walked into a room in an aged care facility and saw an 83-year-old male with dementia having sex with an 86-year-old male amputee how would you respond? Discuss the ethical and legal implications of this.

Scenarios

1. Bhuvan is a registered nurse and has recently commenced employment at a Queensland nursing home. During his shifts he is the only registered nurse in charge of 98 residents, 45 of whom have high care needs. The majority of high care residents have been diagnosed with dementia or related disorders. Most of his shift involves completing medication rounds through various wards and documenting records. The nursing home is constantly plagued with understaffing issues. Bhuvan has little time to attend to the individual needs of residents. Assistants in Nursing provide most of the care to the residents in both the low care and high care wards.

   During his first week at the nursing home he has witnessed the following incidents in the 12-bed high care dementia ward:

   ➤ At any given time up to eight 'mobile' residents in the ward are restrained in chairs (the other four are restricted to bed) for lengthy periods of time. Two of the more alert residents display signs of psychological distress as a result of the restraint. One of the patients continually asks to have the restraint removed. Bhuvan has been told the restraints are necessary to prevent falls as there is not enough staff to watch the residents and ensure their safety.

   ➤ One aggressive and noisy resident is restrained at all times and is often moved to a secured room for long periods of time, particularly during peak visiting hours. Bhuvan has been told that visitors have complained about the resident's constant screaming and that his noise also upsets other residents in the ward and therefore the seclusion of this patient is necessary for the comfort of others.

   Apply the decision-making framework to this problem.

2. Aasha is a registered nurse and is providing wound care to a 92-year-old patient who lives alone in his home. She observes that the patient appears dishevelled and he and the room he was in smelt, although the wound is clean. A carer from another agency provides home care, specifically assistance with showering and hygiene. During one visit the patient appeared particularly distressed as he had just received a

notice he had an overdrawn bank account and several bills had not been automatically paid due to a lack of funds. He tells Aasha he had given his account card and PIN to the carer to get him some cash as he was unable to leave his home due to his wound.

Apply the decision-making framework to this problem.

11

End-of-life issues

Introduction

Situations at the end of a patient's life present special ethical and legal challenges for health professionals. Whether your patient is elderly and the end of life has been anticipated for some time, or has unexpectedly suffered trauma and is not expected to survive, or is an infant whose life expectancy is short, similar issues arise regarding what is legally and ethically most appropriate for those patients. In addition, dealing with dying and death can be personally challenging for nurses and midwives, with every person responding to these significant events in different ways. As noted by Freegard:

> The dying and death of a client can be confronting. It challenges our professional confidence related to healing and rehabilitation. It challenges personal values and beliefs about life and death. It demands we work through personal emotions of grief and loss and cope with the emotional response of family and other health professionals. It confronts our own mortality. (Freegard and Isted 2012, p. 332)

Despite this, patients and families will often look to health professionals to offer appropriate support and care during such difficult times. Recognising this complexity, in this chapter we consider a range of issues relevant to the treatment and care of patients at the end of their life. In particular we discuss the ethics and law relating to administration of palliative care, the issue of euthanasia and assisted suicide and the crimes of unlawful killing. We also consider when it is appropriate and lawful to withhold or withdraw life-sustaining treatment from a patient.

Patients are most vulnerable as they near the end of life and rely heavily on health care staff caring for them. In rare and extreme cases, health professionals such as nurses and doctors have taken advantage of this vulnerability and been found guilty of exploiting and abusing the trust their patients had in them by unlawfully ending their lives. Thankfully, such cases are rare; however, the vulnerability of patients at the end of life does place particular ethical obligations on nurses, and in some circumstances midwives, to be sensitive to and respect the wishes of the patient, and engage family members or loved ones in decision-making at the end of life. In addition, the law makes a distinction between actions taken during the final stages of a patient's life which are lawful or which may result in a crime being committed by health professionals. It goes without saying that it is crucial that all health professionals – including nursing and midwifery staff – are aware of what the law allows and prohibits.

This chapter builds on the principles outlined in Chapter 5 regarding the right of competent adults to make decisions regarding their health care and, where a patient has lost capacity, use of advance directives or the ability of others to act as substitute decision-makers on behalf of adult patients. It also considers the situation of child patients at the end of life, so relies on the discussion in Chapter 6 regarding decision-making by, and on behalf, of children.

Ethical importance of end-of-life issues

As well as the four principles approach, with end-of-life issues, often the principle of maintaining the 'sanctity of life' is referred to. The sanctity of life principle is not one of the four principles of autonomy, beneficence, non-maleficence and justice referred to by Beauchamp and Childress (2013); this principle essentially takes the view that life is precious and should be preserved. While the origin of this principle lies in religion (i.e. life is a gift from God and nothing should be done to shorten it), it is often reflected in secular views as well.

Generally, in a health care setting, most consider that yielding to this principle above all others would not be appropriate; a strict application of this principle in the health care setting may result in the inability to provide palliative medication (where there is a risk of death from respiratory depression) or the need to maintain life-sustaining treatment indefinitely, even when such interventions are considered inappropriate and futile (i.e. considered to be of no medical benefit).

It is recognised that different people will view end-of-life situations from different perspectives depending on how prominently they see the, often competing, principles of the 'sanctity of life', autonomy, beneficence and maleficence. Religious and cultural factors will significantly influence how individual patients and families navigate end-of-life issues. Understanding that there is no single 'correct view' is an important aspect of dealing with these difficult situations.

The principles approach

Autonomy

The concept of autonomy is equally important for patients at the end of life as it is during any other time when they are receiving health care. Adult patients who have capacity to make decisions regarding their treatment and care at the end of their life are entitled to be given information about their condition, have their questions answered and their wishes respected just as any other patient does. They certainly have a right to refuse or accept any treatment or care that is offered to them. However, limits exist on a competent patient's right to autonomy; a patient cannot, for example, demand that they receive treatment that has not been offered to them by their health care team. In addition, a patient cannot demand that staff assist them to end their own life, regardless of their personal circumstances.

For those patients who have lost capacity – and many patients who are near death do lose the ability to make decisions for themselves – the question of how their autonomy can be respected re-emerges. Recognition of a patient's previously expressed views regarding what they would like to happen at the end of their life is another way autonomy is recognised in this circumstance. This may be through respecting a patient's previously executed advance directive (see below at 'Legislation – adults lacking decision-making capacity'), which outlines what treatment the patient wanted and did not want at the end of their life. Or it may be through allowing the person chosen by the patient (before they lost capacity) to make decisions regarding end-of-life care consistent with what the patient would have wanted. For those who have never had capacity, for example infants, autonomy is less relevant and the principles of beneficence and the 'sanctity of life' become more prominent.

Beneficence and non-maleficence

The principles of beneficence and non-maleficence often come into conflict when discussing issues at the end of life. This is because often what may be considered to be benefiting a patient can also be viewed as harming them if the action taken is likely to result in the patient dying sooner than they might have otherwise.

Many consider that acting in the best interests of a patient (i.e. in accordance with beneficence) means following that patient's wishes regarding what they want or do not want at the end of their life (if known) thus providing them with what they consider to be a 'good' or 'dignified' death, as well as easing a patient's suffering. However, where the patient's wishes mean that they reject treatment that may prolong their life, or where pain relief given may result in increased risks of respiratory depression, others may argue that those actions may 'harm' the patient by potentially shortening their lives and, as such, be against the principle of non-maleficence.

The 'harms' at the end of a patient's life can variously be viewed as:

➢ The suffering of a patient

➢ A failure to respect their wishes (where known) regarding care and treatment at the end of life

➢ The potential for a patient's life to be shortened through inaction (for example, failure to intervene/treat) or action (for example, through administering pain relief which risks respiratory depression)

➢ Preventing a patient from dying with 'dignity' (that is, in the way they wished to die).

On the flipside, the 'benefits' for a patient at the end of life can be seen as:

➢ Taking steps to alleviate a patient's suffering at the end of life (for example, through administering sufficient pain relief)

➢ Respecting a patient's wishes as to what care and treatment they should receive at the end of life (where known)

➢ Ensuring a patient is allowed to die with 'dignity' (that is, in the way they wished to die).

Clearly some conduct, like health professionals taking unilateral action to intentionally, maliciously and unlawfully end the life of their patients, is clearly contrary to the principle of maleficence and does not have a countervailing 'benefit' attributed to a patient.

Justice

As already identified in Chapter 5, the concept of justice is crucial to the notion of consent as it relates to a key 'right' of competent adult patients to consent to or refuse treatment within the health care system. This also applies in end-of-life situations regarding the right to choose treatment and care. Where adults lose the ability to make decisions themselves, justice is also important to ensure that substitute decision-makers acting on a patient's behalf fully understand their ethical and legal obligations in making decisions at the end of the patient's life. This is equally important for people – most often parents – making decisions on behalf of child patients who are dying or close to death. The law relating to end-of-life issues can be complex and it is important that health professionals, including nurses and midwives, understand their legal obligations and be in a position to help others understand.

Another aspect of justice more relevant at a societal level is the ability of health departments to fund palliative care services. Unfortunately the money to fund such services or some life-sustaining treatments can be in short supply. These macroeconomic issues require consideration by governments around Australia.

Similarly, issues relating to the rationing or distribution of funding for life-prolonging medical interventions at the end of life are relevant to justice. It has been questioned whether providing high-cost life-prolonging interventions to individuals, in situations which are often seen to be futile (i.e. of limited or no medical benefit and which do not change the ultimate prognosis), is sustainable in a health system where there are so many other demands. This aspect is discussed in greater detail in Chapter 10, the context of treating the elderly.

The nursing and midwifery codes

Within the international and national Codes of Ethics and Codes of Conduct there are general and specific principles that provide guidance in relation to care at the end of life. There is also the recognition that nurses and midwives need to develop personal skills to deal with difficult issues such as the dying and the death of patients. The Codes also recognise the role of nurses and midwives in picking up and reporting unethical and unlawful behaviour of others – this may be relevant in relation to the actions of some at the end of a patient's life. Both the Nursing and the Midwifery Codes of Conduct recognise that particular issues arise during end-of-life care, with each devoting a specific principle to issues relating to end-of-life care. The ICM Code of Ethics also implicitly acknowledges that midwives may encounter these issue too, noting in the preamble that midwifery care 'may encompass the reproductive life cycle of a woman from pre-pregnancy stage right through menopause and to the end of life'.

Principle 3.6 of the national Codes of Conduct of both professions acknowledges the limitations in the care that may be available for patients. It states that nurses and midwives 'have a vital role in helping the community to deal with the reality of death and its consequences' but that in the provision of appropriate end-of-life care the 'limits of healthcare in prolonging life' must be understood, with it also being recognised that some efforts to prolong a patient's life 'may not be in the best interests' of the patient. As part of this, it goes on to state that even in situations where it is not possible to provide an outcome that the patient or their families want, nurses and midwives must 'take reasonable steps to ensure support is provided to people, and their families'.

Respect for participation and decision-making

The principles relevant to consent, refusal of consent and decision-making on behalf of patients lacking capacity are also relevant at the end of life when decisions need to be made. This is explicitly recognised at Principles 3.6(a)–(b) of both professional Codes of Conduct where it states that nurses and midwives 'accept that the person has the right to refuse treatment, or to request withdrawal of treatment, while ensuring the person receives relief from distress' and 'respect diverse cultural practices and beliefs related to death and dying'. Similarly, in recognising differing views of patients at the end of life, the ICN Code of Ethics notes that, in providing care, nurses should promote an environment where 'human rights, values, customs and spiritual beliefs of the individual, family and community are respected' (at Element 1).

One way patients may continue to contribute to decisions regarding their own care even when they have lost decision-making capacity is by leaving instructions (in an 'advance directive') for what they would like to happen in such circumstances. The Codes of Conduct recognise that nurses and midwives may have a role to play in this, and should 'facilitate advance care planning and provision of end-of-life care where relevant and in accordance with local policy and legislation' (3.6(d)). Even without an advance directive or full decision-making capacity, some patients with restricted decision-making may still be able to express their preferences for or against treatment which may help to guide decision-making.

As noted in Chapter 5, when dealing with patients who may be relying on substitute decision-makers to make decisions for them, the Codes of Conduct at 2.2(b) and 2.3(c)–(d) recognise the role of others to contribute to decision-making and the role of nurses and midwives in facilitating their involvement where appropriate.

Vulnerability and public trust

At the end of life, patients will necessarily be in a heightened state of vulnerability. The ICN Code of Ethics notes in Element 1 that a nurse 'shares with society the responsibility for initiating and supporting action to meet the health and social needs of the public, in particular those of vulnerable populations'. Also relevant in caring for vulnerable populations is the recognition that nurses (and midwives) ought to always demonstrate professional values of 'compassion' and 'integrity'.

It is also crucial that the public maintains its trust in nurses and midwives. This requires all nurses and midwives to act appropriately when dealing with patients who are vulnerable and at the end of their lives. The ICN Code of Ethics notes that a nurse 'maintains standards of personal conduct which reflect well on the profession and enhance ... public confidence' (Element 2). Principle 1.2 in both professions' Codes of Conduct emphasises this by stating that unethical or unlawful actions by nurses and midwives can affect 'the reputation of the profession'.

Respect for the law

A number of principles in both professions' Codes of Conduct also highlight nurses' and midwives' obligations to follow the law and question the conduct of others which they regard as unlawful or unethical. Principle 1.2 clearly states that nurses and midwives 'must practise honestly and ethically and should not engage in unlawful behaviour'. The need for nurses and midwives to understand the law relating to end-of-life issues is very important given the severe legal consequences that may result if the law is not complied with.

Where nurses or midwives observe cases of inappropriate conduct by others at the end of a patient's life this gives rise to obligations to act to protect the patient, and also act on the unethical conduct. This is recognised in both international and national Codes. The ICN Code of Ethics recognises the need to pick up on and report unethical and unlawful behaviour of others, and this may be relevant in relation to the actions of some at the end of a patient's life. Nurses should 'challenge unethical practices and settings' (at Element 3) and take 'appropriate action to safeguard individuals, families and communities when their health is endangered by a co-worker or any other person' (at Element 4). In the national Codes of Conduct, at 2.1 (c), it notes that nurses and midwives must 'document and report concerns if they believe the practice environment is compromising the health and safety of people receiving care' and 1.3 acknowledges the mandatory reporting requirements that exist to protect the vulnerable. Acting in circumstances where unethical conduct is observed by others is essential in maintaining appropriate and ethical care for vulnerable patients at the end of their lives who continue to be engaged in the health system through, for example, hospitals, nursing homes and hospices.

Caring for oneself

Both the nursing and midwifery Codes of Conduct comment on the importance of nurses and midwives maintaining their mental health. At 7.1 in both Codes of Conduct, it states that nurse and midwives have a 'responsibility to maintain their physical and mental health' and 'act to reduce the effect of ... stress on their health'. This relevantly applies to nurses and midwives developing competence in communication and emotional health to enable them to deal effectively with the dying and death of their patients. Emotional development in this area is important, together with the technical skills of the profession (Freegard and Isted 2012, p. 333). (For a discussion of coping with professional anxiety in death and dying, see Freegard and Isted 2012, pp. 332–334.)

The law relating to end-of-life issues

In this section we look at the main legal issues that health professionals, including nurses and midwives, are likely to encounter when dealing with an adult or child patient at the end of their life. These issues relate to:

➤ The provision of palliative medication and what is known as the legal doctrine of 'double effect'

➤ The issue of euthanasia, assisted suicide and unlawful killing

➤ The circumstances when it is lawful to withhold or withdraw life-sustaining treatment from a patient.

Palliative medication and the doctrine of double effect

The World Health Organization (WHO) describes palliative care as:

> an approach that improves the quality of life of patients and their families facing the problem associated with life-threatening illness, through the prevention and relief of suffering by means of early identification and impeccable assessment and treatment of pain and other problems, physical, psychosocial and spiritual. (WHO 2018)

In the health care context, palliative medication often refers to the provision of pain relief, particularly in those patients who may be entering the final stages of their life. However, as the WHO definition shows, the term 'palliative care' can be used more broadly to encompass a range of planned care which focuses on the social and emotional side of dying and death (Freegard and Isted 2012, p. 324). In this part of the chapter the focus is on the administration of palliative medication (i.e. the provision of pain relief) where there is a risk that pain relief may increase the risk of respiratory depression.

The provision of appropriate palliative care, including palliative medication, at the end of life for adult or child patients is an aim supported by society; it is seen as a positive thing to ease the suffering of those who are dying. Given that the provision of pain relief at high levels is sometimes accompanied by risks of respiratory depression, the concern is whether such palliative medication can be provided, despite the potentially fatal consequences. Recognition of the legitimate policy aim of relieving suffering at the end of life has resulted in a legal principle which allows palliative medication – in the form of pain relief – to be provided as long as the intention is to relieve pain and not to shorten a patient's life. This principle is known as the doctrine of 'double effect'. While some clinicians find its application ethically complex, given the outcome may be to hasten death (Quill et al. 1997, p. 1769), it is a recognised legal principle in Australia. Case law and, in some States in Australia, legislation reflects this principle.

It is crucial that health professionals understand the law regarding when palliative medication can be provided. A failure to understand these principles could result in health professionals failing to provide adequate pain relief – when it would be appropriate to do so – due to fears that they may be held legally responsible for a patient's death. Here we discuss the common law principle and then the legislation in certain States relating to the provision of palliative medication.

States and Territories without legislation

Most States and Territories around Australia do not have specific legislation dealing with palliative medication and rely on the common law doctrine of double effect. In New South Wales, the Northern Territory, Tasmania and Victoria reliance is placed on the common law.

While there are no Australian cases that have dealt specifically with the doctrine of double effect, it is assumed that the principles from English cases, like *R v Cox* (1992) 12 BMLR 38 (see box), are an accurate representation of the law in these Australian States and Territories.

R v Cox (1992) 12 BMLR 38

In this English case the doctor in question was prosecuted for attempted murder when he administered potassium chloride to a patient who was in a terminal condition and suffering great pain. The doctor in this case was found guilty of attempted murder by a jury who were satisfied that his purpose in administering the potassium chloride was to hasten her death. The evidence showed that potassium chloride had no curative or pain-relieving properties. However, in summing up to the jury, the judge in that case made the following statement which has been relied on as recognition of the legal principle of the doctrine of double effect. Justice Ognall relevantly said

> There can be no doubt that the use of drugs to reduce pain and suffering will often be fully justified notwithstanding that it will, in fact, hasten the moment of death. What can never be lawful is the use of drugs with the primary purpose of hastening of death.

Where the doctrine of double effect applies, the person administering the palliative medication will not be criminally liable.

States with specific legislation

In Queensland, South Australia and Western Australia, legislation has been enacted that provides for a modified version of the doctrine of double effect. These provisions are discussed below.

Queensland

Section 282A of the *Criminal Code* (Qld) deals specifically with the provision of palliative medication. 'Palliative care' in this context is defined as care that is 'directed at maintaining or improving the comfort of a person who is, or would otherwise be, subject to pain and suffering'. It provides that a person is 'not criminally responsible' for providing palliative medication to a patient, even if an 'incidental effect' of providing it is to hasten the patient's death. This will apply where all the following conditions are satisfied:

➢ The person providing 'palliative care' is doing so in good faith with reasonable care and skill

➢ The provision of it is reasonable (i.e. in accordance with 'Good Medical Practice' as outlined in recognised medical and ethical standards of the medical profession in Australia) – having regard to the patient's state at the time and all the circumstances of the case

➢ Either the person providing it is a doctor or it has been ordered by a doctor who confirms the order in writing.

Therefore, this section protects nurses or midwives who administer palliative medication in accordance with a written order from a doctor.

South Australia

In South Australia section 17 of the *Consent to Medical Treatment and Palliative Care Act 1995* (SA), deals with 'The care of people who are dying'. In this section, although the term 'palliative medication' is not mentioned, the phrase 'administering medical treatment with the intention of relieving pain or distress' is used. This section provides that a doctor or a person under a doctor's supervision (which would include nurses or midwives) will not be civilly or criminally liable when giving such treatment, even though an 'incidental effect' of it is to hasten the death of the patient, if all of the following conditions are satisfied:

➢ The patient is in the 'terminal phase of a terminal illness'

➢ The person providing the treatment does so in good faith and without negligence

➢ The provision of treatment is in accordance with proper professional standards

➢ It is given with the consent of the patient or the patient's substitute decision-maker.

Western Australia

In Western Australia section 259 of the *Criminal Code* (WA) deals with palliative medication. It provides that a person will not be criminally responsible where:

➢ The person providing palliative medication does so in good faith and with reasonable care and skill;

➢ The palliative medication is given to a patient for their benefit; and

➢ The administration is reasonable, having regard to the patient's state at the time and all the circumstances of the case.

Australian Capital Territory

The situation in the Australian Capital Territory is a little different from the other States with specific legislation. There, section 17 of the *Medical Treatment (Health Directions) Act 2006* (ACT) and section 86 of the *Powers of Attorney Act 2006 (ACT)* give patients a right to receive 'relief from pain, suffering and discomfort to the maximum extent that is reasonable in the circumstances'. This will apply when the patient is under the care of a health professional and has given an advance directive that treatment be withheld or withdrawn, or where a person's attorney, acting as a substitute decision-maker, has made this decision on behalf of the patient. The effect of the law here is less clear than in other States but is likely to reflect the common law doctrine of double effect.

Euthanasia, assisted suicide and unlawful killing

We now go on to consider the controversial issue of euthanasia and assisted suicide. We also consider the related criminal offences. Understanding these issues, and how they differ significantly from the provision of palliative medication and the withholding and withdrawing of life-sustaining treatment, is very important for health professionals, including nurses and midwives.

Euthanasia and assisted suicide

The term 'euthanasia' is not a legal term and while the meaning of the word derives from the Greek words meaning 'good death', it does not have a set definition. As such, discussions about euthanasia, and assisted suicide, in society or in the media can become confusing (see, for example, the discussion in Freegard and Isted 2012, pp. 326–330). Confusingly, the terms 'voluntary euthanasia', 'physician-assisted suicide', 'voluntary assisted suicide' and 'active euthanasia' have all been used interchangeably at times. However, generally a distinction is made between where the patient themselves does the final act that causes death compared with where another person's actions cause the death.

To be clear then, when mentioned in this chapter, the term 'euthanasia' is intended to mean the intentional ending of a competent patient's life, at their request, where another person's actions causes the death of the patient. 'Assisted suicide' is intended to mean the intentional ending of a competent patient's life, at their request, where assistance is provided by another person, but the patient does the final act that causes death.

As already mentioned, the issues of euthanasia and assisted suicide are very different from that of palliative medication discussed earlier. It is also very different from the issues discussed in the section on 'Withholding or withdrawing life-sustaining treatment'.

The euthanasia and assisted suicide debate

Numerous attempts have been made to legalise the practice of euthanasia and/or assisted suicide in Australia, and studies frequently demonstrate that sections of the community, in principle, support allowing some of these practices. In 2019 Victoria will become the only jurisdiction in Australia where patients may take part in a legal process of undertaking 'voluntary assisted dying' – a form of assisted suicide (see further discussion below).

The rationale that exists in support of allowing euthanasia and assisted suicide to be lawful is that competent persons should be able to exercise their autonomy and gain assistance in ending their lives in the way they want, and at the time of their choosing. Such an argument strongly relies on the principle of autonomy and allowing a person to 'die with dignity' (i.e. in the way they wished to die). This may be particularly relevant for people who are suffering greatly and for whom medical intervention is not working or not an option. These reasons were accepted in the Northern Territory in 1995 when controversial legislation was passed to legalise euthanasia and assisted suicide. However, these laws faced opposition and were overturned by the Australian Government in 1997. Since that time and until the passing of Victoria's legislation in 2017, the practice of euthanasia and assisted suicide was unlawful throughout Australia. Currently, there are a range of jurisdictions around the world that have legislation allowing certain regulated forms of euthanasia or assisted suicide to take place (e.g. the Netherlands; the US states of Oregon, Washington, Vermont, Colorado and the District of Columbia; Switzerland; Belgium; Canada; and Colombia).

On the other hand many people (including many health professionals) argue that euthanasia and assisted suicide should never be allowed. They believe that to assist a person to end their life goes against the principles of non-maleficence and the sanctity of life. There is also the argument that there is the potential for any regulated euthanasia or assisted suicide practice to be abused by those in power, with the consequence that some people may have their life ended in circumstances which would not otherwise occur. Additionally, the 'slippery slope' argument suggests that once you allow euthanasia/assisted suicide to be available for some patients, what's stopping us from extending it to other patients – for example, patients with depression who want to end their lives, patients under 18 years of age, elderly patients with dementia? Others suggest that allowing health professionals to be involved in such practices may result in a lack of trust in the professions and damage the integrity of the health professions (Stewart 2018).

Law reform in Victoria legalising assisted suicide

In 2017 Victoria passed the *Voluntary Assisted Dying* Act 2017 (Vic). This provides that, from June 2019, voluntary assisted dying for competent adults nearing death – with

▶

◀

the involvement of a health practitioner – will be legal in accordance with the scheme provided for under the legislation. The scheme strictly outlines eligibility criteria, the process by which patients approach health professionals, the information they are to receive, how medications will be administered, and includes stringent safeguards such as the establishment of a Voluntary Assisted Dying Review Board to monitor and report on compliance.

The issue of euthanasia and assisted suicide is therefore clearly an emotionally charged and controversial social issue. It is possible that we will see more legal reform in this area around Australia. However, currently the legal position in all States and Territories – except Victoria (from June 2019) – is very clear: euthanasia and assisted suicide is unlawful. Those who carry out euthanasia or assisted suicide can be prosecuted, for example for murder or manslaughter or other offences (such as failure to provide the necessaries of life). Here we discuss the main offence provisions.

Offence of assisted suicide

Although a person does not commit a crime by committing suicide (or attempting to commit suicide), any person who 'assists' them may be committing a crime. This is because legislation exists in all States and Territories that makes 'aiding' another person to commit suicide a crime (*Crimes Act 1900* (ACT), s 17; *Criminal Code Act* (NT), s 162; *Crimes Act 1900* (NSW), s 31C; *Criminal Code* (Qld), s 311; *Criminal Law Consolidation Act 1935* (SA), s 13A(5); *Criminal Code Act 1924* (Tas), s 163; *Crimes Act 1958* (Vic) s 6B(2); *Criminal Code* (WA), s 288). From June 2019 this offence will not apply to health professionals who act in accordance with the scheme provided for under the *Voluntary Assisted Dying Act 2017* (Vic).

Therefore, in some circumstances, where a health professional provides assistance to a patient to commit suicide, they may be prosecuted for assisted suicide. It will be up to the prosecution to decide whether to charge someone with unlawful killing (i.e. murder or manslaughter) or assisted suicide. This will often depend on the degree of assistance given by the accused to the person who committed suicide.

Offences of unlawful killing (murder and manslaughter)

Where a person has 'unlawfully killed' another (sometimes referred to as a 'homicide'), they may ultimately be found guilty of murder or manslaughter. Murder is the most serious charge, but sometimes there may be circumstances that justify the lesser charge of manslaughter. While health professionals being charged with such offences is extremely rare, it is not unheard of.

The Beverley Allitt Inquiry

In 1993 enrolled nurse Beverley Allitt was convicted of four murders and three attempted murders (among other crimes) of child patients on the ward she worked at in an English hospital. Suspicions in the hospital were initially raised as a child's blood sugar had fallen dramatically on a number of occasions and it was discovered the child had been wrongly and intentionally injected with insulin. Allitt was sentenced to life imprisonment for each charge.

The case described here is a rare and truly shocking account of a nurse who intentionally killed her patients and was found guilty of murder and attempted murder. In this case the driving motivation was not related to wanting to provide a 'good death' (as is often the case in those involved with euthanasia) but something far more sinister.

In the Northern Territory, Queensland, Tasmania and Western Australia the criminal law offences relating to murder and manslaughter are contained in legislation. In the remaining States and Territories the relevant law comes from a combination of case law (i.e. the common law) and legislation.

In Australia, in order to be found guilty of murder, there is generally a need to prove the following:

➤ *Intention*: the accused intended to cause death or grievous bodily harm

➤ *Causation*: the accused caused the death of the victim (the accused's actions were the main foreseeable cause of death, or a substantial cause of death).

(See *Crimes Act 1900* (ACT), ss 12, 15; *Criminal Code Act* (NT), ss 156, 160; *Crimes Act 1900* (NSW), s 18; *Criminal Code* (Qld), ss 300, 302, 303; *Criminal Law Consolidation Act 1935* (SA), ss 11, 13; *Criminal Code Act 1924* (Tas), ss 156–159; *Crimes Act 1958* (Vic), ss 3, 5; *Criminal Code* (WA), ss 277, 279, 280.)

The accused's motive for committing the unlawful killing is irrelevant to whether or not a crime has been committed. Therefore, even where a person acts with the best of intentions – as may be the case in relation to a person who participates in euthanasia to ease the suffering of a patient – this does not excuse the act. A crime will still be committed.

Alternatively, the law also recognises that a person can be guilty of unlawful killing without having the requisite 'intention' if death results through reckless action (i.e. through knowingly carrying out acts or omissions which will probably cause death or serious bodily harm). In the case of *R v Crabbe* (1985) 156 CLR 464, the High Court stated:

> The conduct of a person who does an act, knowing that death or grievous bodily harm is a probable consequence, can naturally be regarded for the purposes of the criminal law as just as blameworthy as the conduct of one who does an act intended to kill or to do grievous bodily harm.

If this is the charge made against a health professional the prosecution will need to prove that the health professional knew or believed that death or serious bodily harm would be a likely consequence of their actions. Once again it must be shown that this reckless action caused the death of the person. For example, if a nurse practitioner were to recklessly administer medication in excess of the recommended dose and this caused the death of a patient, it may be argued that the nurse practitioner knew or believed that death or bodily injury would be a likely result of their actions.

Also, the law is clear that a patient consenting to the ending of his or her life is not relevant. In the Northern Territory, Queensland, Tasmania and Western Australia this is made clear in legislation (*Criminal Code Act* (NT), s 26(3); *Criminal Code* (Qld), s 284; *Criminal Code Act 1924* (Tas), s 53; *Criminal Code* (WA), s 261). And in the remaining States and Territories, the common law can be relied on for the same principle.

The less serious charge of manslaughter can result in relation to murder when the accused is found not to have the required 'intention' but still caused the death of the person who died. In addition, when some mitigating factors are present the charge of manslaughter can result.

Withholding or withdrawing life-sustaining treatment

The withholding or withdrawal of life-sustaining treatment in patients will generally result in a patient's death, this is because 'life-sustaining treatments' are those medical interventions which are acting to keep a patient alive – that is, the life-sustaining treatment is prolonging the life of the patient. The law regarding withholding or withdrawing life-sustaining treatment differs from the legal principles of the doctrine of double effect (palliative medication) and unlawful killing. This is because the doctrine of double effect relates to *providing* treatment in the form of palliative medication, and here we are concerned with *withholding* or *withdrawing* treatment. Also, while euthanasia and assisted suicide remain against the law in the majority of Australia, withholding or withdrawing life-sustaining treatment can be lawful in some circumstances and is an accepted part of medical practice. In this section of the chapter we discuss the circumstances when withholding or withdrawing life-sustaining treatment from an adult or child patient will be considered lawful.

What is a 'life-sustaining treatment'?

Where the term 'life-sustaining treatment' is used it refers to a medical intervention or treatment which is keeping a patient alive, without which they are likely to die relatively quickly. Life-sustaining treatments can therefore include:

- Artificial ventilation

- Artificial nutrition and hydration

- The provision of cardiopulmonary resuscitation

- The provision of antibiotics (in some circumstances)

- Blood transfusions (in some circumstances).

Withholding or withdrawing life-sustaining treatments from patients with decision-making capacity – adults and children

Adults with capacity

As described in Chapter 5, competent adult patients are entitled to consent to or refuse consent to any health care or medical treatment offered to them. As the cases of *Re B (adult: refusal of medical treatment)* [2002] 2 All ER 449 and *Brightwater Care Group (Inc) v Rossiter* (2009) 40 WAR 84 made clear (see the section 'Competent adult patients have the right to refuse health care' in Chapter 5), this extends to refusals of consent for life-sustaining treatment. In those cases Ms B and Mr Rossiter, respectively, were granted declarations by the court that continuing to provide treatment against their wishes was unlawful. Therefore, the law is quite simple here: a competent adult patient can refuse life-sustaining treatment that is offered to them, even if it results in their death.

Gillick-competent children

The situation in relation to *Gillick*-competent children is more complex. As discussed in Chapter 6, even if a child has been assessed as being *Gillick*-competent, a child's decision to refuse life-sustaining medical treatment can be overridden by the courts. In the case of *Minister for Health v*

AS (2004) 33 Fam LR 223 (see the section 'Refusal of consent by *Gillick*-competent children' in Chapter 6), the Court authorised blood transfusions despite the fact that the 15-year-old *Gillick*-competent boy refused such treatment. That case demonstrates that the court can override a competent child's decision where it considers it to be in the child's best interests. This contrasts with the position in relation to competent adults where the law respects the autonomy of the individual. For child patients the principles of beneficence and the 'sanctity of life' have more influence at law.

Withholding or withdrawing life-sustaining treatment from patients lacking decision-making capacity

The law relating to how decisions are made to withhold or withdraw life-sustaining treatment from patients who lack decision-making capacity relies on case law and, in some States and Territories, specific legislation. The types of patients in this category include adults lacking decision-making capacity and also some children.

The common law – adults and children lacking decision-making capacity

Where an adult or child who lacks decision-making capacity is seriously ill, a question may arise as to whether life-sustaining treatment ought to be provided or continued. Sometimes this question arises where a patient's decline and eventual death are inevitable and interventions are seen as no longer providing any medical benefit, or are seen to be placing too much of a burden (pain, indignity) on the patient. While normally decisions to withhold or withdraw life-sustaining medical treatment are decided collectively without conflict between those close to the patient and the treating team – taking into account what the patient would have wanted (if known) – sometimes there can be disagreement between these parties. When disagreement arises, tribunals and courts can be called on to resolve the issue by deciding what is in the patient's best interests. The 'best interests' of the patient legal test – discussed in Chapters 5 and 6 – is usually applied by courts and tribunals making decisions about end-of-life treatment for children and adults who lack capacity.

A key case in this area of law is the English case of Tony Bland (*Airedale NHS Trust v Bland* [1993] AC 789 (*Bland's case*)). We outline some of key findings made by the court in that case (see box). This influential case has also been followed in Australia as shown in the case of *Messiha v South East Health* [2004] NSWSC 1061 (see box).

Airedale NHS Trust v Bland [1993] AC 789 (*Bland's case*)

This English case dealt with the case of 17-year-old Tony Bland who, following a crushing injury which deprived his brain of oxygen, was diagnosed as being in a persistent vegetative state (post-coma unresponsiveness). Tony had no higher brain functions and was unable to see, hear or feel anything. He was kept alive through artificial nutrition and hydration for more than three years. After this time, the hospital authority, with the support of Tony's family and treating team, applied to the court for a declaration that they be allowed to cease medical treatment except for that needed to make Tony comfortable. It was understood that this would ultimately mean Tony would die.

For our purposes, it is important to note that the House of Lords (the United Kingdom's highest court) made clear that a duty only exists to provide medical treatment in a patient's best interests. As such, where treatment is futile, it cannot be considered to be in the patient's best interests and there is no duty provide it. One of the judges, Lord Goff stated:

> I cannot see that medical treatment is appropriate or requisite simply to prolong a patient's life, when such treatment has no therapeutic purpose of any kind, as where it is futile because the patient is unconscious and there is no prospect of any improvement in his condition.

As such, it was recognised that where the provision of life-sustaining measures is not in a patient's best interests, the withholding or withdrawing of that measure is lawful.

Messiha v South East Health [2004] NSWSC 1061

In this New South Wales case the principles outlined in *Bland's case* were applied. The patient in this case was a 75-year-old male who had suffered a cardiac arrest, brain damage and remained unconscious. At the time of the application, the patient was being artificially ventilated and being provided with artificial nutrition and hydration. The treating consultant doctor considered that the current treatment should cease and the patient be given palliative care.

In this case the family disagreed with the medical opinion about the patient and approached the court seeking a finding that it would be in the patient's best interests for the current treatment to continue. After receiving medical evidence, Justice Howie made the finding that, 'Apart from extending the patient's life for some relatively brief period, the current treatment is futile. I believe that it is also burdensome and will be intrusive to a degree.' As such, the application of the family, to have the treatment continue, was denied by the Court.

Therefore, where treatment is considered to offer no benefit to the patient or their quality of life, or is considered to be very intrusive or burdensome for the patient, then courts will generally find such life-sustaining treatment to not be in the patient's best interests.

For sick children at the end of life, decisions about the provision of life-sustaining treatment will normally be made by parents together with the treating team. If disagreements or questions as to the lawfulness of a request to not provide treatment arise then an application to a Supreme Court or Family Court may be made. The court will apply the 'best interests' test and decide what is in the child's best interests. We saw examples of such cases in Chapter 6.

The case of *Re Baby D (No 2)* (2011) 45 Fam LR 313 (see box) is an Australian case where the court was asked to decide on the issue of withdrawing life-sustaining treatment – in the form of removal of an endotracheal intubation – from a prematurely born infant.

Re Baby D (No 2) (2011) 45 Fam LR 313

Baby D was born prematurely at 27 weeks and had suffered severe brain damage after an incident in which she was deprived of oxygen. At the time of the application to the Family Court she had an endotracheal intubation; a number of failed attempts had been made to remove the tube prior to this and the option of a tracheostomy was considered to be too painful and burdensome for a child in Baby D's condition. It was the agreed view of the parents, the clinical ethics committee and the treating team that the withdrawal of intensive care support – via the removal of the endotracheal tube and possible provision of palliative care to prevent distress, should it be needed – was in the best interests of Baby D. The parents approached the court seeking authorisation for withdrawal of intensive care support, or a declaration that the parents could make the decision on behalf of their child. Evidence was given by a number of medical professionals who agreed that this course of action was in the best interests of Baby D.

Justice Young in the Family Court decided that the decision to withdraw life-sustaining treatment for Baby D came within the scope of parental decision-making and acknowledged that parents making such a decision in this case would be acting in the best interests of Baby D.

However, the judge made clear in that case that the scope of parental authority to make decisions to withhold or withdraw life-sustaining treatment was dependent on the individual patient and circumstances.

Legislation – adults lacking decision-making capacity

Around Australia, legislation exists which specifically applies to adults who lack capacity. The common law principles (discussed in the previous section) apply alongside the legislation discussed in this section.

Generally speaking, despite the existence of the specific legislation, the option of approaching the State and Territory Supreme Courts to resolve an issue remains open.

This section builds on the discussion of how decisions regarding medical treatment are made on behalf of adult's lacking decision-making capacity described in Chapter 5. The principles that substitute decision-makers have to observe in making decisions discussed in Chapter 5 (at see section on 'Obligations on substitute decision-makers acting on behalf of adult patients lacking capacity) generally apply in this context as well. These principles offer important guidance to difficult decisions that need to be made on behalf of vulnerable patients. Chapter 5 also provides explanations of some key terms used in this section.

Here, we expand on that discussion by examining specifically how decisions about withholding or withdrawing life-sustaining treatment can lawfully be made on behalf of an adult lacking decision-making capacity. It should be noted that the law in this area remains uncertain in some jurisdictions.

The Australian Capital Territory

In the Australian Capital Territory, section 7 of the *Medical Treatment (Health Directions) Act 2006* (ACT) allows a person to make an advance directive called a 'health direction'. This can be used to provide instructions in advance to indicate when a person wants to refuse treatment in the future when they have lost decision-making capacity. Where the health direction is valid, has not been superseded by later appointments, and applies in the circumstances, generally the refusal of treatment must be respected by treating medical staff.

If no health direction exists then a decision to withhold or withdraw life-sustaining treatment from the adult patient must be made by someone else (a substitute decision-maker). Where an enduring power of attorney has been appointed by the adult patient before he or she lost capacity, the person appointed as the enduring attorney can make a decision regarding whether life-sustaining treatment should be withheld or withdrawn. However, section 46(2) of the *Powers of Attorney Act 2006* specifies that an enduring attorney must not ask for life-sustaining treatment to be withheld or withdrawn from the patient unless the enduring attorney:

➢ Has consulted a doctor about the nature of the patient's illness and any alternative forms of treatment available and the consequences to the patient of remaining untreated; and

➢ Believes, on reasonable grounds, that the patient, if able to make a rational judgement and give serious consideration to their own health and wellbeing, would ask for the medical treatment to be withheld or withdrawn.

If a guardian has been appointed for the patient, then depending on what powers are given to the guardian by the ACT Civil and Administrative Tribunal, the guardian may be able to make a decision to withhold or withdraw life-sustaining treatment from the patient (*Guardianship and Management of Property Act 1991* (ACT), s. 7).

If no enduring attorney or guardian has been appointed then a 'health attorney' would normally have power to make health decisions on behalf of a patient (for who is a 'health attorney', see the subsection 'The Australian Capital Territory' under the section 'How do decisions get made if an adult patient lacks the capacity to make a health care decision?' in Chapter 5). In the case of end-of-life decisions, the situation is slightly different; where a health attorney refuses consent to medical treatment (including life-sustaining treatment) in situations where a health professional believes the refusal is inconsistent with a health direction, the matter will be referred to the Public Trustee and Guardian (a statutory official). If the Public Trustee and Guardian thinks the refusal is reasonable then no further action will be taken and the treatment will not be provided; alternatively, it will seek to be appointed as the patient's guardian (*Guardianship and Management of Property Act 1991* (ACT) s 32H). This provision is also discussed in Chapter 5 in the subsection 'The Australian Capital Territory' under the section 'Other ways of resolving disputes'.

The ACT Civil and Administrative Tribunal may also be approached for advice or recommendations in situations regarding end-of-life decision-making (*Guardianship and Management of Property Act 1991* (ACT), s 18). The Supreme Court can also be approached to make a decision.

New South Wales

While the legislation in New South Wales does not mention advance directives, these would be recognised under the common law. As such, an advance directive that gives instructions to refuse life-sustaining treatment in the future when the patient has lost capacity can be legally recognised (as happened in the case of *Hunter and New England Area Health Service v A* (2009) 74 NSWLR 88).

Under the New South Wales *Guardianship Act 1987* (NSW), it seems that, typically, the following persons who can be identified may make decisions regarding withholding and withdrawing life-sustaining treatment from a patient lacking decision-making capacity:

➤ A guardian that has been appointed by the New South Wales Civil and Administrative Tribunal with 'plenary' (i.e. 'full' or 'complete') power to make decisions or given power to make health care decisions.

➤ An enduring guardian that was appointed by the patient (for health care decisions) before they lost capacity is likely to be able to make decisions regarding withholding or withdrawing life-sustaining treatment.

It seems unlikely that other substitute decision-makers would have lawful power to refuse consent to life-sustaining medical treatment (see Willmott et al. 2018, [14.220]). The Tribunal may also be approached for advice or recommendations in situations regarding end-of-life decision-making (*Guardianship Act 1987* (NSW), ss 6E, 21, 28). The Supreme Court can also be approached to make a decision.

Northern Territory

In the Northern Territory the *Advance Personal Planning Act* (NT) provides for an advance directive known as an 'advance personal plan' to be made by a patient before they lose capacity. This allows them to make advance refusals to life-sustaining treatment in the future.

In the absence of an advance directive, a decision regarding refusal of life-sustaining treatment may be made by a 'decision-maker' appointed by the patient prior to losing capacity, or an 'adult guardian' appointed for the patient by the Northern Territory Civil and Administrative Tribunal who has been given power to make health care decisions. The Supreme Court can also be approached to make a decision. (See *Advance Personal Planning Act* (NT), ss 41, 42, 44; *Guardianship of Adults Act* (NT), s 23.)

Queensland

In Queensland the legislation provides a priority list of ways in which a decision can be made on behalf of an adult patient who lacks decision-making capacity. Typically, this priority list applies in a similar way for decisions made regarding withholding or withdrawing life-sustaining treatment from a patient lacking capacity.

If the adult patient has an advance directive (known as an 'advance health directive') then this will only operate in relation to refusals for life-sustaining treatment if the patient:

➤ Is sufficiently ill – that is, the patient:

- has a terminal illness and is expected to die within a year; or
- is in a persistent vegetative state; or
- is permanently unconscious; or
- has an illness or injury that is so severe that there is no reasonable prospect that the patient will recover to the extent that life-sustaining treatment will not be needed; and
- Has no reasonable prospect of regaining decision-making capacity.

In addition, doctors need *not* follow a refusal in an advance directive where they believe the instructions in the directive to be inconsistent with 'Good Medical Practice' (meaning recognised medical and ethical standards, practices and procedures of the medical profession) (see *Powers of Attorney Act 1998* (Qld), ss 36, 103). However, this limitation has been criticised by some as being unwarranted and as removing patient autonomy at the end of life (see Willmott et al. 2018, [14.170]).

If no advance health directive exists, then the first of the following people who is available to act can make decisions on behalf of the patient in relation to withholding or withdrawing life-sustaining treatment, as long as the treating doctor considers that *providing* the life-sustaining treatment in the patient's circumstances would be *against* 'Good Medical Practice':

➢ A guardian appointed by the Queensland Civil and Administrative Tribunal for health care decisions

➢ An attorney appointed by the patient for health care decisions under an advance directive or under an enduring power of attorney before the patient lost capacity

➢ A 'statutory health attorney' who is the first of the following to apply:

  – the patient's spouse – where the relationship is close and continuing;

  – the person who cares for the patient (without being paid);

  – a close friend or relative of the patient; or

  – the Public Guardian (an independent statutory body in Queensland).

As noted in Chapter 5, where there are concerns that a substitute decision-maker is not acting appropriately in making a decision – including a refusal of life-sustaining treatment on behalf of the patient – the Public Guardian can be approached to resolve disputes (see the subsection 'Queensland' under the section 'Other ways of resolving disputes' in Chapter 5).

The Queensland Civil and Administrative Tribunal or the Supreme Court may also make decisions regarding withholding and withdrawing life-sustaining treatment. (See *Guardianship and Administration Act 2000* (Qld), ss 42, 43, 66, 66A, 81, 240; *Powers of Attorney Act 1998* (Qld), ch 4.)

Tasmania

Similar to New South Wales, the Tasmanian legislation does not mention advance directives. However, these would be recognised under the common law. As such, an advance directive that gives instructions to refuse life-sustaining treatment in the future when the patient has lost capacity can be legally recognised.

Under the *Guardianship and Administration Act 1995* (Tas) it would appear that only the following persons can make decisions refusing life-sustaining treatment on behalf of the adult patient:

➢ A guardian that has been appointed with power to make decisions about health care by the Guardianship and Administration Board.

➢ An enduring guardian that was appointed by the patient (for health care decisions) before they lost capacity.

There is uncertainty regarding whether other substitute decision-makers have lawful power to refuse consent to life-sustaining medical treatment (see Willmott et al. 2018, [14.220]). The Tribunal may also be approached for advice or recommendations in a situation regarding end-of-life decision-making. The Supreme Court can also be approached to make a decision. (See *Guardianship and Administration Act 1995* (Tas), ss 25, 31, 32, pt 6.)

South Australia

In South Australia if a question arises about whether to withhold or withdraw life-sustaining treatment the *Advance Care Directives Act 2013* (SA) and *Consent to Medical Treatment and Palliative Care Act 1995* (SA) govern how a decision is made. If an adult patient lacking decision-making capacity has a valid advance directive (known as an 'advance care directive') containing a refusal of life-sustaining treatment that must generally be followed where it is applicable in the circumstances.

Where no advance directive exists that applies to the situation then the following people may decide whether to withhold or withdraw life-sustaining treatment from the adult patient:

➢ A 'substitute decision-maker' appointed by the patient via an 'advance care directive', before the patient lost capacity.

➢ A 'person responsible' who is the first of the following to apply:

– a guardian appointed by the South Australian Civil and Administrative Tribunal who has power to make decisions about health care;

– a relative of the patient (i.e. spouse, domestic partner, adult related by blood, marriage or adoption, and for an Aboriginal or Torres Strait Islander patients – a person related according to their kinship rules);

- an adult friend of the patient; or

- an adult who is charged with the patient's care and wellbeing.

One restriction that applies to a refusal of treatment by a 'substitute decision-maker' on behalf of the patient is that they are prohibited from refusing the administration of drugs to relieve pain or distress, or the natural provision of food and liquids by mouth.

As noted in Chapter 5, if a dispute arises in relation to an advance care directive the South Australian Public Guardian has power to mediate disputes, make declarations or refer matters to the Tribunal.

The South Australian Civil and Administrative Tribunal may also be approached for advice or recommendations in situations regarding end-of-life decision-making. The Supreme Court can also be approached to make a decision. (See *Guardianship and Administration Act 1993* (SA), s 74; *Consent to Treatment and Palliative Care Act 1995* (SA), pt 2, div 3; *Advance Care Directives Act 2013* (SA), ss 11, 19, 23, pt 7, div 2.)

Victoria

The relevant Victorian legislation is the *Medical Treatment Planning and Decisions Act 2016* (Vic) and the *Guardianship and Administration Act 1986* (Vic). The Victorian version of an advance directive is called a 'advance care directive' and this allows a patient to refuse life-sustaining treatment in advance, to apply at a time when they no longer have decision-making capacity. Where an adult has a valid 'advance care directive' that applies in the circumstances the refusal must be followed.

In the absence of such a directive the first of the following persons, known as a 'medical treatment decision maker', may be able to make a decision regarding withholding or withdrawing life-sustaining treatment from the patient:

➢ A person appointed by the patient as a 'medical treatment decision maker', before the patient lost capacity to make the health care decision

➢ A 'guardian' appointed by the Victorian Civil and Administrative Tribunal with power to make decisions in relation to health care

➢ The patient's spouse or domestic partner – where the relationship is close and continuing

➢ The person who cares for the patient (without being paid)

➤ The patient's relative (being the first of the following who is an adult – child of the patient, parent of the patient or sibling of the patient).

As noted in Chapter 5, a special procedure exists for when there is a refusal by a medical treatment decision to 'significant treatment' – which would include a refusal of life-sustaining treatment – and the wishes of the patient are not known in relation to the treatment. If a doctor believes that the wishes of the person are not known in relation to the treatment, the doctor must notify the Victorian Public Advocate (a public official), who can decide whether or not the refusal is 'not unreasonable in the circumstances'. The Victorian Public Advocate can choose to take the matter to the Victorian Civil and Administrative Tribunal if they think the refusal of treatment by the substitute decision-maker is unreasonable.

The Victorian Civil and Administrative Tribunal may also be approached for advice or recommendations in situation regarding end-of-life decision-making. The Supreme Court can also be approached to make a decision. (See *Guardianship and Administration Act 1986* (Vic), pt 4; *Medical Treatment Planning and Decisions Act 2016* (Vic), pts 2–4.)

Western Australia

In Western Australia the *Guardianship and Administration Act 1990* (WA) provides for adults to execute an advance directive (known as an 'advance health directive') to refuse life-sustaining treatment before they lose capacity. Where no advance directive exists or applies in the circumstances, the legislation provides for others to lawfully make decisions to withhold or withdraw life-sustaining treatment on behalf of the adult patient who lacks decision-making capacity. The first of the following people that can be identified can determine what decision regarding withholding or withdrawing life-sustaining treatment gets made for the patient:

➤ An 'enduring guardian' that was appointed by the patient (for health care decisions) before they lost capacity

➤ A guardian appointed by the State Administrative Tribunal who has power to make decisions about health care

➤ A 'person responsible' who is the first of the following to apply:

  – the patient's spouse or de facto partner – where they live with the patient; or

  – the patient's nearest relative who is an adult (spouse, child, parent or sibling) who maintains a close relationship with the person; or

- the person who is the primary carer for the patient (without being paid); or

- any other person who maintains a close personal relationship with the patient.

The State Administrative Tribunal may be approached for advice and directions and the Supreme Court in Western Australia may also make decisions regarding withholding or withdrawing life-sustaining treatment for an adult patient lacking decision-making capacity. (See *Guardianship and Administration Act 1990* (WA), pts 5, 9A–9D.)

Legislation – all children

As noted in Chapter 6, some specific legislation exists which cover the provision of certain types of life-sustaining treatment for all children. For example, the provision of blood transfusions (a form of life-sustaining treatment in some circumstances) is specifically provided for in legislation in some States and Territories (see the section on 'Blood transfusions' in Chapter 6).

Demands for treatment that is not clinically indicated

A related issue at the end of life is whether patients, or their substitute decision-makers, have the right to demand treatment that has not been recommended by their treating team. Sometimes requests will be made for treatment that the treating team does not recommend as it is considered 'futile or non-beneficial treatment'. This term has no legal definition but is often used to describe treatment which is of no benefit, that cannot achieve its purpose or is not in the person's best interests. The common law in Australia generally provides that patients and their substitute decision-makers do not have a legal right to demand treatment that is not recommended by their treating team. This follows the English decision of *R (on the application of Burke) v The General Medical Council* ([2006] QB 273) where the court was of the opinion that even if a patient had decision-making capacity, they did not have a right to demand treatment. The court said 'a patient cannot demand that a doctor administer a treatment which the doctor considers is adverse to the patient's clinical needs'. The court emphasised that while health professionals should discuss requested treatment with patients, if they consider it is not appropriate in the circumstances they should offer to arrange a second opinion.

Where disputes arise between patients, substitute decision-makers and the treating team in relation to end-of-life treatment and care, the mechanisms outlined in Chapter 5 regarding resolution of disputes can apply.

Overview

In this chapter we have covered a range of complex situations and issues that arise at the end of life for both paediatric and adult patients. Decision-making at the end of life is ethically challenging and requires us to consider a number of often competing ethical principles such as beneficence and non-maleficence, or autonomy and the sanctity of life. Having an understanding of these competing interests is necessary to allow you to act in an ethically sensitive manner in dealing with patients at the end of life. It is also recognised that the death or dying of patients in your care may affect you emotionally or spiritually and that this should not be ignored. Development of personal coping qualities are important alongside the technical skills you learn.

We have also covered a range of legal issues that arise at the end of life, from when administration of palliative medication will be lawful to understanding the distinction between euthanasia and assisted suicide, and circumstances when it is lawful to withhold or withdraw life-sustaining treatment from a patient.

Figure 11.1 highlights the interactions between the ethical principles and the legal principles relevant to the end-of-life issues discussed in this chapter.

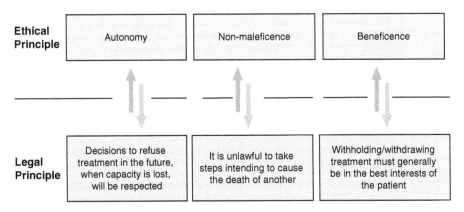

Figure 11.1 Ethical and legal principles relevant to end-of-life issues

Further reading

➤ Freegard, H. 2012, 'End of life' in H. Freegard & L. Isted, eds. *Ethical Practice for Health Professionals*, 2nd edn, Cengage Learning: Sydney.

➤ Australian Commission on Safety and Quality in Health Care. 2015, *National Consensus Statement: Essential elements for safe high quality end of life care*, Sydney, available at www.safetyandquality.gov.au/wp-content/uploads/2015/05/National-Consensus-Statement-Essential-Elements-forsafe-high-quality-end-of-life-care.pdf

➤ End of Life Law in Australia website: https://end-of-life.qut.edu.au

Questions

In 2019 Victoria will allow 'voluntary assisted dying' within a highly regulated legal framework. What are the arguments for and against legalising euthanasia in other States and Territories in Australia?

1. Why does the doctrine of double effect sometimes evoke ethical unease in health professionals?

Scenario

Mr Lam is 30 years old and suffers from metastatic bone cancer. He has frequently attended the oncology unit over the past six months, initially for chemotherapy, but he is now likely to die soon. Mr Lam is popular with nursing staff who have gotten to know him well.

In recent days his condition has deteriorated significantly and he has been moaning in pain and distress. Cancerous growths in his spine are causing him intense pain while metastases in his brain stem threaten death. The goal of Mr Lam's nursing care is now to keep him as comfortable as possible so he has been prescribed a grasby driver with a continuous infusion of morphine. The rate of infusion can be varied by nursing staff but not by the patient.

Finally, Mr Lam pleads to the nurses to do something about the pain, saying 'Please, just make it stop'. A review of his chart shows that the rate of morphine can still be increased; however, nurses note that when he falls asleep his respiratory rate drops and they are concerned that any increase in dose may result in respiratory depression. When he wakes up he is still clearly in pain with the morphine providing inadequate relief. One of the nursing staff says, 'We've got to do something, it's inhumane to leave him like this'.

Apply the ethical decision-making framework to this problem.

12

Issues relevant to reproduction, pregnancy and the birth of a child

Introduction

Planning for children, conceiving and preparing for the birth of a child are significant events in the lives of many individuals, couples and families. Sometimes, individuals and couples will present as patients while going through these events. As such, midwives and nurses may face a myriad of issues relating to reproduction, pregnancy and the birth of a child. In this chapter we look at the legal and ethical issues facing such patients, including the use of assisted reproductive technologies and surrogacy, abortion, prenatal reporting and issues of negligence that relate to conception and birth. (Patient safety and negligence generally are dealt with in Chapter 8 and issues that arise once a child is born are dealt with in Chapter 6.)

During pregnancy nurses and midwives must offer care to pregnant patients but also respect, within limits, the decision that such patients make regarding their own and their developing foetus's wellbeing. Religious, cultural and personal views about their bodies, having children and parenting will guide pregnant women to make different choices. Nurses and midwives are often in a unique position, able to offer information and advice to patients about aspects of their own health and that of their foetus. Pregnancy, birth or the loss of a pregnancy are significant events in the lives of women and their families; often the provision of information and advice will be gratefully received. However, such advice should not become patronising or dictate absolutely what patients can or should do. Such care and respect extends to decisions made during the birthing process, but once a child is born the wellbeing of the child will generally take precedence (see generally Chapter 6).

Ethical issues relating to reproduction, pregnancy and birth

The principles approach

Autonomy and non-maleficence

In the vast majority of circumstances the decisions that a pregnant woman makes will be consistent with their own wellbeing and that of their developing foetus. However, sometimes the decisions of a pregnant patient may be seen to be causing harm to their own health and that of their foetus. For example, decisions about smoking, drinking alcohol or the consumption of certain drugs during pregnancy have known detrimental implications for children once born, as well as impacting on the woman's health. In some cases a pregnant woman may decide to intentionally terminate a pregnancy, that is, have an abortion, whether for medical or social reasons.

Nurses and midwives need to balance the respect for female patients' decision-making autonomy with their ethical obligations of non-maleficence (to prevent harm). Some consider that there is an ethical obligation to interfere with a pregnant woman's conduct where it will harm the foetus so as to protect the foetus from harm (non-maleficence). One example of such conduct is where a woman opts to have an abortion; it also arises where a pregnant woman takes illicit drugs or consumes excessive amounts of alcohol during pregnancy. However, to interfere with a woman's decision as to what happens to her body privileges the interests of the developing foetus over the interests of the pregnant woman. To subordinate the pregnant woman's interests to the developing foetus is to potentially ignore a woman's human right to bodily integrity, privacy and dignity (Royal Commission on New Reproductive Technologies 1993). There is, however, recognition that some health professionals may not be able to reconcile the principles of non-maleficence with such conduct, particularly where they are asked to assist in cases of abortion. As such, health professionals are generally permitted to conscientiously object to taking part in such procedures (see discussion at 'Conscientious objection').

Another area considered in this chapter is the situation where individuals or couples seek help to reproduce. However, the provision of assisted reproductive technologies (ART) and surrogacy services is also an area where autonomy is constrained to some extent. While there are no limitations placed on ordinary procreation, where third parties must assist (such as IVF specialists or surrogates) regulation is often present that limits the options available to people seeking such health services.

There is often an argument that the state has an interest in regulating the provision of such services and that this justifies the incursion on the autonomy of those seeking such services.

Beneficence

The way nurses and midwives maximise beneficence for both a pregnant female and her developing foetus will usually be through the provision of adequate care, support and information for the patient. Nurses and midwives play an important role in giving such support and providing information to promote both the mother's and the developing foetus's health and wellbeing. This may be especially important for some pregnant women who may not be able to easily access such information, whether due to language barriers, lack of services in their local area or lower levels of education about such issues.

There are a number of other situations where nurses and midwives may be particularly important in acting in the best interests of female patients through offering information, care and support. For example, women who are seeking to become pregnant and are undergoing IVF or other forms of fertility services – often an emotionally and physically demanding time – may benefit from such support. For those who become pregnant, information and support from nurses or midwives may be welcome as patients undergo prenatal tests, particularly where abnormalities are detected. Where women suffer a loss of a pregnancy, nurses and midwives may also play an important role. With spontaneous termination of pregnancies being a relatively common, but often traumatic, situation it is likely that nurses and midwives may be in a position to offer care and support to patients suffering such a loss. Women who undergo abortions are also entitled to such care and support from their treating health professionals. In addition, following the birth of a child, midwives and nurses are often in a unique position to help mothers who wish to establish breastfeeding in the period immediately following birth and assist to identify and support women suffering from postpartum depression.

Nurses and midwives also have an important role in working collaboratively with others to ensure that patients and their families receive adequate support. In this context, this will often mean working closely with social workers. Having a good working relationship with other professions is essential in maximising the benefits to the patient and her family.

Justice

One issue relating to justice is the provision of assisted reproductive services. Ideally, the fair distribution of such services would suggest that all persons would have equal access to such services. However, this is not the case in Australia. Many fertility services are primarily available through private practitioners and as such the cost of such services may place them out of reach of many. In the past individuals have been denied access to services based on their marital status or sexual orientation. This position has since changed in relation to IVF but some limitations still exist in relation to accessing surrogacy services in Australia.

Anti-discrimination in the context of provision of fertility services

The provision of fertility services in Australia has been an area where access has historically been limited to certain persons. The position in Victoria and South Australia formerly limited certain fertility services to women who were married or in de facto relationships. Legislation existed in both jurisdictions which meant that single females were essentially denied access to fertility services. However, this situation has changed following successful actions brought by single women in both jurisdictions that found the legislation to be inconsistent with Commonwealth anti-discrimination legislation. In the Victorian case of *McBain v The State of Victoria & Ors* [2000] 99 FCR 116 and the South Australian case of *Pearce v South Australian Health Commission & Ors* (1996) 66 SASR 486 the courts found that legislation limiting access to fertility services to women based on marital status was inconsistent with the *Sex Discrimination Act* 1984 (Cth).

See Szoke, H., Neame, L. & Johnson, L. (2006), pp. 200–203

The nursing and midwifery codes

Informed choice and respect for decisions made

The need to allow pregnant female patients to make informed choices as to their own care and that of their developing foetus is particularly important. This requires the provision of information by health professionals so that pregnant females can make informed choices. Nurses and midwives will often be in a position to provide such information and support to patients. The preamble to the ICN Code of Ethics notes that as part of respecting human rights, the 'right to ... choice' and 'to be treated with respect' must be included. The ICM Code of Ethics is more specific, stating that midwives 'support the right of women/families to participate actively in decisions about their care' (I(b)).

Both international Codes of Ethics importantly refer to the concept of 'informed decision-making' which highlights the importance of health professionals, such as nurses and midwives, disclosing adequate and timely information to patients so that they have sufficient understanding of the choices available to them and so that the decision made by them is ultimately an informed one (ICM Code of Ethics, Principle I(a); ICN Code of Ethics, Element 1). Informed consent is also a key principle in the national Nursing and Midwifery Codes of Conduct (at 2.3). To deny pregnant females the right to make informed decisions about what happens to their bodies is to deny them basic human rights.

Linked to the right of pregnant patients to make decisions is the need to respect the values and beliefs that guide their decision-making. Some patients will be guided by religious, cultural or other personal values which will influence their decisions about accepting medical intervention during pregnancy and birth. The ICM Code of Ethics at II(a) notes that midwives provide care 'with respect for cultural diversity' (but note that they also work to 'eliminate harmful practices within those same cultures'). In addition, I(c) notes midwives' role in empowering women and their families to 'speak for themselves on issues affecting the health of women and families within their culture/society'. The ICN Code of Ethics, at Element 1, states that nurses promote 'an environment in which the human rights, values, customs and spiritual beliefs of the individual, family and community are respected'. Recognising that the patient may embody a particular cultural value or views that influences their choices is important, as is respect for their choice.

Similarly, in Australia, the Codes of Conduct of both professions devote 3.2 to 'culturally safe and respectful practice'. This includes recognising how a nurse's or midwife's own views can influence their interactions with women and families. Principle 3.2(b) and (c) state that nurses and midwives must 'respect diverse cultures' and adopt practices that 'respect diversity'. Principle 3.1 also specifically recognises the importance of Aboriginal and/or Torres Strait Islander Peoples' health in the national context. In dealing with individual patients, Principle 2.2 in the Midwifery Code of Conduct states that midwives must 'take a woman-centred approach to managing' her care which involves, 'supporting the woman in a manner consistent with that woman's values and preferences'. To enable this, requires midwives (and nurses) to develop their knowledge about, and be aware of, different cultural practices. For example, some female patients prefer minimal intervention during pregnancy and childbirth and will opt not to have the usual scans or tests. Others may choose to retain the placenta after birth for cultural or religious reasons. These decisions, while they may seem unusual to some, ought to be respected.

The importance of family

The potential importance of partners and family to the patient in question is recognised in both professions' Codes of Conduct. It is recognised that some patients may wish to involve partners, friends and family, together with nursing, midwifery and other health professionals, in the process of shared decision-making (2.2). Therefore, while the patient is clearly the decision-maker, the potentially important role of her loved ones in helping her to come to decisions, and to help her with issues faced when trying to conceive, when pregnant or during and after labour, is clearly acknowledged. Nurses and midwives may be in a position to assist not only the patient but also their loved ones, in order to benefit the patient.

Conscientious objection

One issue that is particularly relevant for nurses and midwives is where they are asked to be involved in intentional termination of pregnancies in female patients. Some nurses and midwives will see such involvement as no different from taking part in any other care and treatment. However, this is a divisive issue in Australia, particularly when the abortion is not for the pregnant woman's medical wellbeing. Therefore, an acknowledge-ment that some health professionals who are asked to be involved in such procedures may morally object to such acts is contained in the ICM Code of Ethics (at III(c)–(d)) and the national Codes of Conduct (at 4.4 (b)). These statements recognise that nurses and midwives are entitled to conscientiously object to participate in care or treatment they believe on religious or moral grounds to be incompatible with their values, such as abortions. However, they have an explicit obligation to refer patients on to others to ensure they receive appropriate care. As described later in the chapter, this is often something that is reflected in Australian law.

The law relating to reproduction, pregnancy and birth

Laws surrounding reproduction, intervention during pregnancy and issues arising during, or immediately following, birth are varied and com-plex. In this chapter we discuss the key issues that nurses and midwives ought to be aware of in Australia.

Assisted reproductive technologies (ART) and surrogacy

Over 3.6 per cent of births in Australia today are made possible by assisted reproductive technologies (Macaldowie et al. 2010). Or, as noted by the

National Health and Medical Research Council, '1 in 25 individuals who gave birth in Australia in 2012 [used] some form of ART to do so' (NHMRC 2017, p. 13). As such it is becoming increasingly common for couples, or individuals, to seek the assistance of such technologies to conceive children. In addition, the option of engaging a surrogate is also becoming less uncommon.

Procreative autonomy and state regulation

One ethical issue that arises when considering the use of ART and surrogacy relates to whether or not access to such services and treatment ought to be regulated by the government. On the one hand natural reproduction is considered a private issue for individuals to make decisions about. There is no regulation that requires people to be tested as competent parents before conceiving a child. Children are born whether they are conceived while their parents are in a committed relationship or whether sexual intercourse results after a casual encounter – the state does not interfere with the situations in which natural reproduction occurs.

However, the same cannot be said for people who access ART and surrogacy services. In many situations the state does impose some regulation on who can access, and who can provide, such services. As such, there are limits imposed on those individuals' 'procreative autonomy'. Some argue that such interference with a person's procreative autonomy is unjustified – it being a private matter for individuals (Harris 1998, pp. 5–37). On the other hand reasons provided justifying such intervention include:

- Regulation is appropriate where there are concerns about the consequences of conduct (particularly evident when IVF first became available in the 1970s)

- The public has an interest in medical advancement and the availability of services, so it is no longer a strictly private matter between two individuals

- Public money spent on medical advancement in relation to ART justifies state regulation

- The state has a role in ensuring children born using ART will be appropriately cared for.

Szoke (2002), pp. 470–471; Smith and Bennett (2018), [10.20]

The laws relating to assisted reproductive technologies and surrogacy vary throughout Australia. In the following sections a brief overview of the law is provided.

Assisted reproductive technologies (ART)

In this chapter we use the term assisted reproductive technologies (ART) to refer to the 'application of laboratory or clinical techniques to gametes and/or embryos for the purposes of reproduction' (NHMRC 2017, p. 3). This broad term encompasses traditional in vitro fertilisation techniques as well as the less common pre-implantation genetic diagnosis (PGD) (that allows fertilised embryos to be tested for genetic conditions or tissue types).

The scope of ART

The term assisted reproductive technologies refers to an increasingly broad range of interventions to assist in the birth of a healthy child. Traditional IVF refers to fertilisation of a female ovum with male sperm outside the body with the subsequent fertilised ovum then implanted into a woman. In conjunction with this technique (which is used to treat a range of fertility issues) other techniques known as PGD (pre-implantation genetic diagnosis) and PGS (pre-implantation genetic screening) are increasingly being utilised. PGD allows embryos to be genetically tested at a very early stage following fertilisation. It has been used to allow couples to test for known genetic diseases and therefore select embryos without the disease. It has also, more controversially, been used to test for embryos of a particular sex or particular tissue types (to ensure that a resulting child can provide a tissue transplant to an existing patient – usually a sick sibling – suffering from a disease like leukaemia). PGS is a procedure used to test embryos for unspecified genetic abnormalities where there is no known history of genetic disease. This technique is utilised in cases of advanced maternal age or repeated implantation failure (NHMRC 2017). The increasing use of such technologies has led to some fearing that we are on a slippery slope to creating 'designer babies'.

Regulation of ART varies throughout Australia. In New South Wales, South Australia, Victoria and Western Australia there is some legislation that regulates ART (*Assisted Reproductive Technology Act 2007* (NSW); *Assisted Reproduction Treatment Act 1988* (SA); *Assisted Reproductive Treatment Act 2008* (Vic); *Human Reproductive Technology Act 1991* (WA)). The legislation in these states varies but often establishes an authority to oversee ART in that state and generally requires providers to be licensed or registered.

In the other Australian jurisdictions there is no specific legislation. Instead, reliance is placed on National Health and Medical Research Council's *Ethical Guidelines on the Use of Assisted Reproductive Technology in Clinical Practice and Research* (NHMRC 2017) which requires providers of ART to be accredited. The guidelines outline the expected standards regarding use and storage of embryos, use of donated embryos, the provision of information and obtaining consent and record-keeping. In contrast, one issue that is dealt with in a relatively uniform manner in legislation around the country is the prohibition against human cloning.

Surrogacy

Surrogacy generally refers to the situation where a woman (the 'surrogate') agrees with another person or couple (often called the 'commissioning couple' or 'intended parent/s') to become pregnant with the intention of giving the child born to those persons. The surrogate may be the genetic mother of the child (i.e. her ovum has been used to create the embryo) or may be genetically unrelated if an embryo is created using another woman's ovum.

The surrogacy arrangement can be defined as altruistic or commercial surrogacy. Altruistic surrogacy refers to arrangements where no payment is made to the woman acting as a surrogate (other than expenses incurred), whereas in commercial surrogacy arrangements the surrogate is paid a fee for her service in undergoing the pregnancy and birth. In Australia only altruistic surrogacy is lawful. Taking part in a commercial surrogacy is generally an offence, with the perception generally being that such arrangements are too closely associated with the notion of commercialising life that is considered 'unpalatable' (Bennett and Trowse 2018, [12.10]). There are also concerns raised about the exploitation of surrogates. For example, in some countries – such as India – where commercial surrogacy has been allowed, concerns have arisen that 'financially desperate' poorer women are driven to act as surrogates and that the treatment they receive may not be in accordance with international standards (for example, implantation of more embryos than is recommended) (Shetty 2012).

All jurisdictions in Australia except the Northern Territory have legislation which deals to some extent with altruistic surrogacy arrangements (see *Parentage Act 2004* (ACT); *Surrogacy Act 2010* (NSW); *Surrogacy Act 2010* (Qld); *Family Relationships Act 1975* (SA); *Surrogacy Contracts Act 1993* (Tas); *Assisted Reproductive Treatment Act 2008* (Vic); *Surrogacy Act 2008* (WA)).

These laws generally prohibit commercial surrogacy arrangements and advertising of surrogacy services (*Parentage Act 2004* (ACT), pt 4; *Surrogacy Act 2010* (NSW), pt 2, div 2; *Surrogacy Act 2010* (Qld), ch 4, pt 1; *Family Relationships Act 1975* (SA), s 10H; *Surrogacy Act 2012* (Tas), pt 7; *Surrogacy Act 2008* (WA), pt 2, div 2; *Assisted Reproductive Treatment Act 2008* (Vic), ss 44(1), 45). While the legislation in some jurisdictions does not impose conditions on those who wish to enter an altruistic surrogacy arrangement, in New South Wales, South Australia and Victoria conditions do exist. For example, Victoria requires approval from a Patient Review Panel prior to allowing altruistic surrogacy. The Panel must be satisfied of a number of factors, including that the commissioning parent is unlikely to become pregnant or carry a pregnancy to birth, that the surrogate has previously given birth and is at least 25 years old and that all parties have received counselling and legal advice (*Assisted Reproductive Treatment Act 2008* (Vic), s 40).

Typically, as the surrogate is the 'birth' mother of the child, she will be recognised as the legal mother. The majority of jurisdictions (with the exception of the Northern Territory) now have procedures for changing the legally recognised parents specifically in circumstances of surrogacy (see *Family Law Act 1975* (Cth), s 60HB; *Status of Children Act 1974* (Vic), pt IV, div 2, subdiv 1; *Surrogacy Act 2010* (Qld), ch 3, pt 2; *Surrogacy Act 2008* (WA), pt 3, div 3; *Parentage Act 2004* (ACT), pt 2, div 2.5; *Family Relationships Act 1975* (SA), s 10HB; *Surrogacy Act 2010* (NSW), s 12; *Surrogacy Act 2012* (Tas), pt 4, div 1). Alternatively, an application for adoption, or to the Family Court (in relation to who has parental responsibility for the child), can be made.

Abortion

The issue of abortion is an ethically fraught and emotional issue. Here we use the term abortion to mean the intentional termination of pregnancy by drugs or surgical procedure. Abortion is a matter on which polarising views exist in our society.

The abortion debate

The issue of terminating pregnancies and whether or not such actions should be available on demand or criminalised is a very contentious issue. Societal views on abortion may depend on an individual's religion, their views on the status of an embryo or their views on women's rights to choice.

There are various views reflected in society about the morality of abortion. Often this will depend on a person's perspective of when the developing foetus should be recognised as a separate person entitled to protection. Over the years the following positions have emerged regarding when a foetus has its own 'life'. Some consider that abortion after these stages in development of the foetus are morally wrong (Gillon 2001). Gillon notes that some argue that the foetus should be protected from:

▶

◄

- the point of fertilisation; or

- 14 days post-fertilisation when the 'primitive streak' develops; or

- the point of 'ensoulment' (traditionally 40 days for boys and 90 days for girls); or

- the time of 'quickening' – when the pregnant woman first feels the foetus move; or

- the development of 'brain life', that is, a functioning brain; or

- the point of capacity for sentience (i.e. consciousness) which is usually proposed as being around 20–24 weeks; or

- the point of 'viability' – the stage at which the foetus can survive independently of the mother. (This is a point in time which continues to reduce with technological medical advancement – currently around 22 weeks in western nations such as Australia. The point at which a foetus becomes viable and able to survive independent of the mother is often a time which people find significant. However, the issue of viability is determined by what medical treatment and technology are available and as such would differ in a highly resourced hospital in Australia as compared with a rural hospital in a developing country where health care resources are very limited. It is not, therefore, a point that can be accurately determined for all developing foetuses.)

Others consider that the foetus should only be protected from birth. Given this diversity of views regarding the status of the foetus it is not surprising that the issue of abortion, and when it is or is not appropriate, is an ethically complex one. While most people would acknowledge that a developing foetus has certain interests, the scope of those interests and whether they are deserving of protection varies. Some may equate a foetus's rights to protection to those of an adult, while others consider the foetus's interests are not equivalent to the fully fledged rights that individuals – such as the pregnant mother – have. One perspective, which is reflected in the approach of the law, is that the rights of the pregnant woman to choose what should be done to her own body, including the developing foetus within her, remain paramount (Royal Commission on New Reproductive Technologies 1993).

A further issue which complicates the abortion debate is that some laws allow for abortion on the grounds of foetal disability. With increased availability and specificity of prenatal tests available for pregnant woman, the detection of conditions – such as Down's Syndrome – has become increasingly common. This has resulted in disability rights advocates suggesting that abortion on the grounds of foetal abnormality devalues the worth of a disabled life and, as such, is disrespectful to disabled people (Mcguinness 2013).

In some countries, particularly Asian countries and India, sex-selective abortion has also been used as a method to ensure the birth of male children where sons are preferred. This appears to be a contributing factor to the social problem of gender imbalance which is becoming more prevalent in these countries (Hesketh and Xing 2006).

Given the variety of issues and diversity of views on this topic it is not surprising that existing laws regarding abortion and law reform in this area remain controversial.

The law in Australia regarding abortion has historically been complex and confusing, with each State and Territory having different laws. Previously, the act of carrying out an abortion was considered a criminal act; however, there is now a clear trend towards removing abortion from the criminal law. Most States and Territories have modernised their legal approach by decriminalising abortion, while only a minority have kept the old model. As discussed in the sections that follow, this has resulted in more 'modern' laws in the majority of jurisdictions and, in general, a common approach to this issue in most of Australia. Here we discuss the law that applies in each State and Territory in Australia.

The Australian Capital Territory

In the Australian Capital Territory the only legal limitations on abortions being carried out are contained in part 6 of the *Health Act 1993* (ACT). This legislation states that it is an offence for a person other than a doctor to carry out an abortion or for an abortion to be carried out in an unapproved facility. Offences relating to abortion were removed in 2002 following the enactment of the *Crimes (Abolition of the Offence of Abortion) Act 2002* (ACT).

The legislation makes clear in the Australian Capital Territory that a person can refuse to assist in carrying out an abortion (*Health Act 1993* (ACT), s 84).

New South Wales

The law in New South Wales regarding the legality of abortion is complex and relies on both the criminal law and the common law. Unlike the other jurisdictions, New South Wales has not modernised their laws regarding abortion.

The *Crimes Act 1900* (NSW) has provisions (ss 82–84) which state that a pregnant women who 'unlawfully administers to herself any drug or noxious thing, or unlawfully uses any instrument or other means' and who intends to procure a miscarriage shall be guilty of a crime. Similarly, any person who causes an abortion in a woman or supplies the drugs that causes an abortion will be subject to the criminal law. While these provisions would appear to make any woman who has an abortion, or any doctor who provides an abortion, to be guilty of a crime, these provisions must be read in light of the interpretation given to them by case law.

The cases of *R v Wald* (1971) 3 DCR (NSW) and *CES v Superclinics (Australia) Pty Ltd* (1995) 38 NSWLR 47 interpreted provisions of the *Crimes Act 1900* (NSW) such that where a doctor forms an honest belief on reasonable grounds (economic, social or medical grounds) that the abortion is necessary to preserve a woman's life or health (including psychological health), they will not be guilty of an offence. This interpretation was confirmed in the case *R v Sood* [2006] NSWSC 1141 (see box).

R v Sood [2006] NSWSC 1141

In this New South Wales case Dr Sood was found guilty and convicted of administering and supplying a drug with intent to procure a miscarriage in a patient under the *Crimes Act* 1900 (NSW). The pregnant patient had sought a late-term abortion from Dr Sood who administered prostaglandin tablets to the patient and supplied further tablets to induce labour without physically examining the patient. The woman later gave birth to a baby boy who died; there was conflicting evidence regarding whether the baby was born alive.

It was accepted on the evidence that Dr Sood did not honestly and genuinely hold the belief that the abortion was necessary in order to protect the mother from serious danger to her life or health, whether physical or mental. As such, the abortion was unlawful. The penalty imposed by the court was a two-year good behaviour bond. (In separate disciplinary action Dr Sood was also banned from practising medicine for ten years.)

Northern Territory

The law in the Northern Territory was modernised in 2017 with the introduction of the *Termination of Pregnancy Law Reform Act* (NT). The new legislation provides that abortions can be performed by doctors up to 14 weeks of pregnancy if considered appropriate, having regard to all the circumstances. This encompasses the woman's medical circumstances and her current and future psychological and social circumstances, and includes consideration of professional guidelines and standards (s 7).

Importantly, the legislation provides that authorised Aboriginal and Torres Strait Islander health practitioners, midwives and nurses may supply or administer a termination drug when directed by a doctor where the woman is not more than 14 weeks' pregnant (s 8).

Where the pregnancy is between 14 and 23 weeks' duration, the doctor must consult with at least one other doctor and they must both consider the termination to be appropriate in circumstances – taking into account the same factors (i.e. medical circumstances, current and future psychological and social circumstances, and consideration of professional guidelines and standards) (s 9).

One exception to these provisions is where a doctor considers the abortion is 'necessary to preserve the life of the woman', in which case an abortion can be performed (s 10).

Any health professional (including nurses and midwives) can conscientiously object to taking part in an abortion procedure. In that circumstance the doctor must direct other health professionals, who do not object, to assist. However, if an emergency abortion is necessary to save the woman's life, then a nurse or midwife is legally obligated to assist (ss 11–13).

Where abortions are carried out by unqualified persons (i.e. persons other than authorised health professionals), then they commit an offence (*Criminal Code Act* (NT), s 208A).

Queensland

The situation in Queensland was recently reformed with the introduction of the *Termination of Pregnancy Act 2018* (Qld). Prior to this, Queensland was similar to New South Wales, being governed by sections of the criminal law and cases which had interpreted those sections. However, following a review by the Queensland Law Reform Commission (QLRC 2018), new laws were introduced to decriminalise abortion in Queensland.

The legislation states that a termination may be performed by a medical practitioner on a woman who is not more than 22 weeks pregnant (s 5). After 22 weeks, termination can only occur if two medical practitioners consider that the termination should be performed, taking into account the woman's 'current and future physical, psychological and social circumstances' and the relevant 'professionals standards and guidelines' (s 6). A nurse, midwife or Aboriginal and Torres Strait Islander health practitioner may assist a medical practitioner in performing the termination (s 7).

The legislation allows health professionals to not participate in abortions where they conscientiously object. But health professionals are required by section 8 to refer the woman requesting an abortion to another health professional. One circumstance where nurses and midwives are unable to act on a conscientious objection is when a termination needs to be performed in an emergency. In this circumstance nurses and midwives are under a legal duty to assist.

South Australia

Section 82A of the *Criminal Law Consolidation Act 1935* (SA) outlines the circumstances where an abortion is lawful. Abortions can be carried out in hospitals when two doctors who have examined the woman form an opinion in good faith that:

➤ the continuance of the pregnancy would involve greater risk to the life of the pregnant woman, or greater risk of injury to the physical or mental health of the pregnant woman, than if the pregnancy were terminated; or

➤ that there is a substantial risk that, if the pregnancy were not terminated and the child were born to the pregnant woman, the child would suffer from such physical or mental abnormalities as to be seriously handicapped.

It is also lawful to carry out an abortion where one doctor considers that it is necessary to save the life, or to prevent grave injury to the physical or mental health, of the pregnant woman. However, it is an offence to carry out abortions outside of these circumstances (ss 81–82).

Tasmania

In Tasmania, the *Reproductive Health (Access to Termination) Act 2013* (Tas) outlines the circumstances where it is lawful for abortion to occur. It states that abortion can be performed by a doctor up to 16 weeks with the consent of the pregnant woman (s 4).

For abortions after 16 weeks, additional conditions need to be fulfilled. A doctor must:

➤ reasonably believe that the continuation of the pregnancy would involve greater risk of injury to the physical or mental health of the pregnant woman (taking into account physical, psychological, economic and social circumstances) than if the pregnancy were terminated; and another doctor agrees with the assessment (s 5).

Like some of the other jurisdictions, the legislation states that a person who has a conscientious objection to participating in an abortion need not take part or assist in such a procedure. However, this does not affect a nurse or midwife who 'has a duty to assist' a doctor in performing an abortion 'in an emergency if the termination is necessary to save the life of a pregnant woman or to prevent her serious physical injury' (s 6).

Victoria

For women not more than 24 weeks' pregnant the *Abortion Law Reform Act 2008* (Vic) states:

➢ that a doctor is able to perform an abortion on a woman (s 4); and

➢ that a registered nurse or midwife who is authorised to supply drugs can supply or administer drugs to cause an abortion in a woman (s 6).

However, for abortions after 24 weeks there are further conditions that need to be satisfied for the abortion to be lawful. Abortions can only be performed after 24 weeks when two doctors reasonably believe that abortion is appropriate in all the circumstances, having regard to all relevant medical circumstances and the woman's current and future physical, psychological and social circumstances (s 5). In addition, registered nurses or midwives can supply or administer drugs to cause an abortion in a woman who is more than 24 weeks' pregnant if they:

➢ are employed by a hospital; and

➢ have a written direction from a doctor (who has satisfied themselves that the abortion is appropriate in the circumstances) to do so (s 7).

Abortions performed by an unqualified person remains an offence under the *Crimes Act 1958* (Vic) (s 65).

The legislation allows health professionals to not participate in abortions where they conscientiously object. But health professionals are required by section 8 to refer the woman requesting an abortion to another health professional. One circumstance where nurses and midwives are unable to act on a conscientious objection is where their assistance is required when a doctor performs an abortion in an emergency to preserve the life of the pregnant woman. In this circumstance section 8 states that nurses and midwives are under a legal duty to assist.

Western Australia

The circumstances in which abortions can be carried out lawfully in Western Australia are outlined in section 334 of the *Health Act 1911* (WA). It provides that for woman less than 20 weeks' pregnant abortions are lawful where:

➢ the woman concerned has given informed consent; or

➢ the woman concerned will suffer serious personal, family or social consequences if the abortion is not performed; or

➢ serious danger to the physical or mental health of the woman concerned will result if the abortion is not performed; or

➤ the pregnancy of the woman concerned is causing serious danger to her physical or mental health.

For women over 20 weeks' pregnant, the legislation requires that two doctors from a panel of doctors appointed by the Minister 'have agreed that the mother, or the unborn child, has a severe medical condition that, in the clinical judgment of those two doctors, justifies the procedure' and the abortion is performed in an approved facility (s 334(7)). The legislation also states that no person is under a duty to assist or to perform an abortion (s 334(2)).

If abortions are performed that do not comply with section 334 of the *Health Act 1911* (WA), then this results in an offence being committed (*Criminal Code* (WA), s 199).

Prenatal reporting

Most jurisdictions in Australia have laws which allow concerned persons to make a report, and officials to act on information, where there is significant concern that a child to be born may require care and assistance after birth. The purpose of such provisions is generally to allow support to be given to the pregnant woman to reduce 'risky behaviours' that can affect the foetus or newborn (e.g. substance abuse or family violence), therefore reducing the likelihood of risk to the child when born (Taplin 2017). It also provides early information that a child who is not yet born may be at risk of harm following birth. Midwives and nurses may be in a position to view such circumstances given their unique relationship with women during pregnancy.

Such provisions exist in some form in the Australian Capital Territory, New South Wales, Queensland, South Australia, Tasmania, Victoria and Western Australia (*Children and Young People Act 2008* (ACT), pt 11.1, div 11.1.3; *Children and Young Persons (Care and Protection) Act 1998* (NSW), s 25; *Child Protection Act 1999* (Qld), s 21A; *Children and Young People (Safety) Act 2017* (SA), s 31(3)-(4); *Children, Young Persons and Their Families Act 1997* (Tas), s 13(1A); *Children, Youth and Families Act 2005* (Vic), ss 29, 30, 32, 33; *Children and Community Services Act 2004* (WA), s 33A, 33B).

While these reporting obligations are generally voluntary, the situation in Tasmania is different. In Tasmania the obligation to report is mandatory if a person suspects on reasonable ground that the child of a pregnancy once born is 'reasonably likely' to suffer abuse or neglect or require treatment or other intervention due to the behaviour of the woman or others she lives with (*Children, Young Persons and Their Families Act 1997* (Tas), s 13(1A)).

Consent and emergency caesareans

While an ethical conflict can arise between the rights of the woman to complete control over what happens to her body during pregnancy and labour and the interests of the unborn foetus, in law, resolving these issues is relatively clear.

Legally, the unborn foetus is not considered an individual person until they are born alive. Regardless of a person's ethical view as to when the developing foetus should be given the same rights as other persons (see discussion at 'Autonomy and non-maleficence'), at law, until they are born they are not viewed as an independent person from the pregnant woman and have no independent legal rights. Where a pregnant woman is competent, she can decide what treatment to have or not have. This can cause controversy when, for example, an emergency caesarean section is recommended but the pregnant woman refuses. In these circumstances, the woman's health and that of the unborn child are at risk. Despite this, the law is quite clear that a competent pregnant woman retains the legal right to make decisions to consent or refuse consent to treatment.

If a woman is not deemed competent to make decisions about her own health care, then it may be possible to legally override her refusal of recommended procedures (such as emergency caesarean sections). This may occur under the guardianship legislation (see Chapter 5) or under the mental health legislation (see Chapter 9), depending on the situation of the pregnant woman. The British case of *St George's Healthcare NHS Trust v S, R v Collins, ex p S* [1998] 3 All ER 673 (see box) demonstrates these legal principles.

St George's Healthcare NHS Trust v S, R v Collins, ex p S [1998] 3 All ER 673

In this British case the patient was suffering from pre-eclampsia and had been advised that a caesarean section was required. The patient wanted to have a natural birth and refused to be admitted to hospital for a caesarean. She was fully aware of the risks to herself and her unborn child. The hospital utilised mental health legislation to keep the patient in hospital despite her being competent to refuse consent to treatment. The hospital also sought an order from the court to require the patient to have a caesarean section to safeguard the foetus. The court granted the order and the caesarean was performed despite the patient's refusal.

After the caesarean was performed, the patient appealed the court order and was successful. The Court of Appeal found that the treatment imposed was unlawful (it being a trespass to her person; see the discussion in Chapter 5 on 'Civil trespass').

▶

The Court of Appeal concluded that the woman should not have been made to undergo a caesarean section and criticised the use of the mental health legislation to detain her. The Court made clear that a competent pregnant woman has the absolute right to refuse medical intervention regardless of the risks to herself or her foetus.

Negligence actions relating to pregnancy and birth

While midwives and nurses may be found to be generally negligent in their conduct when providing care to a patient (and we discuss in detail the law relating to medical negligence in Chapter 8), three specific negligence actions against health professionals (usually doctors) arise in relation to conception and birth which are useful to highlight here. These three negligence actions have become known as 'wrongful conception', 'wrongful birth' and 'wrongful life' actions. Table 12.1 summarises these three actions and outlines the person bringing the action against the health professional in each case.

Wrongful conception

As shown in Table 12.1, an action in negligence against a health professional for 'wrongful conception' refers to a negligence action in performing a sterilisation procedure which resulted in the birth of a child. The parent or parents are the individuals seeking compensation from the health professional in this case. The key Australian case is High Court case of *Cattanach v Melchior* (2003) 215 CLR 1 (see box). That case confirmed

Table 12.1   Negligence actions in relation to conception and birth

Type of negligence action	Description of the action	Who brings the action
Wrongful conception	An action for monetary compensation (damages) for the birth of an unplanned child usually following an unsuccessful sterilisation procedure.	Parent
Wrongful birth	An action for monetary compensation (damages) for the birth of an unplanned child due to failure to diagnose a pregnancy.	Parent
Wrongful life	An action for monetary compensation (damages) for the birth of a disabled child following negligent care of the pregnant mother.	Disabled child who is born

that where negligence is found on the part of the health professional in performing a sterilisation, and a child is subsequently born, the costs of raising that child were recoverable.

Cattanach v Melchior (2003) 215 CLR 1

In this case Dr Cattanach, an obstetrician and gynaecologist, was negligent in providing advice regarding the effectiveness of a sterilisation procedure that he performed on Mrs Melchoir. Mrs Melchior believed that her right fallopian tube had been removed as a child. It was found that Dr Cattanach had too readily accepted Mrs Melchior's assertion that her right fallopian tube had been removed. Instead he should have advised her to have that specifically investigated, and he should have warned her that, if she was wrong, there was a risk that she might become pregnant. Following the procedure, Mrs Melchior became pregnant and gave birth to a healthy child.

The Australian High Court case dealt with the question of whether parents of a healthy child born due to the negligence of a doctor were entitled to recover from the negligent doctor the costs of raising the child. The majority of the High Court agreed that the parents were entitled to money for the reasonable costs of raising and maintaining their child.

A number of States have passed legislation to alter the common law principle allowing parents to receive compensation for the cost of raising a child in actions for wrongful conception (see, for example, *Civil Liability Act 2002* (NSW), s 71; *Civil Liability Act 2003* (Qld), ss 49A, 49B; *Civil Liability Act 1936* (SA), s 67). In these jurisdictions a court is unable to award damages for the cost of raising a healthy child.

Wrongful birth

This action refers to negligence on the part of a health professional in failing to diagnose a pregnancy which then results in the undesired birth of a child. The argument here is that the negligence removes the pregnant women's chance of terminating the pregnancy. Here the action is taken by the parent against the health professional. In one case of wrongful birth, a woman sued due to the repeated failure of doctors to diagnose her pregnancy despite her repeated consultations with them. The New South Wales Court of Appeal found that while damages were recoverable by the female patient those damages did not extend to the cost of raising the child that was born (*CES v Superclinics (Aust) P/L* (1995) 38 NSWLR 47).

Wrongful life

A wrongful life action is an action taken by a disabled child who was born following negligent care of the mother. The negligent care often denies the mother the opportunity to seek an abortion. Claiming monetary compensation in such circumstances is controversial as the child is essentially claiming compensation for the fact that they are alive as a disabled child, versus not being alive (i.e. they would have been terminated had there been no negligence). This issue came before the Australian High Court in the case of *Harriton v Stephens* (2006) 226 CLR 52. In that case, a female infant, Alexia, had been born with severe disabilities, including spasticity and mental retardation, due to the fact that her mother was incorrectly informed about her rubella status while she was pregnant. Alexia's mother asserted that she would have had an abortion if she had been correctly informed. Alexia brought the action against the doctor who had incorrectly informed her mother. The High Court, while conceding that the doctor had made a mistake, did not allow the action to succeed. One of the reasons why the High Court did not allow recovery was on the basis that allowing Alexia to recover may raise the perception that the law did not value life with a disability.

Notification and registration of birth

In all jurisdictions in Australia there are legal obligations on those present at a birth to notify a government official (known as the Registrar) of the birth of a child. This obligation falls to attending midwives who have the care of the mother, if no doctor is present at the birth. (*Births, Deaths and Marriages Registration Act 1997* (ACT), s 5; *Births, Deaths and Marriages Registration Act* (NT), s 12; *Births, Deaths and Marriages Registration Act 1995* (NSW), s 12; *Births, Deaths and Marriages Registration Act 2003* (Qld), s 5; *Births, Deaths and Marriages Registration Act 1996* (SA), s 12; *Births, Deaths and Marriages Registration Act 1999* (Tas), s 11; *Births, Deaths and Marriages Registration Act 1996* (Vic), s 12; *Births, Deaths and Marriages Registration Act 1998* (WA), s 12.)

Overview

In this chapter we have covered a variety of legal and ethical issues relating to reproduction, pregnancy and birth. Often we have seen a tension arise between the autonomy of individuals and the interest of

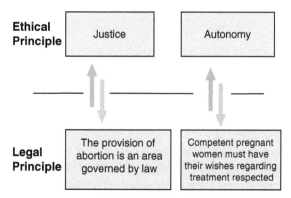

Figure 12.1   Ethical and legal principles relevant to reproduction, pregnancy and birth

government in regulating aspects of reproduction (particularly in relation to ART, surrogacy and abortion). These issues are ethically complex and nurses and midwives need to be cognisant of the variety of views on these issues. They need to offer adequate care and support to their patients – whether this is a woman who was formerly pregnant (but lost the pregnancy via spontaneous miscarriage or intentional abortion), a currently pregnant female or persons seeking to become pregnant through ART or surrogacy.

We have also seen that the law is often complex and varied in approaching these issues throughout Australia. Given the pace of technological development and society's evolving views on these issues, legal reform in these areas seems inevitable in the future.

Further reading

Bennett, B. & Douglas, H. 2018, 'Abortion' in B. White, F. McDonald & L. Willmott, eds. *Health Law in Australia*, 3rd edn, Thomson Reuters: Sydney.
Meredith, S. 2005, *Policing Pregnancy: The Law and Ethics of Obstetric Conflict*, Ashgate: London.

Questions

1. Consider how the interests of a pregnant patient and the developing foetus can be balanced in circumstances where the patient may be acting in a manner contrary to both the patient's health and the developing foetus's health.

2. Should assisted reproductive technologies be freely available and not subject to any form of regulation or is this a matter in which governments are justified in intervening? Provide reasons for your view.

Scenarios

1. Bella is a 25-year-old patient who presented to a public hospital suffering from extreme anxiety. She had a history of bipolar disorder and was found to be 13 weeks' pregnant. On being told of her pregnancy Bella became upset and requested an abortion. She was assessed by her treating doctor as being likely to suffer extreme mental stress if her pregnancy was allowed to continue and she was to give birth.
   Oskar is a registered nurse who has recently begun working at the hospital. He is asked to assist by caring for Bella while she attends the hospital for her procedure to induce a termination of the pregnancy. While Oskar is committed to his patients he disagrees from a moral perspective with aborting a developing foetus. Oskar is unsure what to do but does not want to take any part in the care of Bella when it involves terminating her pregnancy.

Apply the ethical decision-making framework to this scenario.

2. Lee Lin is a midwife who provides prenatal care and assessments to pregnant women in her small regional town. One of her patients, Ellen, has attended on a number of occasions and has said she is suffering hardship at home. She confided with Lee Lin that her boyfriend – with whom she lives – has been difficult about the pregnancy and initially wanted her to get an abortion. Ellen is adamant that she wants to keep the baby and is looking forward to being a mother. One day she attended for an appointment and admitted that her boyfriend had hit her. Ellen says she's worried about him hurting her baby and, while she wants to leave her boyfriend, she cannot see how she can do it.

Apply the ethical decision-making framework to this scenario.

13

Ethics, law and Aboriginal and Torres Strait Islander patients

Introduction

Aboriginal and/or Torres Strait Islander peoples are parts of the longest continuous practising cultures on Earth. They have been custodians of the land and islands that are now called Australia since the Dreamtime or over 60,000 years. Aboriginal and Torres Strait Islanders comprise, as of 2016, 3.3 per cent of the population (ABS 2018). There are hundreds of vibrant nations or language groups, although many languages are now endangered. The values and traditions among these nations or groups will differ and are not static. There are complex kinship practices and social roles and responsibilities among each nation and language group. In the context of health care these nations and groups have their own ancient healing practices and healers.

Aboriginal and/or Torres Strait Islanders have lesser life expectancy than non-Indigenous Australians and are generally less healthy (Commonwealth of Australia 2017a). They also experience significant disadvantage in other areas that are social determinants for good health, such as education, employment, housing and income. The Aboriginal and Torres Strait Islander Social Justice Commissioner (2005) attributed the health inequalities experienced by Aboriginal and Torres Strait Islander peoples to systematic discrimination through the inaccessibility of health services and the inadequate provision of health-related infrastructure (including clean drinking water, sewerage systems and healthy housing). Others have noted more generally the powerlessness of Aboriginal and/or Torres Strait Islander peoples (Uluru Declaration 2017) and intergenerational trauma and grief resulting from many factors, including colonisation, massacres, alienation from land, destruction of culture, racism and racist policies and the Stolen Generations (Griffiths et al. 2016). In working with Aboriginal and/or Torres Strait Islanders it is critical to acknowledge this history of oppression.

There is often a consequent lack of trust by Aboriginal and/or Torres Strait Islander peoples in the institutions of the state, including health services and health professionals. Nurses and midwives have been perceived by Aboriginal and/or Torres Strait Islanders as implementers of discriminatory government policies aimed at Aboriginal and/or Torres Strait Islanders, such as sterilising Aboriginal women without consent, separation of children from parents, enforcing segregated wards (Commonwealth of Australia 1997), the mandatory medical checks of the Northern Territory intervention and so on. Additionally, health professionals, including nurses and midwives, have contributed to and some continue to contribute to the development of racist, pejorative and disempowering stereotypes of Aboriginal and/or Torres Strait Islander peoples. For example, much early research undertaken by health professionals and scientists aimed to prove Aboriginal and Torres Strait Islander peoples were racially inferior to those of European descent (Kerridge et al. 2013).

Health professionals and scientists have considerable influence over the eventual abandonment of negative stereotypes of Aboriginal and/or Torres Strait Islander peoples. Sometimes these stereotypes are deeply embedded into the consciousness of some non-Indigenous Australians and are not recognised as shaping their practices and relationships. Western cultural practices are privileged in Australia generally, and in the health system, and the knowledge, beliefs and values of Aboriginal and/or Torres Strait Islander peoples may be devalued or ignored as a consequence. The challenge going forward is how to ensure 'the health system is safe, accessible and responsive for Aboriginal and Torres Strait Islander people and cultural values, strengths and differences are respected' (Australian Health Ministers' Advisory Council 2016, p. 5).

We acknowledge that there is an ethical question about whether it is respectful for non-Indigenous persons, such as the authors of this book, to write about, and hence appropriate, the health status and values of Aboriginal and/or Torres Strait Islanders peoples and to construct another non-Aboriginal representation of the values or needs of Aboriginal and/or Torres Strait Islander peoples (Kerridge et al. 2013). We are sensitive to these concerns. Our analysis reflects the fact that we are not Indigenous and therefore we cannot and do not truly understand the lived experiences of Aboriginal and/or Torres Strait Islander peoples. In this chapter we examine some ethical responsibilities and issues for nurses and midwives in providing care to Aboriginal and/or Torres Strait Islander patients, their families and communities by examining ethical principles and the relevant sections of the Codes of Ethics and Conduct. We also examine relevant law.

Ethics and nursing and midwifery practice

The principles approach

It should not be assumed that ethical models derived from a western individualistic viewpoint can or should be automatically applied to Aboriginal and/or Torres Strait Islander individuals and communities. The principles model was developed in the United States in the context of acute tertiary-level hospital care. It was not designed to consider the needs of persons from less individualistic cultures. That is not to say that the principles model is not useful; it is more that parts of it, in some circumstances, may need to be discarded or greatly modified.

Justice

The principle of justice is very relevant to providing health care to Aboriginal and/or Torres Strait Islander peoples. Rights-based justice is important as there is recognition at the international level that Indigenous peoples have specific collective human rights associated with their status as First Peoples. The United Nations *Declaration on the Rights of Indigenous Persons* is discussed later in this chapter but recognises that Indigenous persons have rights associated with accessing health services, having the highest attainable standard of health, and retaining their traditional medicines and health practices.

Distributive justice is also important. Reducing health inequalities is about fairness and social justice (Marmot et al. 2010). There is a significant disparity in life expectancy between Indigenous and non-Indigenous Australians. Life expectancy for Aboriginal and/or Torres Strait Islander men is 12.4 years less than for non-Indigenous men and 10.9 years less for Aboriginal and/or Torres Strait Islander women (Australian Bureau of Statistics 2012). Chronic conditions are the major cause of death and illness among Aboriginal and/or Torres Strait Islander peoples, accounting for two-thirds of the life expectancy gap (AIHW 2015). Aboriginal and/or Torres Strait Islander peoples experience greater disparities in health outcomes and have lower life expectancies than Indigenous populations in New Zealand, Canada and the United States (Commonwealth of Australia 2008). There are a number of elements to access to health services, which includes physical proximity to services, such as distance or drive time (availability); financial aspects (affordability); and cultural aspects (acceptability). In 2012–13, 30 per cent of Aboriginal and/or Torres Strait Islanders surveyed reported that they needed to but did not access a health professional or hospital in the previous 12 months. Reasons varied across types of services being accessed (but data on nurses and midwives were not analysed). Reasons for not going to a doctor included being too busy (30 per cent); waiting too long/service not available at time required (22 per cent); transport/distance (14 per cent); dislikes service/professional or is embarrassed/afraid (14 per cent); cost of service (13 per cent); felt service would be inadequate (9 per cent); does not trust service provider (6 per cent); service not available in area (5 per cent); and discrimination/not culturally appropriate/language problem (3 per cent) (Commonwealth of Australia 2017a).

Beneficence and non-maleficence

Beneficence (acting in the best interests of the patient) is a problematic principle when applied to Aboriginal and/or Torres Strait Islander patients and communities. This is because there is a long history of policies and practices which have systematically diminished the values and decisions of Aboriginal and/or Torres Strait Islanders in all aspects of their lives, including health-related choices. This is in part a legacy of colonial policies that considered Aboriginal and/or Torres Strait Islanders to be racially inferior and therefore in need of protection and of 'civilising'. Also given the structural disadvantages (for example, poverty) faced by some Aboriginal and/or Torres Strait Islanders, there may be a tendency by some that Aboriginal and/or Torres Strait Islanders need to be protected and steered into 'good' decisions. But as Henry and colleagues (2004) note:

> Lack of respect by white Australians for Aboriginal values, the discounting of these values by those who have sought, patronisingly and paternalistically, to 'do good' to Aboriginal people (according to a 'good' defined by white fellas), leads to further erosion of trust.

Conversely, it would be very much in the interests of Aboriginal and/or Torres Strait Islanders to receive care that is respectful of them and their culture and seeks to build relationships based on a partnership model of care. There is evidence to suggest that patient outcomes improve when patients' emotional and personal concerns are taken into account (Levinson et al. 2000).

Non-maleficence is the duty to do no needless harm. The harm to a patient as perceived by nurses and midwives will often be framed around clinical concerns, and the broader harms associated with ignoring or diminishing the values of the person, their family and their community may be overlooked. In addition, racist attitudes towards Aboriginal and/or Torres Strait Islanders peoples have the potential to cause significant harm immediately or in the long term.

> ## Quote from a participant in research conducted by Durey and Thompson (2012)
>
> *'One thing I would say about racism in hospitals is that sometimes things seem racist from the patient perspective even when they are not. And I suspect the feeling of racism is as bad as the real thing – in terms of flow on effects. Recently, a patient of mine walked out of an oncology clinic because "other people were being taken in ahead of her". As a result, she was refusing to continue her medication, refusing all further follow up and was in a really bad way. When I followed this up with the clinic, they said that my patient had arrived 30 minutes early and the patients seen before her had earlier bookings. My patient's interpretation of this "innocent" situation was based on her life-long experience of manifest indisputable racism. And she was especially vulnerable because of the nature and severity of her illness. Sadly, the outcome could have been very bad as she had been responding well to treatment.'*

Another element of beneficence is the duty to take professional development and training. In this instance nurses and midwives should be identifying their need for, and actively seeking out, advice, assistance and input in building care partnerships with Aboriginal and/or Torres Strait Islander patients and their families and communities. This input could be from taking advantage of professional development opportunities, participating in Aboriginal and/or Torres Strait Islander cultural events and seeking advice from Aboriginal and Torres Strait Islander staff.

Autonomy

Autonomy is a core value in western health systems and is premised on an individual making decisions in their best interest. This premise does not necessarily hold for all Aboriginal and/or Torres Strait Islander peoples whose decision-making practices may have a more collective orientation, or may be delegated to specific people within their family or community (see Chapter 5). This does not mean to say that autonomy is not important, but that it might manifest in other ways. One challenge is that legal processes in Australia require individual consent, which can cause tension between the desire to respect the decision-making processes of the individual and their particular family or community practices, and the need to meet legal and institutional requirements.

There are three requirements for consent to be legally valid – that the patient has capacity; is informed (which includes effective communication); and makes a voluntary decision (see Chapters 5 and 8). In terms of capacity or competence this may be difficult. The presumption specified in Australian law is that a person has capacity unless there is a good reason to suspect they do not. However, sometimes stereotypes of Aboriginal and/or Torres Strait Islanders can give rise to an unfair and unlawful presumption that an Aboriginal and/or Torres Strait Islander is not competent. Additionally, criteria for capacity assessment were developed on the basis of the norms of non-Indigenous persons. Also, if English is not the person's first language, this will affect the validity of the assessment. In the absence of capacity assessment processes that have been validated against that person's first language, there needs to be greater reliance on translators, Aboriginal and/or Torres Strait Islander health workers, and families to assist in assessing capacity. 'Normalcy' of behaviour will be assessed and these norms vary between cultures. A faith in practices, such as sorcery, may be seen as a sign of mental illness, for example, by those who do not share those beliefs. Similarly silence may be taken as a symptom of not understanding, when it is simply a different style of communication.

Consent must be informed. This relies on effective communication and so a translator may be required if English is not the person's first language. But if the person speaks a number of languages it is important that the translator can translate into the person's first language, instead of their second or third language, but this relies on nurses and midwives, or other health professionals, taking the time to understand where the person comes from to access the most appropriate translator. The legal test for informed consent includes the provision of information that the particular patient would consider important. This may require, in addition to respectful engagement with the patient, support from an Aboriginal and/or Torres Strait Islander liaison or the use of other supports, such as family, to better understand that person's specific context and to better communicate with that patient and their family. There may come a point where health professionals and patients talk past each other as there may be no shared understandings of concepts of health or disease (McGrath and Phillips 2008), but family and Aboriginal and/or Torres Strait Islander health workers may also be able to assist with this.

That the person's decision is voluntary is also important. One factor that is often examined when thinking about voluntariness is whether the family, or other people, are placing pressure on the person to make a decision in a certain way. However, what may be perceived as familial pressure can be normal dynamics if consent processes are not individually focused. Kerridge and colleagues (2013) have also noted that the institution of the hospital can place pressure on Aboriginal and/or Torres Strait Islander patients to make decisions that health professionals are perceived as wanting them to make. The emphasis on efficient processes to enable a volume of patients to be assessed and treated may create an expectation by health professionals that communication and decision-making will occur quickly to meet organisational needs. However, longer, more supportive processes that enable Aboriginal and Torres Strait Islander patients to consult with family and community leaders, who may be some distance away, in a less coercive environment may minimise the possibility of duress. There is some research that suggests that Aboriginal and Torres Strait Islander patients are likely to be less 'compliant' with a course of treatment than non-Indigenous patients on aggregate (Kerridge et al. 2013). This could be characterised as a form of resistance, perhaps to consent obtained under (unintentional) institutional duress, or because the offered treatment does not fit with the way the patient lives their life and their values as a member of a particular community. This then is not a compliance issue but an autonomous choice to refuse treatment. Other reasons could be educational, communication and systemic faults in health care delivery or in social supports more generally (Kerridge et al. 2013). Research has also indicated that Aboriginal and/or Torres Strait Islander patients are more likely not to withdraw from treatment if supported by family when decisions are made (Kerridge et al. 2013).

All of these factors mean that if nurses and midwives are truly committed to the principle of autonomy, then they will need to understand that autonomy can manifest in different ways with less focus on the individual. Nurses and midwives will need to listen, be sensitive and use appropriate supports to endeavour to effectively communicate with patients and families, acknowledging and accepting that this may take time and extensive consultation.

Respect

A core principle that sits behind the four principles that are discussed above, and which is a key tenet of international and domestic human rights law, is respect for human dignity. Article 1 of the *United Nation's Universal Declaration of Human Rights* states:

> All human beings are born free and equal in dignity and rights. They are endowed with reason and conscience and should act towards one another in a spirit of brotherhood.

The Declaration, as a whole, emphasises the dignity and worth of the human person. The *United Nations Declaration on the Rights of Indigenous Peoples* also notes in its preamble:

> that indigenous peoples are equal to all other peoples, while recognizing the right of all peoples to be different, to consider themselves different, and to be respected as such.

These principles, and others like them in other INTERNATIONAL human rights instruments, underline the ethical importance of respecting both the dignity of Aboriginal and/or Torres Strait Islanders individually and collectively and their right to have their culture respected. In the health context this requires participation, partnership, respect, negotiation, a willingness to learn and a respect for the rich and ancient culture and history of Aboriginal and/or Torres Strait Islanders. Importantly, it also requires an absence of racism and other discriminatory practices, including stereotyping. It also involves acknowledging the events in the individual person's life or in their family history that may influence the interaction between the person, their family, health professionals and the health system, including past traumatic events, such as being part of the Stolen Generations and/or experiencing institutional abuse, and their day-to-day experiences with racism, discrimination and lack of respect for culture and community. The effects of intergenerational trauma need to be acknowledged.

Respect also involves nurses and midwives being aware of and acknowledging their own cultural assumptions. This awareness can support effective and empathic communication, particularly given the asymmetry of power that is often amplified in interactions between nurses and/or midwives and Aboriginal and/or Torres Strait Islander peoples. But it is also important for nurses and midwives to understand that it is not Aboriginal and/or Torres Strait Islander cultures that are a problem that make practice difficult, but to acknowledge that health care has its own distinct culture that may be problematic for Aboriginal and/or Torres Strait Islander peoples.

The nursing and midwifery codes

As international codes, the Codes of Ethics do not directly address ethical practice when providing care to Aboriginal and/or Torres Strait Islanders, but do, to some extent, address culturally respectful practices more generally. As the Codes of Conduct are authored by the Nursing and Midwifery Board of Australia they have a specific principle – Principle 3: Cultural practice and respectful relationships – that addresses issues in respect of culturally respectful practice in general, as well a sub-principle focused specifically on Aboriginal and/or Torres Strait Islander peoples' health.

Both Codes of Conduct at 3.1 state:

> Australia has always been a culturally and linguistically diverse nation. Aboriginal and/or Torres Strait Islander peoples have inhabited and cared for the land as the first peoples of Australia for millennia, and their histories and cultures have uniquely shaped our nation. Understanding and acknowledging historic factors

such as colonisation and its impact on Aboriginal and/or Torres Strait Islander peoples' health helps inform care. In particular, Aboriginal and/or Torres Strait Islander peoples bear the burden of gross social, cultural and health inequity.

The Codes go on (at 3.2.c) to say nurses and midwives must 'acknowledge the social, economic, cultural, historic and behavioural factors influencing health, both at the individual, community and population levels'.

Human rights

International and nationally recognised human rights for Aboriginal and/or Torres Strait Islander peoples are discussed in the next section of this chapter. However, the Codes of Ethics also recognise the importance of human rights. The ICM Code of Ethics states: 'The Code acknowledges women as persons with human rights, seeks justice for all people and equity in access to health care, and is based on mutual relationships of respect, trust and the dignity of all members of society' (preamble). Similarly, the ICN Code of Ethics states: 'Inherent to nursing is respect for human rights, including cultural rights, the right to life and choice, to dignity and to be treated with respect' (preamble). It goes on to note (at 1): 'In providing care, the nurse promotes an environment in which the human rights, values, customs and spiritual beliefs of the individual, family and community are respected.'

Discrimination

One key human right is the right not to be discriminated against on the grounds of race, as well as other characteristics. Non-discrimination is emphasised in all of the Codes. The ICM Code of Ethics (II.d) notes: 'midwives respond to the psychological, physical, emotional and spiritual needs of women seeking health care, whatever the circumstances (non-discrimination).' The ICN Code of Ethics notes in its preamble: 'Nursing care is respectful of and unrestricted by considerations of age, colour, creed, culture, disability or illness, gender, sexual orientation, nationality, politics, race or social status' (which are all forms of prohibited discrimination).

Both Codes of Conduct discuss non-discrimination extensively, both specifically in relation to Aboriginal and/or Torres Strait Islanders and more generally in respect of racial discrimination. The Codes note that nurses and midwives (3.1.a) must 'provide care that is holistic, free of bias and racism, challenges belief based upon assumption and is culturally safe and respectful for Aboriginal and/or Torres Strait Islander peoples'.

The Codes of Conduct (3.2.d) also state that midwives and nurses must 'adopt practices that respect diversity, avoid bias, discrimination and racism, and challenge belief based on assumption (for example, based on gender, disability, race, ethnicity, religion, sexuality, age or political beliefs)'.

More generally the Codes of Conduct recognise that discrimination and racism can be associated with bullying and harassment. The Codes (at 3.4.a and b) state that nurses and midwives must 'never engage in, ignore, or excuse such behaviour [bullying and harassment]' and must 'recognise that bullying and harassment takes many forms, including behaviours such as physical and verbal abuse, racism, discrimination, violence, aggression, humiliation, pressure in decision-making, exclusion and intimidation directed towards peoples or colleagues'. Further, that nurses and midwives must 'be non-judgemental and not refer to people in a non-professional manner verbally or in correspondence/records, including refraining from behaviour that may be interpreted as bullying or harassment and/or culturally unsafe' (3.3.e).

Respect for cultural diversity

The requirement to actively show respect for cultural diversity is also clearly expressed in the ICM Code of Ethics (II.a): 'Midwives provide care for women and childbearing families with respect for cultural diversity while also working to eliminate harmful practices within those same cultures.' Additionally, both Codes of Conduct (at 3.2.b) state that nurses and midwives must 'respect diverse cultures, beliefs, gender identities, sexualities and experiences of people'.

Informed consent

As discussed, informed consent practices based on western values may be lacking in respect for the values and ways of Aboriginal and/or Torres Strait Islanders. The Codes of Conduct (3.1.c) state that nurses and midwives must 'recognise the importance of family, community, partnership and collaboration in the healthcare decision-making of Aboriginal and/or Torres Strait Islander peoples, for prevention strategies and care delivery.' They further state (3.3.b) that nurses and midwives must 'make arrangements, whenever possible, to meet the specific language, cultural, and communication needs of people and their families, through the utilisation of translating and interpreting services where necessary, and be aware of how these needs affect understanding'.

Advocacy and empowerment

The Codes of Conduct also create a positive duty on nurses and midwives to 'advocate for and act to facilitate access to quality and culturally safe health services for Aboriginal and/or Torres Strait Islander peoples' (3.1.b). The ICN Code of Ethics also notes more generally that (1): 'The nurse advocates for equity and social justice in resource allocation, access to health care and other social and economic services.' Given that Aboriginal and/or Torres Strait Islanders have traditionally faced significant barriers to accessing health services, disparities in health outcomes, and access to other key social and economic services connected to the social determinants of health, such as an adequate standard of housing, this advocacy responsibility would apply.

Law

Australia's legal system has, over the centuries, not dealt well with protecting and promoting the interests of Aboriginal and/or Torres Strait Islanders. Aboriginal and/or Torres Strait Islanders were dispossessed of their sovereignty, law and much of their land by the British under the legal doctrine of *terra nullius* – that the continent of Australia was unoccupied. This remained the legal position until 1992 when the Australia High Court overturned this legal fiction. In *Mabo v Queensland (No 2) (1992) 175 CLR 1 at 109* Justices Deane and Gauldron noted:

> The acts and events by which that dispossession in legal theory was carried into practical effect constitute the darkest aspect of the history of this nation. The nation as a whole must remain diminished unless and until there is an acknowledgement of, and retreat from, those past injustices ... The lands of this continent were not terra nullius or 'practically unoccupied' in 1788.

Until 1967 Aboriginal and/or Torres Strait Islander people were effectively excluded from the Australian *Constitution* under section 51(xxvi), which placed responsibility for Aboriginal and/or Torres Strait Islanders in the hands of the states. Section 127 of the *Constitution* also stated that 'Aboriginal natives were not to be counted' in taking a census. The references to Aboriginal and Torres Strait Islanders in section 51 were deleted and section 127 was repealed in a national referendum in 1967. However, there are still sections in the *Constitution* that allow differential treatment on the grounds of race (under s 25 people can be banned from voting on the basis of race; s 51(xxvi) can be used to pass laws that discriminate on the grounds of race). There is a current campaign for a national referendum to repeal the discriminatory sections of the *Constitution* and in the body of the *Constitution* to constitutionally recognise Aboriginal and/or Torres Strait Islanders as Australia's First Peoples and recognise their languages, while preserving English as the official language. The Uluru Statement from the Heart (2017) seeks 'a First Nations Voice enshrined in the Constitution'. At a minimum, reformers are seeking to explicitly recognise Aboriginal and/or Torres Strait Islanders as Australia's First Peoples in the preamble to the *Constitution* which would not have legal, although it would have symbolic, effect.

International human rights law

A starting point for the discussion of law as it relates to Aboriginal and/or Torres Strait Islanders and health services begins by looking at international human rights norms. There are several core International Human Rights treaties which Australia has ratified.

➢ the *International Covenant on Civil and Political Rights* (ICCPR)

➢ the *International Covenant on Economic, Social and Cultural Rights* (ICESCR)

➢ the *International Convention on the Elimination of All Forms of Racial Discrimination* (CERD)

➢ the *Convention on the Elimination of All Forms of Discrimination against Women* (CEDAW)

➢ the *Convention against Torture and Other Cruel, Inhuman or Degrading Treatment or Punishment* (CAT)

➢ the *Convention on the Rights of the Child* (CRC)

➢ the *Convention on the Rights of Persons with Disabilities* (CRPD).

The earliest international human rights treaties focused on individual political and civil rights (i.e. voting, freedom of expression, anti-discrimination, etc). Subsequent 'second generation' rights address economic, social and cultural rights (including the right to the highest attainable standard of health). 'Third generation' rights, which include collectively held group rights, have expressly included Indigenous peoples' rights.

Right to health

The *United Nations Declaration on the Rights of Indigenous Persons* (UNDRIP) was passed in 2007, recognising the collective group rights of Indigenous groups. It is important to note that Australia was one of four nations that voted against the passing of this non-legally binding Declaration (also Canada, New Zealand and the United States). Australia subsequently became a signatory to UNDRIP in 2009, after a change of government. Although it is non-binding in a legal sense, Australia has recognised UNDRIP as a framework to better recognise and enable the rights of Aboriginal and/or Torres Strait Islanders who are recognised as Australia's Indigenous population. Because UNDRIP is non-binding it does not create legal rights; it does create moral rights.

This UNDRIP explicitly addresses the right to health. Article 24 states:

1. Indigenous peoples have the right to their traditional medicines and to maintain their health practices, including the conservation of their vital medicinal plants, animals and minerals. Indigenous individuals also have the right to access, without any discrimination, to all social and health services.

2. Indigenous individuals have an equal right to the enjoyment of the highest attainable standard of physical and mental health. States shall take the necessary steps with a view to achieving progressively the full realization of this right.

In addition to the right to access health and social services and the highest attainable standard of physical and mental health, this human right also states that Indigenous peoples have the right to their traditional medicines and health practices, which would include traditional healers. A broad reading of this right would suggest an obligation to enable this, if it is the patient's choice, while the patient is accessing western health services.

A 2015 review of Australia's implementation of UNDRIP saw 104 countries make not made comments about Australia's human rights record and a number of countries noted concerns about continuing high-level discrimination against Aboriginal and/or Torres Strait Islanders and a need for greater efforts to protect and promote the rights of Aboriginal and/or Torres Strait Islanders (Reconciliation Australia n.d.). This can be seen in the health context, given the continuing significant differences in life expectancy and health outcomes between Indigenous and non-Indigenous Australians and ongoing concerns about inequalities in access to health services, as discussed earlier in the chapter.

In 2008 the Commonwealth Government re-acknowledged it needed to work with Aboriginal and/or Torres Strait Islander communities to improve health outcomes. It entered into a Statement of Intent to work with Aboriginal and/or Torres Strait Islander communities to achieve equality in health status and life expectancy for Indigenous Australians by 2030 (Australian Human Rights Commission 2008). A number of similar commitments had been previously made. Six Closing the Gaps Targets were subsequently established, two of which relate to health:

> To close the life expectancy gap within a generation

> To halve the gap in mortality rates for Indigenous children under five within a decade (Council of Australian Governments 2012).

In 2009 the Commonwealth and the State and Territory governments signed a *National Partnership Agreement on Closing the Gap in Indigenous Health Outcomes*. This Agreement establishes five areas of priority for addressing and significantly improving health outcomes for Indigenous Australians:

> Prevention (smoking, and drug and alcohol abuse)

> Primary health (expand access and improve co-ordination)

> Hospital services (improving service quality and the delivery of culturally appropriate services)

> Patient experiences (broader access to culturally competent care delivered in partnership with the community and that is accountable for the needs of its users)

> Sustainability (increase the Aboriginal and Torres Strait Islander health workforce, create sustainable and responsive systems and programmes, and evaluate those programmes).

However, it is not only governments who must enable the right to health. Nurses and midwives also play a significant role in enabling access to health services by Aboriginal and/or Torres Strait Islander peoples through their personal attitudes, involvement in institutional practices and advocacy.

Racial discrimination

In Australian law treaties do not have the force of law unless they are given effect by statute. The *International Covenant on Civil and Political Rights* put into effect internationally accepted principles of equality and non-discrimination. These principles were reinforced in the *International Convention on the Elimination of All Forms of Racial Discrimination*, which focuses on discrimination on the basis of race. Australia must report regularly to the United Nations about its implementation of these treaties. A Committee operating under the auspices of the *International Convention on the Elimination of All Forms of Racial Discrimination*, for example, undertakes specific monitoring of Indigenous issues. Australia has ratified

Table 13.1 Anti-discrimination legislation across all Australian jurisdictions

Jurisdiction	Legislation
Commonwealth	*Racial Discrimination Act 1975* (Cth) s 9
Australian Capital Territory	*Discrimination Act 1991* (ACT) s 7
New South Wales	*Anti-Discrimination Act 1977* (NSW) s 7
Northern Territory	*Anti-Discrimination Act 1996* (NT) s 19
Queensland	*Anti-Discrimination Act 1991* (Qld) s 7
South Australia	*Equal Opportunity Act 1984* (SA) Pt 4
Tasmania	*Anti-Discrimination Act 1998* (Tas) s 16
Victoria	*Equal Opportunity Act 2010* (Vic) Pt 2
Western Australia	*Equal Opportunity Act 1984* (WA) Pt III

the anti-discrimination provisions in both treaties through the passing of anti-discrimination legislation in Australia (see Table 13.1).

All anti-discrimination legislation has 'race' as a prohibited ground of discrimination (others include age, gender, marital status, disability, religion and many more). Discrimination occurs when a person is treated less favourably, or not given the same opportunities, as others in a similar situation, because of their race. The Acts apply to many areas of public life, including employment, health, education, getting or using goods or services, accommodation, and accessing public places. There are usually exceptions for special measures aimed at remedying long-standing inequalities for groups who face or have faced entrenched discrimination – for example, the funding and provision of health services that primarily provide health care to Aboriginal and/or Torres Strait Islanders. The purpose of these services is to achieve improved health outcomes for Aboriginal and/or Torres Strait Islander peoples, who have faced entrenched discrimination, through the delivery of comprehensive and culturally appropriate health services.

Livermore v New Children's Hospital Westmead [2002] NSWADT 111

Parents of a child who had died in a neonatal intensive care unit claimed they had been racially discriminated against. Both parents were Aboriginal. The parents alleged racial discrimination on three grounds:

1. Failure to provide an Aboriginal liaison officer at all times (the liaison officer went on leave at the critical time)

▶

◄

2. The parents were not provided with help to overcome language difficulties

3. Hospital staff had discussed matters with the wife, who was caucasian in appearance, rather than the husband and this had humiliated him within his cultural framework.

The Tribunal found (at 28): 'To show discrimination on the grounds of race the onus is on the Applicants to show that the aggrieved person has been treated "less favourably". It is not less favourable treatment to speak to the more assertive person and/ or the mother of a new born. The treatment must be looked at from an objective view rather than how the Applicants would like to have been treated. What constitutes discrimination is where the treatment received by the aggrieved person is different or less favourable than the treatment given to others. In this case the treatment received by the Livermores is treatment that would be given to all couples that come in with a critically ill baby.'

The fact that the liaison was on leave was not held to be discrimination as there was no obligation (at that time) to provide a liaison. The court found that both parents were fluent in English, despite the mother speaking a number of different Aboriginal languages.

There are a number of ways in which Aboriginal and/or Torres Strait Islanders experience outright racism and/or racial discrimination within the health system and from health professionals, including nurses and midwives. Kelahar and colleagues (2014) surveyed 755 Aboriginal participants from Victoria about their experience of racism in health settings. Almost a third of participants (221) reported racism within health settings within the preceding 12-month period, including name-calling, teasing and comments based on racial stereotypes, being ignored, left out, verbally abused, or told they do not belong in Australia. The research showed that experiencing racism in health settings is associated with Aboriginal and/or Torres Strait Islander peoples experiencing psychological distress. Also, that racism in health settings may be experienced more negatively than racism in other settings. Racism in health settings may contribute to poorer health through psychological distress, as well as through reduced quality of health care and barriers to access to health services. There are several other studies that report similar findings where Aboriginal and/or Torres Strait Islanders report experiencing racism in health settings and associated psychological distress.

There have also been a number of cases indicating that Aboriginal and/or Torres Strait Islanders experience less overt forms of racism or discrimination which affect how health professionals, including nurses and midwives, provide or do not provide appropriate health services to them. Research has indicated that Aboriginal and/or Torres Strait Islander patients are less likely to be referred for testing or treatments than non-Indigenous Australians. For example, in South Australia Aboriginal and/or Torres Strait Islanders have a 40 per cent lower rate of angiography and percutaneous coronary interventions than other Australians (Tavella et al. 2016). Recent research has indicated that Aboriginal and/or Torres Strait Islanders who are undergoing dialysis are substantially less likely than non-Indigenous Australians to be placed on the transplantation waiting list (Khanal et al. 2018).

There have also been a large number of Coronial hearings who have investigated less overt forms of racial discrimination against Aboriginal and/or Torres Strait Islander patients. One of these is described in the box 'Inquest into the death of Ms DHU (11020–14) Ref no: 47/15 Western Australia'.

Inquest into the death of Ms DHU (11020–14) Ref no: 47/15 Western Australia

Ms Dhu was a 22-year-old Aboriginal woman from the Yamatji Nanda family group on her mother's side and the Bunjima family group on her father's side. She died at Hedland Health Campus (HHC) on 4 August 2014 while she was in the custody of the Western Australia Police Service. She had been arrested for unpaid fines and costs totalling $3,622.34. The focus of the inquest into Ms Dhu's death was on the quality of her supervision, treatment and care by the police, as well as her medical treatment. On two occasions during her two-day detention she had been escorted by the police to HHC for medical assessment and then returned to custody. The two doctors who assessed Ms Dhu did not find evidence of illness or injury. Ms Dhu died as a result of an overwhelming staphylococcal infection. She had complained of ill health and asked for help from a number of health professionals and police officers. However, the Coroner found that the majority of the persons responsible for Ms Dhu's care formed the view that she was exaggerating or feigning symptoms of being unwell and was feigning her final collapse. This assumption persisted up until she died.

The Coroner found: 'I do not find that any of the HHC staff or police were motivated by conscious deliberations of racism in connection with their treatment of Ms Dhu, nor does Ms Dhu's family make that submission. ... However, it would be naïve to deny the existence of societal patterns that lead to assumptions being formed in relation to Aboriginal persons. This is not a matter only for HHC, or its staff or the police. It is a community wide issue and until there is a seismic shift in the understanding that is extended towards the plight of Aboriginal persons, the risk of unfounded

▶

◀

assumptions being made without conscious deliberation continues, with the attendant risk of errors' (paras 859–860).

Media have reported Ms Dhu's family made a formal complaint in June 2018 to the Australian Human Rights Commissioner of racial discrimination in respect of her treatment by police and health professionals.

Nothing had changed from 1991 when the Royal Commission into Aboriginal Deaths in Custody noted (para 31.3.38):

> The case of Mark Quayle is perhaps best known, owing to media publicity, as one where responsibility for the death fell on nursing and medical personnel as well as on police officers. Commissioner Wootten, in his report on the case, referred to the 'shocking and callous disregard' for Quayle's welfare on the part of the staff, and pointed out that this unacceptable behaviour reflected 'the dehumanising stereotype of Aboriginals so common in Australia'.

Overview

Figure 13.1 highlights the interactions between the ethical principles and the legal principles relevant to nursing practice.

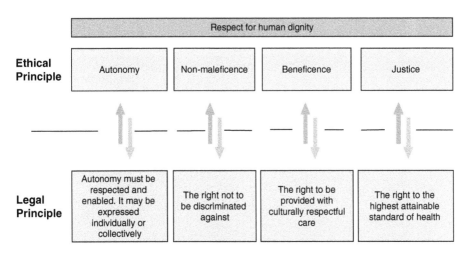

Figure 13.1   Ethical and legal principles relevant to the care of Aboriginal and/or Torres Strait Islander patients

Further reading

Australian Indigenous Health*InfoNet*: https://healthinfonet.ecu.edu.au/

Best, O. & Fredericks, B. eds. 2018, *Yatdjuligin: Aboriginal and Torres Strait Islander Nursing and Midwifery Care*, Cambridge University Press: Cambridge.

Questions

1. What should nurses and/or midwives do to improve access to health services for Aboriginal and/or Torres Strait Islander peoples?
2. What should nurses and/or midwives do if they see racism in the workplace?

Scenario

Donna is a Murri woman who is five and a half months pregnant. She has presented to the small local hospital's emergency department eight times with nausea and vomiting, and sometimes diarrhoea and dehydration. On Donna's ninth presentation with these symptoms, Tracey, a newly employed nurse, is assessing Donna. She notes that on six previous occasions the emergency department has referred Donna to either drug and alcohol services or mental health services. Each time the services have said Donna has no issues of dependence. On this presentation Donna's blood pressure and temperature are elevated. Tracey consults with a registered midwife, Tara, who said, 'Her again. She's one of our frequent flyers as she's an alco. She's just putting it on. Give her a few Panadol and send her home.'

Apply the decision-making framework to this problem.

Appendix A – Code of conduct for nurses

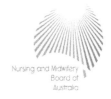

Nursing and Midwifery
Board of
Australia

Code of conduct for nurses

Foreword

The Nursing and Midwifery Board of Australia (NMBA) undertakes functions as set by the Health Practitioner Regulation National Law (the National Law), as in force in each state and territory. The NMBA regulates the practice of nursing and midwifery in Australia, and one of its key roles is to protect the public. The NMBA does this by developing standards, codes and guidelines that together establish the requirements for the professional and safe practice of nurses and midwives in Australia.

In developing the *Code of conduct for nurses*, and consistent with its commitment to evidence-based structures, systems and processes, the NMBA carried out a comprehensive review that was informed by research and by the profession. The research included an international and national literature review of other codes and similar publications, a comparative analysis of the predecessor code of conduct to other codes and an analysis of notifications (complaints) made about the conduct and behaviour of nurses. Input was extensively sought in the form of focus groups, workshops, an expert working group and other consultation strategies which included the profession, the public and professional organisations.

The *Code of conduct for nurses* (the code) sets out the legal requirements, professional behaviour and conduct expectations for nurses in all practice settings, in Australia. The code is written in recognition that nursing practice is not restricted to the provision of direct clinical care. Nursing practice settings extend to working in a non-clinical relationship with clients, working in management, leadership, governance, administration, education, research, advisory, regulatory, policy development roles or other roles that impact on safe, effective delivery of services in the profession and/or use of the nurse's professional skills.

The code is supported by the NMBA Standards for practice and, with the other NMBA standards, codes and guidelines, underpins the requirements and delivery of safe, kind and compassionate nursing practice.

Associate Professor Lynette Cusack, RN

Chair
Nursing and Midwifery Board of Australia

Contents

Introduction

The *Code of conduct for nurses* sets out the legal requirements, professional behaviour and conduct expectations for all nurses, in all practice settings, in Australia. It describes the principles of professional behaviour that guide safe practice, and clearly outlines the conduct expected of nurses by their colleagues and the broader community.

Individual nurses have their own personal beliefs and values. However, the code outlines specific standards which all nurses are expected to adopt in their practice. The code also gives students of nursing an appreciation of the conduct and behaviours expected of nurses. Nurses have a professional responsibility to understand and abide by the code. In practice, nurses also have a duty to make the interests of people their first concern, and to practise safely and effectively.

The code is consistent with the National Law. It includes seven principles of conduct, grouped into domains, each with an explanatory value statement. Each value statement is accompanied by practical guidance to demonstrate how to apply it in practice. Underpinning the code is the expectation that nurses will exercise their professional judgement to deliver the best possible outcomes in practice.

This code applies to all nurses

The principles of the code apply to all types of nursing practice in all contexts. This includes any work where a nurse uses nursing skills and knowledge, whether paid or unpaid, clinical or non-clinical. This includes work in the areas of clinical care, clinical leadership, clinical governance responsibilities, education, research, administration, management, advisory roles, regulation or policy development. The code also applies to all settings where a nurse may engage in these activities, including face-to-face, publications, or via online or electronic means.

Using the code of conduct

The code will be used:

- to support individual nurses in the delivery of safe practice and fulfilling their professional roles
- as a guide for the public and consumers of health services about the standard of conduct and behaviour they should expect from nurses
- to help the NMBA protect the public, in setting and maintaining the standards set out in the code and to ensure safe and effective nursing practice
- when evaluating the professional conduct of nurses. If professional conduct varies significantly from the values outlined in the code, nurses should be prepared to explain and justify their decisions and actions. Serious or repeated failure to abide by this code may have consequences for nurses' registration and may be considered as unsatisfactory professional performance, unprofessional conduct or professional misconduct[1], and
- as a resource for activities which aim to enhance the culture of professionalism in the Australian health system. These include use, for example, in administration and policy development by health services and other institutions; in nursing education, in management and for the orientation, induction and supervision of nurses and students.

The code is not a substitute for requirements outlined in the National Law, other relevant legislation, or case law. Where there is any actual or perceived conflict between the code and any law, the law takes precedence. Nurses also need to understand and comply with all other NMBA standards, codes and guidelines.

---

[1] As defined in the National Law, with the exception of NSW where the definitions of unsatisfactory professional conduct and professional misconduct are defined in the Health Practitioner Regulation National Law (NSW).

Nursing and Midwifery
Board of
Australia

Code of conduct for nurses: domains, principles and values

These domains, principles and values set out legal requirements, professional behaviour and conduct expectations for all nurses. The principles apply to all areas of practice, with an understanding that nurses will exercise professional judgement in applying them, with the goal of delivering the best possible outcomes.

(To note: **Person** or **people** is used to refer to those individuals who have entered into a therapeutic and/or professional relationship with a nurse. See the glossary for further detail.)

Domain: Practise legally

1. **Legal compliance**
    Nurses respect and adhere to their professional obligations under the National Law, and abide by relevant laws.

Domain: Practise safely, effectively and collaboratively

2. **Person-centred practice**
    Nurses provide safe, person-centred and evidence-based practice for the health and wellbeing of people and, in partnership with the person, promote shared decision-making and care delivery between the person, nominated partners, family, friends and health professionals.

3. **Cultural practice and respectful relationships**
    Nurses engage with people as individuals in a culturally safe and respectful way, foster open and honest professional relationships, and adhere to their obligations about privacy and confidentiality.

Domain: Act with professional integrity

4. **Professional behaviour**
    Nurses embody integrity, honesty, respect and compassion.

5. **Teaching, supervising and assessing**
    Nurses commit to teaching, supervising and assessing students and other nurses, in order to develop the nursing workforce across all contexts of practice.

6. **Research in health**
    Nurses recognise the vital role of research to inform quality healthcare and policy development, conduct research ethically and support the decision-making of people who participate in research.

Domain: Promote health and wellbeing

7. **Health and wellbeing**
    Nurses promote health and wellbeing for people and their families, colleagues, the broader community and themselves and in a way that addresses health inequality.

Code of conduct for nurses

Domain: Practise legally

Principle 1: Legal compliance

Value
Nurses respect and adhere to professional obligations under the National Law, and abide by relevant laws[2].

1.1   Obligations

It is important that nurses are aware of their obligations under the National Law, including reporting requirements and meeting registration standards. Nurses must

a. abide by any reporting obligations under the National Law and other relevant legislation. Please refer to sections 129, 130, 131 and 141 of the National Law and the NMBA Guidelines for mandatory notifications

b. inform the Australian Health Practitioner Regulation Agency (AHPRA) and their employer(s) if a legal or regulatory entity has imposed restrictions on their practice, including limitations, conditions, undertakings, suspension, cautions or reprimands, and recognise that a breach of any restriction would place the public at risk and may constitute unprofessional conduct or professional misconduct

c. complete the required amount of CPD relevant to their context of practice. See the NMBA Registration standard: Continuing professional development, Policy: Exemptions from continuing professional development for nurses and midwives and Fact sheet: Continuing professional development for these requirements

d. ensure their practice is appropriately covered by professional indemnity insurance (see the NMBA Registration standard: Professional indemnity insurance arrangements and Fact sheet: Professional indemnity insurance arrangements), and

e. inform AHPRA of charges, pleas and convictions relating to criminal offences (see the NMBA Registration standard: Criminal history).

1.2   Lawful behaviour

Nurses practise honestly and ethically and should not engage in unlawful behaviour as it may affect their practice and/or damage the reputation of the profession. Nurses must

a. respect the nurse-person professional relationship by not taking possessions and/or property that belong to the person and/or their family

b. comply with relevant poisons legislation, authorisation, local policy and own scope of practice, including to safely use, administer, obtain, possess, prescribe, sell, supply and store medications and other therapeutic products

c. not participate in unlawful behaviour and understand that unlawful behaviour may be viewed as unprofessional conduct or professional misconduct and have implications for their registration, and

d. understand that making frivolous or vexatious complaints may be viewed as unprofessional conduct or professional misconduct and have implications for their registration.

---

[2] The code does not address in detail the full range of legal and ethical obligations that apply to nurses. Examples of legal obligations include, but are not limited to, obligations arising in Acts and Regulations relating to privacy, the aged and disabled, child protection, bullying, anti-discrimination and workplace health and safety issues. Nurses should ensure they know all of their legal obligations relating to professional practice, and abide by them.

1.3   Mandatory reporting

Caring for those who are vulnerable brings legislative responsibilities for nurses, including the need to abide by relevant mandatory reporting requirements as they apply across individual states and territories. Nurses must:

a. abide by the relevant mandatory reporting legislation that is imposed to protect groups that are particularly at risk, including reporting obligations about the aged, child abuse and neglect and remaining alert to the newborn and infants who may be at risk, and

b. remain alert to other groups who may be vulnerable and at risk of physical harm and sexual exploitation and act on welfare concerns where appropriate.

Domain: Practise safely, effectively and collaboratively

Principle 2: Person-centred practice

> **Value**
> Nurses provide safe, person-centred, evidence-based practice for the health and wellbeing of people and, in partnership with the person, promote shared decision-making and care delivery between the person, nominated partners, family, friends and health professionals.

2.1   Nursing practice

Nurses apply person-centred and evidence-based decision-making, and have a responsibility to ensure the delivery of safe and quality care. Nurses must:

a. practise in accordance with the standards of the profession and broader health system (including the NMBA Standards, codes and guidelines, the Australian Commission on Safety and Quality in Health Care and Standards for aged care)

b. provide leadership to ensure the delivery of safe and quality care and understand their professional responsibility to protect people, ensuring employees comply with their obligations, and

c. document and report concerns if they believe the practice environment is compromising the health and safety of people receiving care.

2.2   Decision-making

Making decisions about healthcare is the shared responsibility of the person (who may wish to involve their nominated partners, family and friends), the nurse and other health professionals. Nurses should create and foster conditions that promote shared decision-making and collaborative practice. To support shared decision-making, nurses must:

a. take a person-centred approach to managing a person's care and concerns, supporting the person in a manner consistent with that person's values and preferences

b. advocate on behalf of the person where necessary, and recognise when substitute decision-makers are needed (including legal guardians or holders of power of attorney)

c. support the right of people to seek second and/or subsequent opinions or the right to refuse treatment/care

d. recognise that care may be provided to the same person by different nurses, and by other members of the healthcare team, at various times

e. recognise and work within their scope of practice which is determined by their education, training, authorisation, competence, qualifications and experience, in accordance with local policy (see also the NMBA Decision-making framework)

f. recognise when an activity is not within their scope of practice and refer people to another health practitioner when this is in the best interests of the person receiving care

g. take reasonable steps to ensure any person to whom a nurse delegates, refers, or hands over care has the qualifications, experience, knowledge, skills and scope of practice to provide the care needed (see also the NMBA Decision-making framework), and

h. recognise that their context of practice can influence decision-making. This includes the type and location of practice setting, the characteristics of the person receiving care, the focus of nursing activities, the degree to which practice is autonomous and the resources available.

2.3   Informed consent

Informed consent is a person's voluntary agreement to healthcare, which is made with knowledge and understanding of the potential benefits and risks involved. In supporting the right to informed consent, nurses must:

a. support the provision of information to the person about their care in a way and/or in a language/dialect they can understand, through the utilisation of translating and interpreting services, when necessary. This includes information on examinations and investigations, as well as treatments

b. give the person adequate time to ask questions, make decisions and to refuse care, interventions, investigations and treatments, and proceed in accordance with the person's choice, considering local policy

c. act according to the person's capacity for decision-making and consent, including when caring for children and young people, based on their maturity and capacity to understand, and the nature of the proposed care

d. obtain informed consent or other valid authority before carrying out an examination or investigation, providing treatment (this may not be possible in an emergency), or involving people in teaching or research, and

e. inform people of the benefit, as well as associated costs or risks, if referring the person for further assessment, investigations or treatments, which they may want to clarify before proceeding.

2.4   Adverse events and open disclosure

When a person is harmed by healthcare (adverse events), nurses have responsibilities to be open and honest in communicating with the person, to review what happened, and to report the event in a timely manner, and in accordance with local policy. When something goes wrong, nurses must:

a. recognise and reflect on what happened and report the incident

b. act immediately to rectify the problem if possible, and intervene directly if it is needed to protect the person's safety. This responsibility includes escalating concerns if needed

c. abide by the principles of open disclosure and non-punitive approaches to incident management

d. identify the most appropriate healthcare team member to provide an apology and an explanation to the person, as promptly and completely as possible, that supports open disclosure principles

e. listen to the person, acknowledge any distress they experienced and provide support. In some cases it may be advisable to refer the person to another nurse or health professional

f. ensure people have access to information about how to make a complaint, and that in doing so, not allow a complaint or notification to negatively affect the care they provide, and

g. seek advice from their employer, AHPRA, their professional indemnity insurer, or other relevant bodies, if they are unsure about their obligations.

See also the Australian Commission on Safety and Quality in Health Care's Australian Open Disclosure Framework.

Value
Nurses engage with people as individuals in a culturally safe and respectful way, foster open, honest and compassionate professional relationships, and adhere to their obligations about privacy and confidentiality.

3.1   Aboriginal and/or Torres Strait Islander peoples' health

Australia has always been a culturally and linguistically diverse nation. Aboriginal and/or Torres Strait Islander peoples have inhabited and cared for the land as the first peoples of Australia for millennia, and their histories and cultures have uniquely shaped our nation. Understanding and acknowledging historic factors such as colonisation and its impact on Aboriginal and/or Torres Strait Islander peoples' health helps inform care. In particular, Aboriginal and/or Torres Strait Islander peoples bear the burden of gross social, cultural and health inequality. In supporting the health of Aboriginal and/or Torres Strait Islander peoples, nurses must:

   a.   provide care that is holistic, free of bias and racism, challenges belief based upon assumption and is culturally safe and respectful for Aboriginal and/or Torres Strait Islander peoples

   b.   advocate for and act to facilitate access to quality and culturally safe health services for Aboriginal and/or Torres Strait Islander peoples, and

   c.   recognise the importance of family, community, partnership and collaboration in the healthcare decision-making of Aboriginal and/or Torres Strait Islander peoples, for both prevention strategies and care delivery.

See the National Aboriginal and Torres Strait Islander Health Plan 2013-2023.

See also Congress of Aboriginal and Torres Strait Islander Nurses and Midwives.

3.2   Culturally safe and respectful practice

Culturally safe and respectful practice requires having knowledge of how a nurse's own culture, values, attitudes, assumptions and beliefs influence their interactions with people and families, the community and colleagues. To ensure culturally safe and respectful practice, nurses must:

   a.   understand that only the person and/or their family can determine whether or not care is culturally safe and respectful

   b.   respect diverse cultures, beliefs, gender identities, sexualities and experiences of people, including among team members

   c.   acknowledge the social, economic, cultural, historic and behavioural factors influencing health, both at the individual, community and population levels

   d.   adopt practices that respect diversity, avoid bias, discrimination and racism, and challenge belief based upon assumption (for example, based on gender, disability, race, ethnicity, religion, sexuality, age or political beliefs)

   e.   support an inclusive environment for the safety and security of the individual person and their family and/or significant others, and

   f.   create a positive, culturally safe work environment through role modelling, and supporting the rights, dignity and safety of others, including people and colleagues.

3.3   Effective communication

Positive professional relationships are built on effective communication that is respectful, kind, compassionate and honest. To communicate effectively, nurses must:

   a.   be aware of health literacy issues, and take health literacy into account when communicating with people

b. make arrangements, whenever possible, to meet the specific language, cultural, and communication needs of people and their families, through the utilisation of translating and interpreting services where necessary, and be aware of how these needs affect understanding

c. endeavour to confirm a person understands any information communicated to them

d. clearly and accurately communicate relevant and timely information about the person to colleagues, within the bounds of relevant privacy requirements, and

e. be non-judgemental and not refer to people in a non-professional manner verbally or in correspondence/records, including refraining from behaviour that may be interpreted as bullying or harassment and/or culturally unsafe.

3.4   Bullying and harassment

When people repeatedly and intentionally use words or actions against someone or a group of people, it causes distress and risks their wellbeing. Nurses understand that bullying and harassment relating to their practice or workplace is not acceptable or tolerated and that where it is affecting public safety it may have implications for their registration. Nurses must:

a. never engage in, ignore or excuse such behaviour

b. recognise that bullying and harassment takes many forms, including behaviours such as physical and verbal abuse, racism, discrimination, violence, aggression, humiliation, pressure in decision-making, exclusion and intimidation directed towards people or colleagues

c. understand social media is sometimes used as a mechanism to bully or harass, and that nurses should not engage in, ignore or excuse such behaviour

d. act to eliminate bullying and harassment, in all its forms, in the workplace, and

e. escalate their concerns if an appropriate response does not occur.

For additional guidance see the Australian Human Rights Commission Fact sheet.

See also Nurse & Midwife Support, the national health support service for nurses, midwives and students.

3.5   Confidentiality and privacy

Nurses have ethical and legal obligations to protect the privacy of people. People have a right to expect that nurses will hold information about them in confidence, unless the release of information is needed by law, legally justifiable under public interest considerations or is required to facilitate emergency care. To protect privacy and confidentiality, nurses must:

a. respect the confidentiality and privacy of people by seeking informed consent before disclosing information, including formally documenting such consent where possible

b. provide surroundings to enable private and confidential consultations and discussions, particularly when working with multiple people at the same time, or in a shared space

c. abide by the NMBA Social media policy and relevant Standards for practice, to ensure use of social media is consistent with the nurse's ethical and legal obligations to protect privacy

d. access records only when professionally involved in the care of the person and authorised to do so

e. not transmit, share, reproduce or post any person's information or images, even if the person is not directly named or identified, without having first gained written and informed consent. See also the NMBA Social media policy and Guidelines for advertising regulated health services

f. recognise people's right to access information contained in their health records, facilitate that access and promptly facilitate the transfer of health information when requested by people, in accordance with local policy, and

g. when closing or relocating a practice, facilitating arrangements for the transfer or management of all health records in accordance with the legislation governing privacy and health records.

3.6   End-of-life care

Nurses have a vital role in helping the community to deal with the reality of death and its consequences. In providing culturally appropriate end-of-life care, nurses must:

a. understand the limits of healthcare in prolonging life, and recognise when efforts to prolong life may not be in the best interest of the person

b. accept that the person has the right to refuse treatment, or to request withdrawal of treatment, while ensuring the person receives relief from distress

c. respect diverse cultural practices and beliefs related to death and dying

d. facilitate advance care planning and provision of end-of-life care where relevant and in accordance with local policy and legislation, and

e. take reasonable steps to ensure support is provided to people, and their families, even when it is not possible to deliver the outcome they desire.

See also the Australian Commission on Safety and Quality in Health Care - End-of-Life Care.

Domain: Act with professional integrity

Principle 4: Professional behaviour

Value
Nurses embody integrity, honesty, respect and compassion.

4.1   Professional boundaries

Professional boundaries allow nurses, the person and the person's nominated partners, family and friends, to engage safely and effectively in professional relationships, including where care involves personal and/or intimate contact. In order to maintain professional boundaries, there is a start and end point to the professional relationship and it is integral to the nurse-person professional relationship. Adhering to professional boundaries promotes person-centred practice and protects both parties. To maintain professional boundaries, nurses must:

a. recognise the inherent power imbalance that exists between nurses, people in their care and significant others and establish and maintain professional boundaries

b. actively manage the person's expectations, and be clear about professional boundaries that must exist in professional relationships for objectivity in care and prepare the person for when the episode of care ends

c. avoid the potential conflicts, risks, and complexities of providing care to those with whom they have a pre-existing non-professional relationship and ensure that such relationships do not impair their judgement. This is especially relevant for those living and working in small, regional or cultural communities and/or where there is long-term professional, social and/or family engagement

d. avoid sexual relationships with persons with whom they have currently or had previously entered into a professional relationship. These relationships are inappropriate in most circumstances and could be considered unprofessional conduct or professional misconduct

e. recognise when over-involvement has occurred, and disclose this concern to an appropriate person, whether this is the person involved or a colleague

f. reflect on the circumstances surrounding any occurrence of over-involvement, document and report it, and engage in management to rectify or manage the situation

g. in cases where the professional relationship has become compromised or ineffective and ongoing care is needed, facilitate arrangements for the continuing care of the person to another health practitioner, including passing on relevant clinical information (see also 3.3 Effective communication)

h. actively address indifference, omission, disengagement/lack of care and disrespect to people that may reflect under-involvement, including escalating the issue to ensure the safety of the person if necessary

i. avoid expressing personal beliefs to people in ways that exploit the person's vulnerability, are likely to cause them unnecessary distress, or may negatively influence their autonomy in decision-making (see the NMBA Standards for practice), and

j. not participate in physical assault such as striking, unauthorised restraining and/or applying unnecessary force.

4.2   Advertising and professional representation

Nurses must be honest and transparent when describing their education, qualifications, previous occupations and registration status. This includes, but is not limited to, when nurses are involved in job applications, self-promotion, publishing of documents or web content, public appearances, or advertising or promoting goods or services. To honestly represent products and regulated health services, and themselves, nurses must:

a. comply with legal requirements about advertising outlined in the National Law (explained in the NMBA Guidelines for advertising regulated health services), as well as other relevant Australian state and territory legislation

b. provide only accurate, honest and verifiable information about their registration, experience and qualifications, including any conditions that apply to their registration (see also Principle 1: *Legal compliance*)

c. only use the title of nurse if they hold valid registration and/or endorsement (see also the NMBA Fact sheet: The use of health practitioner protected titles), and

d. never misrepresent, by either a false statement or an omission, their registration, experience, qualifications or position.

4.3   Legal, insurance and other assessments

Nurses may be contracted by a third party to provide an assessment of a person who is not in their care, such as for legal, insurance or other administrative purposes. When this occurs the usual nurse-person professional relationship does not exist. In this situation, nurses must:

a. explain to the person their professional area of practice, role, and the purpose, nature and extent of the assessment to be performed

b. anticipate and seek to correct any misunderstandings the person may have about the nature and purpose of the assessment and report, and

c. inform the person and/or their referring health professional of any unrecognised, serious problems that are discovered during the assessment, as a matter of duty-of-care.

4.4   Conflicts of interest

People rely on the independence and trustworthiness of nurses who provide them with advice or treatment. In nursing practice, a conflict of interest arises when a nurse has financial, professional or personal interests or relationships and/or personal beliefs that may affect the care they provide or result in personal gain.

Such conflicts may mean the nurse does not prioritise the interests of a person as they should, and may be viewed as unprofessional conduct. To prevent conflicts of interest from compromising care, nurses must:

a. act with integrity and in the best interests of people when making referrals, and when providing or arranging treatment or care

b. responsibly use their right to not provide, or participate directly in, treatments to which they have a conscientious objection. In such a situation, nurses must respectfully inform the person, their employer and other relevant colleagues, of their objection and ensure the person has alternative care options

c. proactively and openly inform the person if a nurse, or their immediate family, has a financial or commercial interest that could be perceived as influencing the care they provide

d. not offer financial, material or other rewards (inducements) to encourage others to act in ways that personally benefit the nurse, nor do anything that could be perceived as providing inducements, and

e. not allow any financial or commercial interest in any entity providing healthcare services or products to negatively affect the way people are treated.

4.5 Financial arrangements and gifts

It is necessary to be honest and transparent with people. To ensure there is no perception of actual or personal gain for the nurse, nurses must:

a. when providing or recommending services, discuss with the person all fees and charges expected to result from a course of treatment in a manner appropriate to the professional relationship, and not exploit people's vulnerability or lack of knowledge

b. only accept token gifts of minimal value that are freely offered and report the gifts in accordance with local policy

c. not accept, encourage or manipulate people to give, lend, or bequeath money or gifts that will benefit a nurse directly or indirectly

d. not become financially involved with a person who has or who will be in receipt of their care, for example through bequests, powers of attorney, loans and investment schemes, and

e. not influence people or their families to make donations, and where people seek to make a donation refer to the local policy.

Principle 5: Teaching, supervising and assessing

Value
Nurses commit to teaching, supervising and assessing students and other nurses in order to develop the nursing workforce across all contexts of practice.

5.1 Teaching and supervising

It is the responsibility of all nurses to create opportunities for nursing students and nurses under supervision to learn, as well as benefit from oversight and feedback. In their teaching and supervisor roles, nurses must:

a. seek to develop the skills, attitudes and practices of an effective teacher and/or supervisor

b. reflect on the ability, competence and learning needs of each student or nurse who they teach or supervise and plan teaching and supervision activities accordingly, and

c. avoid, where possible, any potential conflicts of interest in teaching or supervision relationships that may impair objectivity or interfere with the supervised person's learning outcomes or experience. This includes, for example, not supervising somebody with whom they have a pre-existing non-professional relationship.

5.2   Assessing colleagues and students

Assessing colleagues and students is an important part of making sure that the highest standard of practice is achieved across the profession. In assessing the competence and performance of colleagues or students, nurses must:

a. be honest, objective, fair, without bias and constructive, and not put people at risk of harm by inaccurate and inadequate assessment, and

b. provide accurate and justifiable information promptly, and include all relevant information when giving references or writing reports about colleagues.

See also the NMBA Supervision guidelines for nursing and midwifery.

Principle 6: Research in health

Value
Nurses recognise the vital role of research to inform quality healthcare and policy development, conduct research ethically and support the decision-making of people who participate in research.

6.1   Rights and responsibilities

Nurses involved in design, organisation, conduct or reporting of health research have additional responsibilities. Nurses involved in research must:

a. recognise and carry out the responsibilities associated with involvement in health research

b. in research that involves human participants, respect the decision-making of people to not participate and/or to withdraw from a study, ensuring their decision does not compromise their care or any nurse-person professional relationship(s), and

c. be aware of the values and ethical considerations for Aboriginal and/or Torres Strait Islander communities when undertaking research.

See also the National Health and Medical Research Council publication: Values and Ethics - Guidelines for Ethical Conduct in Aboriginal and Torres Strait Islander Health Research.

See also Principle 2 on the application of evidence-based decision-making for delivery of safe and quality care.

Domain: Promote health and wellbeing

Principle 7: Health and wellbeing

Value
Nurses promote health and wellbeing for people and their families, colleagues, the broader community and themselves and in a way that addresses health inequality.

7.1   Your and your colleagues' health

Nurses have a responsibility to maintain their physical and mental health to practise safely and effectively. To promote health for nursing practice, nurses must:

a. understand and promote the principles of public health, such as health promotion activities and vaccination

b. act to reduce the effect of fatigue and stress on their health, and on their ability to provide safe care

c. encourage and support colleagues to seek help if they are concerned that their colleague's health may be affecting their ability to practise safely, utilising services such as the national health support service for nurses, midwives and students

d. seek expert, independent and objective help and advice, if they are ill or impaired in their ability to practise safely. Nurses must remain aware of the risks of self-diagnosis and self-treatment, and act to reduce these, and

e. take action, including a mandatory or voluntary notification to AHPRA, if a nurse knows or reasonably suspects that they or a colleague have a health condition or impairment that could adversely affect their ability to practise safely, or put people at risk (see Principle 1: Legal compliance).

7.2 Health advocacy

There are significant disparities in the health status of various groups in the Australian community. These disparities result from social, historic, geographic, environmental, legal, physiological and other factors. Some groups who experience health disparities include Aboriginal and/or Torres Strait Islander peoples, those with disabilities, those who are gender or sexuality diverse, and those from social, culturally and linguistically diverse backgrounds, including asylum seekers and refugees. In advocating for community and population health, nurses must:

a. use their expertise and influence to protect and advance the health and wellbeing of individuals as well as communities and populations

b. understand and apply the principles of primary and public health, including health education, health promotion, disease prevention, control and health screening using the best available evidence in making practice decisions, and

c. participate in efforts to promote the health of communities and meet their obligations with respect to disease prevention including vaccination, health screening and reporting notifiable diseases.

See also the NMBA Position statement on nurses, midwives and vaccination.

Glossary

These meanings relate to the use of terms in the *Code of conduct for nurses*.

Advance care planning is an on-going process of shared planning for current and future healthcare. It allows an individual to make known their values, beliefs and preferences to guide decision-making, even after when the individual cannot make or communicate their preferences and decisions (See <u>Advance Care Planning Australia</u>).

Bullying and harassment is 'when people repeatedly and intentionally use words or actions against someone or a group of people to cause distress and risk to their wellbeing. These actions are usually done by people who have more influence or power over someone else, or who want to make someone else feel less powerful or helpless'.[3]

Competence is the possession of required skills, knowledge, education and capacity.

Cultural safety concept was developed in a First Nations' context and is the preferred term for nursing and midwifery. Cultural safety is endorsed by the Congress of Aboriginal and Torres Strait Islander Nurses and Midwives (CATSINaM), who emphasise that cultural safety is as important to quality care as clinical safety. However, the "presence or absence of cultural safety is determined by the recipient of care; it is not defined by the caregiver" (CATSINaM 2014, p. 9[4]). Cultural safety is a philosophy of practice that is about how a health professional does something, not [just] what they do. It is about how people are treated in society, not about their diversity as such, so its focus is on systemic and structural issues and on the social determinants of health. Cultural safety represents a key philosophical shift from providing care regardless of difference, to care that takes account of peoples' unique needs. It requires nurses and midwives to undertake an ongoing process of self-reflection and cultural self-awareness, and an acknowledgement of how a nurse's/midwife's personal culture impacts on care. In relation to Aboriginal and Torres Strait Islander health, cultural safety provides a de-colonising model of practice based on dialogue, communication, power sharing and negotiation, and the acknowledgment of white privilege. These actions are a means to challenge racism at personal and institutional levels, and to establish trust in healthcare encounters (CATSINaM 2017b, p. 11[5]). In focusing on clinical interactions, particularly power inequity between patient and health professional, cultural safety calls for a genuine partnership where power is shared between the individuals and cultural groups involved in healthcare. Cultural safety is also relevant to Aboriginal and Torres Strait Islander health professionals. Non-Indigenous nurses and midwives must address how they create a culturally safe work environment that is free of racism for their Aboriginal and Torres Strait Islander colleagues (CATSINaM 2017a[6]).

Delegation is the relationship that exists when a nurse devolves aspects of nursing practice to another person. Delegations are made to meet the person's health needs. The nurse who is delegating retains accountability for the decision to delegate. The nurse is also accountable for monitoring of the communication of the delegation to the relevant persons and for the practice outcomes. Both parties share the responsibility of making the delegation decision, which includes assessment of the competence and risks. For further details see the NMBA <u>National framework for the development of decision-making tools for nursing and midwifery practice</u>.

Discrimination is the unjust treatment of one or more person/s based on factors such as race, religion, sex, disability or other grounds specified in anti-discrimination legislation.[7]

Handover is the process of transferring all responsibility for the care of one or more people to another health practitioner or person.

---

[3] Australian Human Rights Commission, '*What is bullying?*' <u>https://www.humanrights.gov.au/what-bullying-violence-harassment-and-bullying-fact-sheet</u>.

[4] CATSINaM, 2014, *Towards a shared understanding of terms and concepts: strengthening nursing and midwifery care of Aboriginal and Torres Strait Islander peoples*, CATSINaM: Canberra.

[5] CATSINaM, 2017b, *The Nursing and Midwifery Aboriginal and Torres Strait Islander Health Curriculum Framework (Version 1.0)*, CATSINaM: Canberra.

[6] CATSINaM, 2017a, *Position statement: Embedding cultural safety across Australian nursing and midwifery*, CATSINaM: Canberra.

[7] Australian Human Rights Commission, '*Discrimination*' <u>www.humanrights.gov.au/quick-guide/12030</u>.

Health literacy 'is about how people understand information about health and healthcare, how they apply that information to their lives, use it to make decisions and act on it'.[8]

Local policy refers to the policies that apply to decision-making, relevant to the specific location and/or organisation where practice is being undertaken.

Mandatory notification is the requirement under the National Law for registered health practitioners, employers and education providers to report certain conduct (see Guidelines for mandatory notifications).

Mandatory reporting is a state and territory legislative requirement imposed to protect at-risk ? groups such as the aged, children and young people.

National law means the Health Practitioner Regulation National Law that is in force in each state and territory in Australia and applies to those professions regulated under that law (see Australian Health Practitioner Regulation Agency).

Nominated partners, family and friends include people in consensual relationships with the person, as identified by the person receiving care.

Nurse refers to a registered nurse, enrolled nurse or nurse practitioner. The term is reserved in Australia, under law, for a person who has completed the prescribed training, demonstrates competence to practise, and is registered as a nurse under the National Law.

Open disclosure 'is an open and honest discussion with a person about any incident(s) that caused them harm while they were receiving healthcare. It includes an apology or expression of regret (including the word 'sorry'), a factual explanation of what happened, an opportunity for the patient to describe their experience, and an explanation of the steps being taken to manage the event and prevent recurrence'[9] (Australian Commission on Safety and Quality in Health Care).

Over-involvement is when the nurse confuses their needs with the needs of the person in their care and crosses the boundary of a professional relationship. Behaviour may include favouritism, gifts, intimacy or inappropriate relationships with the partner or family member of a person in the nurse's care.

Person or people refers to those individuals who have entered into a therapeutic and/or professional relationship with a nurse. These individuals will sometimes be healthcare consumers, at other times they may be colleagues or students, this will vary depending on who is the focus of practice at the time. Therefore, the words person or people include all the patients, clients, consumers, families, carers, groups and/or communities, however named, that are within the nurse's scope and context of practice.

Person-centred practice is collaborative and respectful partnership built on mutual trust and understanding through good communication. Each person is treated as an individual with the aim of respecting people's ownership of their health information, rights and preferences while protecting their dignity and empowering choice. Person-centred practice recognises the role of family and community with respect to cultural and religious diversity.

Practice means any role, whether remunerated or not, in which the individual uses their skills and knowledge as a nurse. Practice is not restricted to the provision of direct clinical care. It also includes working in a direct nonclinical relationship with clients, working in management, administration, education, research, advisory, regulatory or policy development roles, and any other roles that impact on safe, effective delivery of services in the profession and/or use their professional skills.

Professional boundaries allow a nurse and a person to engage safely and effectively in a therapeutic and/or professional relationship. Professional boundaries refers to the clear separation that should exist between professional conduct aimed at meeting the health needs of people, and behaviour which serves a nurse's own personal views, feelings and relationships that are not relevant to the professional relationship.

---

[8] Australian Commission on Safety and Quality in Health Care, *Health literacy:* https://www.safetyandquality.gov.au/our-work/patient-and-consumer-centred-care/health-literacy/.
[9] Australian Commission on Safety and Quality in Health Care, *Australian Open Disclosure Framework:* https://www.safetyandquality.gov.au/wp-content/uploads/2013/03/Australian-Open-Disclosure-Framework-Feb-2014.pdf.

Professional misconduct includes conduct by a health practitioner that is substantially below the expected standard, and which, whether connected to practice or not, is inconsistent with being a fit and proper person to be registered in the profession.

Professional relationship is an ongoing interaction that observes a set of established boundaries or limits deemed appropriate under governing standards. The nurse is sensitive to a person's situation and purposefully engages with them using knowledge and skills with respect, compassion and kindness. In the relationship, the person's rights and dignity are recognised and respected. The professional nature of the relationship involves recognition of professional boundaries and issues of unequal power.

Referral involves a nurse sending a person to obtain an opinion or treatment from another health professional or entity. Referral usually involves the transfer (all or in part) of responsibility for the care of the person, usually for a defined time and for a particular purpose, such as care that is outside the referring practitioner's expertise or scope of practice.

Social media describes the online and mobile tools that people use to share opinions, information, experiences, images, and video or audio clips. It includes websites and applications used for social networking. Common sources of social media include, but are not limited to, social networking sites such as Facebook and LinkedIn, blogs (personal, professional and those published anonymously), WOMO, True Local, microblogs such as Twitter, content-sharing websites such as YouTube and Instagram, and discussion forums and message boards.

Substitute decision-maker is a general term for a person who is either a legally appointed decision-maker for a person, or has been nominated to make healthcare decisions on behalf of a person whose decision-making capacity is impaired.

Supervision includes managerial supervision, professional supervision and clinically focused supervision as part of delegation. For details see the NMBA Supervision guidelines for nursing and midwifery.

Therapeutic relationships are different to personal relationships. In a therapeutic relationship the nurse is sensitive to a person's situation and purposefully engages with them using knowledge and skills in respect, compassion and kindness. In the relationship the person's rights and dignity are recognised and respected. The professional nature of the relationship involves recognition of professional boundaries and issues of unequal power.

Unprofessional conduct includes conduct of a lesser standard that might reasonably be expected by the public or professional peers.

Bibliography

The Australian Commission on Safety and Quality in Health Care website www.safetyandquality.gov.au provides relevant guidance on a range of safety and quality issues. Information of particular relevance to nurses includes:

- end-of-life care
- hand hygiene
- healthcare rights
- health literacy
- medication administration, and
- open disclosure and incident management

The Australian Health Practitioner Regulation Agency (AHPRA) works in partnership with the NMBA to regulate nurses and midwives in Australia.

The Australian Human Rights Commission also provides resources that promote and protect human rights. Resources on workplace bullying include a fact sheet and a 'get help' section at https://www.humanrights.gov.au.

The Congress of Aboriginal and Torres Strait Islander Nurses and Midwives (CATSINaM) website (http://catsinam.org.au/) 'promotes, supports and advocates for Aboriginal and Torres Strait Islander nurses and midwives and to close the gap in health for Aboriginal and Torres Strait Islander peoples'.

The National Aboriginal and Torres Strait Islander Health Plan 2013 – 2023 provides an evidence-based framework for a coordinated approach to improving Aboriginal and/or Torres Strait Islander peoples' health. For additional information go to www.health.gov.au/NATSIHP.

The National Health and Medical Research Council website www.nhmrc.gov.au provides relevant information on informed consent and research issues.

The national Nurse & Midwife Support service provides 24 hour access to health support anywhere in Australia.

The Therapeutic Goods Administration website www.tga.gov.au provides relevant information on therapeutic goods.

The Nursing and Midwifery Board of Australia website is the best place to find up to date information, standards and guidelines for nurses and midwives (www.nursingmidwiferyboard.gov.au).

Appendix B – Code of conduct for midwives

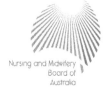

Nursing and Midwifery
Board of
Australia

Code of conduct for midwives

Nursing and Midwifery Board of Australia
G.P.O. Box 9958 | Melbourne VIC 3001 | www.nursingmidwiferyboard.gov.au

Foreword

The Nursing and Midwifery Board of Australia (NMBA) undertakes functions as set by the Health Practitioner Regulation National Law (the National Law), as in force in each state and territory. The NMBA regulates the practice of nursing and midwifery in Australia, and one of its key roles is to protect the public. The NMBA does this by developing standards, codes and guidelines that together establish the requirements for the professional and safe practice of nurses and midwives in Australia.

In developing the *Code of conduct for midwives,* and consistent with its commitment to evidence-based structures, systems and processes, the NMBA carried out a comprehensive review that was informed by research and by the profession. The research included an international and national literature review of other codes and similar publications, a comparative analysis of the predecessor code of conduct to other codes and an analysis of notifications (complaints) made about the conduct and behaviour of midwives. Input was extensively sought in the form of focus groups, workshops, an expert working group and other consultation strategies which included the profession, the public and professional organisations.

The *Code of conduct for midwives* (the code) sets out the legal requirements, professional behaviour and conduct expectations for midwives in all practice settings, in Australia. The code is written in recognition that midwifery practice is not restricted to the provision of direct clinical care. Midwifery practice settings extend to working in a non-clinical relationship with women, working in management, leadership, governance, administration, education, research, advisory, regulatory, policy development roles or other roles that impact on safe, effective delivery of services in the profession and/or use of the midwife's professional skills.

The code is supported by the NMBA Standards for practice and, with the other NMBA standards, codes and guidelines, underpins the requirements and delivery of safe, kind and compassionate midwifery practice.

Associate Professor Lynette Cusack, RN

Chair
Nursing and Midwifery Board of Australia

Contents

Introduction

The *Code of conduct for midwives* sets out the legal requirements, professional behaviour and conduct expectations for all midwives, in all practice settings, in Australia. It describes the principles of professional behaviour that guide safe practice, and clearly outlines the conduct expected of midwives by their colleagues and the broader community.

Individual midwives have their own personal beliefs and values. However, the code outlines specific standards which all midwives are expected to adopt in their practice. The code also gives students of midwifery an appreciation of the conduct and behaviours expected of midwives. Midwives have a professional responsibility to understand and abide by the code. In practice, midwives have a duty to make the interests of women their first concern, and to practise safely and effectively.

The code is consistent with the National Law. It includes seven principles of conduct, grouped into domains, each with an explanatory value statement. Each value statement is accompanied by practical guidance to demonstrate how to apply it in practice. Underpinning the code is the expectation that midwives will exercise their professional judgement to deliver the best possible outcomes in practice.

This code applies to all midwives

The principles of the code apply to all types of midwifery practice in all contexts. This includes any work where a midwife uses midwifery skills and knowledge, whether paid or unpaid, clinical or non-clinical. This includes work in the areas of clinical care, clinical leadership, clinical governance responsibilities, education, research, administration, management, advisory roles, regulation or policy development. The code also applies to all settings where a midwife may engage in these activities, including face-to-face, publications, or via online or electronic means.

Using the code of conduct

The code will be used:

- to support individual midwives in the delivery of safe practice and fulfilling their professional roles
- as a guide for the public and consumers of health services about the standard of conduct and behaviour they should expect from midwives
- to help the NMBA protect the public, in setting and maintaining the standards set out in the code and to ensure safe and effective midwifery practice
- when evaluating the professional conduct of midwives. If professional conduct varies significantly from the values outlined in the code, midwives should be prepared to explain and justify their decisions and actions. Serious or repeated failure to abide by this code may have consequences for midwives' registration and may be considered as unsatisfactory professional performance, unprofessional conduct or professional misconduct[1], and
- as a resource for activities which aim to enhance the culture of professionalism in the Australian health system. These include use, for example, in administration and policy development by health services and other institutions; in midwifery education, in management and for the orientation, induction and supervision of midwives and students.

The code is not a substitute for requirements outlined in the National Law, other relevant legislation, or case law. Where there is any actual or perceived conflict between the code and any law, the law takes precedence. Midwives also need to understand and comply with all other NMBA standards, codes and guidelines.

---

[1] As defined in the National Law, with the exception of NSW where the definitions of unsatisfactory professional conduct and professional misconduct are defined in the Health Practitioner Regulation National Law (NSW).

Nursing and Midwifery
Board of
Australia

Code of conduct for midwives: domains, principles and values

These domains, principles and values set out legal requirements, professional behaviour and conduct expectations for all midwives. The principles apply to all areas of practice, with an understanding that midwives will exercise professional judgement in applying them, with the goal of delivering the best possible outcomes.

(To note: **Woman** or **women** is used to refer to those individuals who have entered into a therapeutic and/or professional relationship with a midwife. See glossary for further detail.)

Domain: Practise legally

1. **Legal compliance**
   Midwives respect and adhere to their professional obligations under the National Law, and abide by relevant laws.

Domain: Practise safely, effectively and collaboratively

2. **Woman-centred practice**
   Midwives provide safe, woman-centred and evidence-based practice for the health and wellbeing of women and, in partnership with the woman, promote shared decision-making and care delivery between the woman, her baby, nominated partners, family, friends and health professionals.

3. **Cultural practice and respectful relationships**
   Midwives engage with women as individuals in a culturally safe and respectful way, foster open and honest professional relationships and adhere to their obligations about privacy and confidentiality.

Domain: Act with professional integrity

4. **Professional behaviour**
   Midwives embody integrity, honesty, respect and compassion.

5. **Teaching, supervising and assessing**
   Midwives commit to teaching, supervising and assessing students and other midwives, in order to develop the midwifery workforce across all contexts of practice.

6. **Research in health**
   Midwives recognise the vital role of research to inform quality healthcare and policy development, conduct research ethically and support the decision-making of women who participate in research.

Domain: Promote health and wellbeing

7. **Health and wellbeing**
   Midwives promote health and wellbeing for women and their families, colleagues, the broader community and themselves and in a way that addresses health inequality.

Code of conduct for midwives

Domain: Practise legally

Principle 1: Legal compliance

Value
Midwives respect and adhere to professional obligations under the National Law, and abide by relevant laws[2].

1.1 Obligations

It is important that midwives are aware of their obligations under the National Law, including reporting requirements and meeting registration standards. Midwives must:

a. abide by any reporting obligations under the National Law and other relevant legislation. Please refer to sections 129, 130, 131 and 141 of the National Law and the NMBA Guidelines for mandatory notifications

b. inform the Australian Health Practitioner Regulation Agency (AHPRA) and their employer(s) if a legal or regulatory entity has imposed restrictions on their practice, including limitations, conditions, undertakings, suspension, cautions or reprimands, and recognise that a breach of any restriction would place the public at risk and may constitute unprofessional conduct or professional misconduct

c. complete the required amount of CPD relevant to their context of practice. See the NMBA Registration standard: Continuing professional development, Policy: Exemptions from continuing professional development for nurses and midwives and Fact sheet: Continuing professional development for these requirements

d. ensure their practice is appropriately covered by professional indemnity insurance (see the NMBA Registration standard: Professional indemnity insurance arrangements and Fact sheet: Professional indemnity insurance arrangements), and

e. inform AHPRA of charges, pleas and convictions relating to criminal offences (see the NMBA Registration standard: Criminal history).

1.2 Lawful behaviour

Midwives practise honestly and ethically and should not engage in unlawful behaviour as it may affect their practice and/or damage the reputation of the profession. Midwives must:

a. respect the midwife-woman professional relationship by not taking possessions and/or property that belong to the woman and/or her family

b. comply with relevant poisons legislation, authorisation, local policy and own scope of practice, including to safely use, administer, obtain, possess, prescribe, sell, supply and store medications and other therapeutic products

c. not participate in unlawful behaviour and understand that unlawful behaviour may be viewed as unprofessional conduct or professional misconduct and have implications for their registration, and

d. understand that making frivolous or vexatious complaints may be viewed as unprofessional conduct or professional misconduct and have implications for their registration.

---

[2] The code does not address in detail the full range of legal and ethical obligations that apply to midwives. Examples of legal obligations include, but are not limited to, obligations arising in Acts and Regulations relating to privacy, the aged and disabled, child protection, bullying, anti-discrimination and workplace health and safety issues. Midwives should ensure they know all of their legal obligations relating to professional practice, and abide by them.

1.3   Mandatory reporting

Caring for those who are vulnerable brings legislative responsibilities for midwives, including the need to abide by relevant mandatory reporting requirements as they apply across individual states and territories. Midwives must:

a. abide by the relevant mandatory reporting legislation that is imposed to protect groups that are particularly at risk, including reporting obligations about child abuse and neglect and remaining alert to the newborn and infants who may be at risk, and

b. remain alert to other groups who may be vulnerable and at risk of physical harm and sexual exploitation and act on welfare concerns where appropriate.

Domain: Practise safely, effectively and collaboratively

Principle 2: Woman-centred practice

> **Value**
> Midwives provide safe, woman-centred, evidence-based practice for the health and wellbeing of women and, in collaboration with the woman, promote shared decision-making and care delivery between the woman and baby, nominated partners, family, friends and health professionals.

2.1   Midwifery practice

Midwives apply woman-centred and evidence-based decision-making, and have a responsibility to ensure the delivery of safe and quality care. Midwives must:

a. practise in accordance with the standards of the profession and broader health system (including the NMBA standards, codes and guidelines and the Australian Commission on Safety and Quality in Health Care)

b. provide leadership to ensure the delivery of safe and quality care and understand their professional responsibility to protect women, ensuring employees comply with their obligations, and

c. document and report concerns if they believe the practice environment is compromising the health and safety of women receiving care.

2.2   Decision-making

Making decisions about healthcare is the shared responsibility of the woman (who may wish to involve her nominated partners, family and friends), the midwife and other health professionals. Midwives should create and foster conditions that promote shared decision-making and collaborative practice. To support shared decision-making, midwives must:

a. take a woman-centred approach to managing a woman's care and concerns, supporting the woman in a manner consistent with that woman's values and preferences

b. advocate on behalf of the woman where necessary, and recognise when substitute decision-makers are needed (including legal guardians or holders of power of attorney)

c. support the right of women to seek second and/or subsequent opinions, or the right to refuse treatment/care

d. recognise that care may be provided to the same woman by different midwives, and by other members of the healthcare team, at various times

e. recognise and work within their scope of practice which is determined by their education, training, authorisation, competence, qualifications and experience in accordance with local policy (see also the NMBA Decision-making framework)

f. recognise when an activity is not within their scope of practice and refer women to another health practitioner when this is in the best interests of the woman receiving care

g. take reasonable steps to ensure any person to whom a midwife delegates, refers, or hands over care has the qualifications, experience, knowledge, skills and scope of practice to provide the care needed (see also the NMBA Decision-making framework), and

h. recognise that their context of practice can influence decision-making. This includes the type and location of practice setting, the characteristics of the woman receiving care, the focus of midwifery activities, the degree to which practice is autonomous and the resources available.

2.3 Informed consent

Informed consent is a woman's voluntary agreement to healthcare, which is made with knowledge and understanding of the potential benefits and risks involved. In supporting the right to informed consent, midwives must:

a. support the provision of information to the woman about her care in a way and/or in a language/dialect she can understand through the utilisation of translating and interpreting services, when necessary. This includes information on examinations and investigations, as well as treatments

b. give the woman adequate time to ask questions, make decisions and to refuse, interventions, investigations and treatments, and proceed in accordance with the woman's choice, considering local policy

c. act according to the woman's capacity for decision-making and consent, including when caring for children and young people, based on their maturity and capacity to understand, and the nature of the proposed care

d. obtain informed consent or other valid authority before carrying out an examination or investigation, provide treatment (this may not be possible in an emergency), or involving women in teaching or research, and

e. inform the woman of the benefit as well as associated costs or risks if referring the woman for further assessment, investigations or treatments, which they may want to clarify before proceeding. (See also the Australian College of Midwives National Midwifery Guidelines for Consultation and Referral).

2.4 Adverse events and open disclosure

When a woman is harmed by healthcare (adverse events), midwives have responsibilities to be open and honest in communicating with the woman, to review what happened, and to report the event in a timely manner and in accordance with local policy. When something goes wrong, midwives must:

a. recognise and reflect on what happened and report the incident

b. act immediately to rectify the problem if possible, and intervene directly if it is needed to protect the woman's safety. This responsibility includes escalating concerns if needed

c. abide by the principles of open disclosure and non-punitive approaches to incident management

d. identify the most appropriate healthcare team member to provide an apology and an explanation to the woman, as promptly and completely as possible, that supports open disclosure principles

e. listen to the woman, acknowledge any distress she experienced and provide support. In some cases it may be advisable to refer the woman to another midwife or health professional

f. ensure women have access to information about how to make a complaint, and that in doing so, not allow a complaint or notification to negatively affect the care they provide, and

g. seek advice from their employer, AHPRA, their professional indemnity insurer, or other relevant bodies, if they are unsure about their obligations.

See also the Australian Commission on Safety and Quality in Health Care's publication <u>Australian Open Disclosure Framework</u>.

Value
Midwives engage with women as individuals in a culturally safe and respectful way, foster open, honest and compassionate professional relationships and adhere to their obligations about privacy and confidentiality.

3.1 Aboriginal and/or Torres Strait Islander peoples' health

Australia has always been a culturally and linguistically diverse nation. Aboriginal and/or Torres Strait Islander peoples have inhabited and cared for the land as the first peoples of Australia for millennia, and their histories and cultures have uniquely shaped our nation. Understanding and acknowledging historic factors such as colonisation and its impact on Aboriginal and/or Torres Strait Islander peoples' health helps inform care. In particular, Aboriginal and/or Torres Strait Islander peoples bear the burden of gross social, cultural and health inequality. In supporting the health of Aboriginal and/or Torres Strait Islander peoples, midwives must:

   a. provide care that is holistic, free of bias and racism, challenges belief based upon assumption and is culturally safe and respectful for Aboriginal and/or Torres Strait Islander peoples

   b. advocate for and act to facilitate access to quality and culturally safe health services for Aboriginal and/or Torres Strait Islander peoples, and

   c. recognise the importance of family, community, partnership and collaboration in the healthcare decision-making of Aboriginal and/or Torres Strait Islander peoples, for both prevention strategies and care delivery.

   See the <u>National Aboriginal and Torres Strait Islander Health Plan 2013–2023</u>.

   See also <u>Congress of Aboriginal and Torres Strait Islander Nurses and Midwives</u>.

3.2 Culturally safe and respectful practice

Culturally safe and respectful practice requires having knowledge of how a midwife's own culture, values, attitudes, assumptions and beliefs influence their interactions with women and families, the community and colleagues. To ensure culturally safe and respectful practice, midwives must:

   a. understand that only the woman and/or her family can determine whether or not care is culturally safe and respectful

   b. respect diverse cultures, beliefs, gender identities, sexualities and experiences of women and others, including among team members

   c. acknowledge the social, economic, cultural, historic and behavioural factors influencing health, both at the individual, community and population levels

   d. adopt practices that respect diversity, avoid bias, discrimination and racism, and challenge belief based upon assumption (for example, based on gender, disability, race, ethnicity, religion, sexuality, age or political beliefs)

   e. support an inclusive environment for the safety and security of the individual woman and her family and/or significant others, and

   f. create a positive, culturally safe work environment through role modelling, and supporting the rights, dignity and safety of others, including women and colleagues.

3.3 Effective communication

Positive professional relationships are built on effective communication that is respectful, kind, compassionate and honest. To communicate effectively, midwives must:

a. be aware of health literacy issues, and take health literacy into account when communicating with women

b. make arrangements, whenever possible, to meet the specific language, cultural, and communication needs of women and their families, through the utilisation of translating and interpreting services where necessary, and be aware of how these needs affect understanding

c. endeavour to confirm the woman understands any information communicated to her

d. clearly and accurately communicate relevant and timely information about the woman to colleagues, within the bounds of relevant privacy requirements, and

e. be non-judgemental and not refer to women in a non-professional manner verbally or in correspondence/records, including refraining from behaviour that may be interpreted as bullying or harassment and/or culturally unsafe.

3.4 Bullying and harassment

When people repeatedly and intentionally use words or actions against someone or a group of people, it causes distress and risks their wellbeing. Midwives understand that bullying and harassment relating to their practice or workplace is not acceptable or tolerated and that where it is affecting public safety, may have implications for their registration. Midwives must:

a. never engage in, ignore or excuse such behaviour

b. recognise that bullying and harassment takes many forms, including behaviours such as physical and verbal abuse, racism, discrimination, violence, aggression, humiliation, pressure in decision-making, exclusion and intimidation directed towards people or colleagues

c. understand social media is sometimes used as a mechanism to bully or harass, and that midwives should not engage in, ignore or excuse such behaviour

d. act to eliminate bullying and harassment, in all its forms, in the workplace, and

e. escalate their concerns if an appropriate response does not occur.

For additional guidance see the Australian Human Rights Commission's Fact sheet on workplace bullying.

See also Nurse & Midwife Support, the national health support service for nurses, midwives and students.

3.5 Confidentiality and privacy

Midwives have ethical and legal obligations to protect the privacy of women. Women have a right to expect that midwives will hold information about them in confidence, unless the release of information is needed by law, legally justifiable under public interest considerations or is required to facilitate emergency care. To protect privacy and confidentiality, midwives must:

a. respect the confidentiality and privacy of the woman by seeking informed consent before disclosing information, including formally documenting such consent where possible

b. provide surroundings to enable private and confidential consultations and discussions, particularly when working with multiple women at the same time, or in a shared space

c. abide by the NMBA Social media policy and relevant Standards for practice, to ensure use of social media is consistent with the midwife's ethical and legal obligations to protect privacy

d. access records only when professionally involved in the care of the woman, and authorised to do so

e. not transmit, share, reproduce or post any woman's information or images even if the woman is not directly named or identified, without having first gained written and informed consent. See also the NMBA <u>Social media policy</u> and <u>Guidelines for advertising regulated health services</u>

f. recognise the woman's right to access information contained in her health records, facilitate that access and promptly facilitate the transfer of health information when requested by the woman in accordance with local policy, and

g. when closing or relocating a practice, facilitating arrangements for the transfer or management of all health records in accordance with the legislation governing privacy and health records.

3.6   End-of-life care

Midwives may have a role in helping the community to deal with the reality of death and its consequences. In providing culturally appropriate end-of-life care, midwives must:

a. understand the limits of healthcare in prolonging life, and recognise when efforts to prolong life may not be in the best interest of the woman

b. accept that the woman, has the right to refuse treatment, or to request withdrawal of treatment, while ensuring the woman receives relief from distress

c. respect diverse cultural practices and beliefs related to death and dying

d. facilitate advance care planning and provision of end-of-life care where relevant and in accordance with local policy and legislation, and

e. take reasonable steps to ensure support is provided to the woman and her family, even when it is not possible to deliver the outcome they desire.

See also the <u>Australian Commission on Safety and Quality in Health Care - End-of-Life Care</u>.

Domain: Act with professional integrity

Principle 4: Professional behaviour

Value
Midwives embody integrity, honesty, respect and compassion.

4.1   Professional boundaries

Professional boundaries allow midwives, the woman and the woman's nominated partners, family and friends to engage safely and effectively in professional relationships, including where care involves personal and/or intimate contact. In order to maintain professional boundaries, there is a start and end point to the professional relationship and it is integral to the midwife-woman professional relationship. Adhering to professional boundaries promotes woman-centred practice and protects both parties. To maintain professional boundaries, midwives must:

a. recognise the inherent power imbalance that exists between midwives, women in their care and significant others and establish and maintain professional boundaries

b. actively manage the woman's expectations, and be clear about professional boundaries that must exist in professional relationships for objectivity in care and prepare the woman for when the episode of care ends

c. avoid the potential conflicts, risks, and complexities of providing care to those with whom they have a pre-existing non-professional relationship, and ensure that such relationships do not impair their judgement. This is especially relevant for those living and working in small, regional or cultural communities and/or where there is long-term professional, social and/or family engagement

d. avoid sexual relationships with the woman, her partner and/or members of the woman's family, with whom they have currently or had previously entered into a professional relationship. These relationships are inappropriate in most circumstances and could be considered unprofessional conduct or professional misconduct

e. recognise when over-involvement has occurred, and disclose this concern to an appropriate person, whether this is the person involved or a colleague

f. reflect on the circumstances surrounding any occurrence of over-involvement, document and report it and engage in management to rectify or manage the situation

g. in cases where the professional relationship has become compromised or ineffective and ongoing care is needed, facilitate arrangements for the continuing care of the woman to another health practitioner, including passing on relevant clinical information (see also 3.3 Effective communication)

h. actively address indifference, omission, disengagement/lack of care and disrespect to women that may reflect under-involvement, including escalating the issue to ensure the safety of the woman if necessary

i. avoid expressing personal beliefs to the woman in ways that exploit the woman's vulnerability, are likely to cause them unnecessary distress, or may negatively influence their autonomy in decision-making (see the NMBA Standards for practice), and

j. not participate in physical assault such as striking, unauthorised restraining and/or applying unnecessary force.

4.2   Advertising and professional representation

Midwives must be honest and transparent when describing their education, qualifications, previous occupations and registration status. This includes, but is not limited to, when midwives are involved in job applications, self-promotion, publishing of documents or web content, public appearances, or advertising or promoting goods or services. To honestly represent products and regulated health services, and themselves, midwives must:

a. comply with legal requirements about advertising outlined in the National Law (explained in the NMBA Guidelines for advertising regulated health services), as well as other relevant Australian state and territory legislation

b. provide only accurate, honest and verifiable information about their registration, experience and qualifications, including any conditions that apply to their registration (see also Principle 1: Legal compliance)

c. only use the title of midwife if they hold valid registration (see the NMBA Fact sheet: The use of health practitioner protected titles), and

d. never misrepresent, by either a false statement or an omission, their registration, experience, qualifications or position.

4.3   Legal, insurance and other assessments

Midwives may be contracted by a third party to provide an assessment of a woman who is not in their care, such as for legal, insurance or other administrative purposes. When this occurs, the usual midwife-woman professional relationship does not exist. In this situation, midwives must:

a. explain to the woman their professional area of practice, role, and the purpose, nature and extent of the assessment to be performed

b. anticipate and seek to correct any misunderstandings the woman may have about the nature and purpose of the assessment and report, and

c. inform the woman and/or her referring health professional of any unrecognised, serious problems that are discovered during the assessment, as a matter of duty-of-care.

4.4   Conflicts of interest

Women rely on the independence and trustworthiness of midwives who provide them with advice or treatment. In midwifery practice, a conflict of interest arises when a midwife has financial, professional or personal interests or relationships and/or personal beliefs that may affect the care they provide or result in personal gain.

Such conflicts may mean the midwife does not prioritise the interests of the woman as they should, and may be viewed as unprofessional conduct. To prevent conflicts of interest from compromising care, midwives must:

a. act with integrity and in the best interests of women when making referrals, and when providing or arranging treatment or care

b. responsibly use their right to not provide, or participate directly in, treatments to which they have a conscientious objection. In such a situation, midwives must respectfully inform the woman, their employer and other relevant colleagues, of their objection and ensure the woman has alternative care options

c. proactively and openly inform the woman if a midwife, or the midwife's immediate family, have a financial or commercial interest that could be perceived as influencing the care they provide

d. not offer financial, material or other rewards (inducements) to encourage others to act in ways that personally benefit the midwife, nor do anything that could be perceived as providing inducements, and

e. not allow any financial or commercial interest in any entity providing healthcare services or products to negatively affect the way the woman is treated.

4.5   Financial arrangements and gifts

It is necessary to be honest and transparent with women. To ensure there is no perception of actual or personal gain for the midwife, midwives must:

a. when providing or recommending services, discuss with the woman all fees and charges expected to result from a course of treatment in a manner appropriate to the professional relationship, and not exploit the woman's vulnerability or lack of knowledge

b. only accept token gifts of minimal value that are freely offered, and report the gift in accordance with local policy

c. not accept, encourage or manipulate the woman to give, lend, or bequeath money or gifts that will benefit a midwife directly or indirectly

d. not become financially involved with a woman who has or who will be in receipt of their care, for example through bequests, powers of attorney, loans and investment schemes, and

e. not influence the woman or their family to make donations and where the woman seeks to make a donation refer to the local policy.

Principle 5: Teaching, supervising and assessing

| **Value** |
| Midwives commit to teaching, supervising and assessing students and other midwives in order to develop the midwifery workforce across all contexts of practice. |

5.1   Teaching and supervising

It is the responsibility of all midwives to create opportunities for midwifery students and midwives under supervision to learn, as well as benefit from oversight and feedback. In their teaching and supervisor roles, midwives must:

a. seek to develop the skills, attitudes and practices of an effective teacher and/or supervisor

b. reflect on the ability, competence and learning needs of each student or midwife who they teach or supervise and plan teaching and supervision activities accordingly, and

c. avoid, where possible, any potential conflicts of interest in teaching or supervision relationships that may impair objectivity or interfere with the supervised person's learning outcomes or experience. This includes, for example, not supervising somebody with whom they have a pre-existing non-professional relationship.

5.2   Assessing colleagues and students

Assessing colleagues and students is an important part of making sure that the highest standard of practice is achieved across the profession. In assessing the competence and performance of colleagues or students, midwives must:

a. be honest, objective, fair, without bias and constructive, and not put women at risk of harm by inaccurate and inadequate assessment, and

b. provide accurate and justifiable information promptly, and include all relevant information when giving references or writing reports about colleagues.

See also the NMBA Supervision guidelines for nursing and midwifery

Principle 6: Research in health

Value
Midwives recognise the vital role of research to inform quality healthcare and policy development, conduct research ethically and support the decision-making of women who participate in research.

6.1   Rights and responsibilities

Midwives involved in design, organisation, conduct or reporting of health research have additional responsibilities. Midwives involved in research must:

a. recognise and carry out the responsibilities associated with involvement in health research

b. in research that involves human participants, respect the decision-making of women to not participate and/or withdraw from a study, ensuring their decision does not compromise their care or any midwife-woman professional relationship(s), and

c. be aware of the values and ethical considerations for Aboriginal and/or Torres Strait Islander communities when undertaking research.

See also the National Health and Medical Research Council publication: Values and Ethics - Guidelines for Ethical Conduct in Aboriginal and Torres Strait Islander Health Research.

See also Principle 2 on the application of evidence-based decision-making for delivery of safe and quality care.

Domain: Promote health and wellbeing

Principle 7: Health and wellbeing

Value
Midwives promote health and wellbeing for women and their families, colleagues, the broader community and themselves and in a way that addresses health inequality.

7.1   Your and your colleagues' health

Midwives have a responsibility to maintain their physical and mental health to practise safely and effectively. To promote health for midwifery practice, midwives must:

a. understand and promote the principles of public health, such as health promotion activities and vaccination

b. act to reduce the effect of fatigue and stress on their health, and on their ability to provide safe care

c. encourage and support colleagues to seek help if they are concerned that their colleague's health may be affecting their ability to practise safely, utilising services such as Nurse & Midwife Support, the national health support service for nurses, midwives and students

d. seek expert, independent and objective help and advice if they are ill or impaired in their ability to practise safely. Midwives must remain aware of the risks of self-diagnosis and self-treatment, and act to reduce these, and

e. take action, including a mandatory or voluntary notification to AHPRA, if a midwife knows or reasonably suspects that they or a colleague have a health condition or impairment that could adversely affect their ability to practise safely, or put women at risk (see also Principle 1: Legal compliance).

7.2   Health advocacy

There are significant disparities in the health status of various groups in the Australian community. These disparities result from social, historic, geographic, environmental, legal, physiological and other factors. Some groups who experience health disparities include Aboriginal and/or Torres Strait Islander peoples, those with disabilities, those who are gender or sexuality diverse, and those from social, culturally and linguistically diverse backgrounds, including asylum seekers and refugees. In advocating for community and population health, midwives must:

a. use their expertise and influence to protect and advance the health and wellbeing of individuals as well as communities and populations

b. understand and apply the principles of primary and public health, including health education, health promotion, disease prevention and control and health screening using the best available evidence in making practice decisions, and

c. participate in efforts to promote the health of communities and meet their obligations with respect to disease prevention including vaccination, health screening and reporting notifiable diseases.

See also the NMBA Position statement on nurses, midwives and vaccination.

Glossary

These meanings relate to the use of the terms in the *Code of conduct for midwives*.

Advance care planning is an on-going process of shared planning for current and future healthcare. It allows an individual to make known their values, beliefs and preferences to guide decision-making, even after when the individual cannot make or communicate their preferences and decisions (see Advance Care Planning Australia).

Bullying and harassment is 'when people repeatedly and intentionally use words or actions against someone or a group of people to cause distress and risk to their wellbeing. These actions are usually done by people who have more influence or power over someone else, or who want to make someone else feel less powerful or helpless'[3] (Australian Human Rights Commission definition).

Competence is the possession of required skills, knowledge, education and capacity.

Cultural safety concept was developed in a First Nations' context and is the preferred term for nursing and midwifery. Cultural safety is endorsed by the Congress of Aboriginal and Torres Strait Islander Nurses and Midwives (CATSINaM), who emphasise that cultural safety is as important to quality care as clinical safety. However, the "presence or absence of cultural safety is determined by the recipient of care; it is not defined by the caregiver" (CATSINaM 2014, p. 9[4]). Cultural safety is a philosophy of practice that is about how a health professional does something, not [just] what they do. It is about how people are treated in society, not about their diversity as such, so its focus is on systemic and structural issues and on the social determinants of health. Cultural safety represents a key philosophical shift from providing care regardless of difference, to care that takes account of peoples' unique needs. It requires nurses and midwives to undertake an ongoing process of self-reflection and cultural self-awareness, and an acknowledgement of how a nurse's/midwife's personal culture impacts on care. In relation to Aboriginal and Torres Strait Islander health, cultural safety provides a de-colonising model of practice based on dialogue, communication, power sharing and negotiation, and the acknowledgment of white privilege. These actions are a means to challenge racism at personal and institutional levels, and to establish trust in healthcare encounters (CATSINaM 2017b, p. 11[5]). In focusing on clinical interactions, particularly power inequity between patient and health professional, cultural safety calls for a genuine partnership where power is shared between the individuals and cultural groups involved in healthcare. Cultural safety is also relevant to Aboriginal and Torres Strait Islander health professionals. Non-Indigenous nurses and midwives must address how they create a culturally safe work environment that is free of racism for their Aboriginal and Torres Strait Islander colleagues (CATSINaM 2017a[6]).

Delegation is the relationship that exists when a midwife devolves aspects of midwifery practice to another person. Delegations are made to meet the woman and her baby's health needs. The midwife who is delegating retains accountability for the decision to delegate. The midwife is also accountable for monitoring of the communication of the delegation to the relevant persons and for the practice outcomes. Both parties share the responsibility of making the delegation decision, which includes assessment of the competence and risks. For further details see the NMBA National framework for the development of decision-making tools for nursing and midwifery practice.

Discrimination is the unjust treatment of one or more person/s based on factors such as race, religion, sex, disability or other grounds specified in anti-discrimination legislation.[7]

Handover is the process of transferring all responsibility for the care of the woman to another health practitioner or person.

---

[3] Australian Human Rights Commission, '*What is bullying*?' https://www.humanrights.gov.au/what-bullying-violence-harassment-and-bullying-fact-sheet.

[4] CATSINaM, 2014, *Towards a shared understanding of terms and concepts: strengthening nursing and midwifery care of Aboriginal and Torres Strait Islander peoples*, CATSINaM: Canberra.

[5] CATSINaM: 2017b, *The Nursing and Midwifery Aboriginal and Torres Strait Islander Health Curriculum Framework (Version 1.0)*, CATSINaM, Canberra.

[6] CATSINaM, 2017a, *Position statement: Embedding cultural safety across Australian nursing and midwifery*, CATSINaM: Canberra.

[7] Australian Human Rights Commission, '*Discrimination*' www.humanrights.gov.au/quick-guide/12030.

Health literacy 'is about how people understand information about health and healthcare, how they apply that information to their lives, use it to make decisions and act on it'[8] (Australian Commission on Safety and Quality in Health Care)

Local policy refers to the policies that apply to decision-making, relevant to the specific location and/or organisation where practice is being undertaken.

Mandatory notification is the requirement under the National Law for registered health practitioners, employers and education providers to report certain conduct (see Guidelines for mandatory notifications).

Mandatory reporting is a state and territory legislative requirement imposed to protect at risk groups such as children and young people.

Midwife is a person with prescribed educational preparation and competence for practice who is registered by the NMBA. The NMBA has endorsed the International Confederation of Midwives definition of a midwife and applied it to the Australian context.

National law means the Health Practitioner Regulation National Law that is in force in each state and territory in Australia and applies to those professions regulated under that law (see Australian Health Practitioner Regulation Agency).

Nominated partners, family and friends include people in consensual relationships with the woman as identified by the woman.

Open disclosure 'is an open and honest discussion with a woman about any incident (s) that caused harm while receiving healthcare. It includes an apology or expression of regret (including the word 'sorry'), a factual explanation of what happened, an opportunity for the woman to describe their experience, and an explanation of the steps being taken to manage the event and prevent recurrence'[9] (Australian Commission on Safety and Quality in Health Care).

Over-involvement is when the midwife confuses their needs with the needs of the woman in their care and crosses the boundary of a professional relationship. Behaviour may include favouritism, gifts, intimacy or inappropriate relationships with the partner or family member of a woman in the midwife's care.

Practice means any role, whether remunerated or not, in which the individual uses their skills and knowledge as a midwife. Practice is not restricted to the provision of direct clinical care. It also includes working in a nonclinical relationship with women, working in management, administration, education, research, advisory, regulatory or policy development roles, and any other roles that impact on safe, effective delivery of services in the profession and/or use their professional skills.

Professional boundaries allow a midwife and a woman and her baby, and any of the woman's significant other persons, to engage safely and effectively in a therapeutic and/or professional relationship. Professional boundaries refers to the clear separation that should exist between professional conduct aimed at meeting the health needs of the woman, and behaviour which serves a midwife's own personal views, feelings and relationships that are not relevant to the professional relationship.

Professional misconduct includes conduct by a health practitioner that is substantially below the expected standard and which, whether connected to practice or not, is inconsistent with being a fit and proper person to be registered in the profession.

Professional relationship is an ongoing interaction that observes a set of established boundaries or limits that is deemed appropriate under governing standards. The midwife is sensitive to a woman's situation and purposefully engages with her using knowledge and skills with respect, compassion and kindness. In the relationship, the woman's rights and dignity are recognised and respected. The professional nature of the relationship involves recognition of professional boundaries and issues of unequal power.

---

[8] Australian Commission on Safety and Quality in Health Care, *Health literacy:* https://www.safetyandquality.gov.au/our-work/patient-and-consumer-centred-care/health-literacy/.
[9] Australian Commission on Safety and Quality in Health Care, *Australian Open Disclosure Framework:* https://www.safetyandquality.gov.au/wp-content/uploads/2013/03/Australian-Open-Disclosure-Framework-Feb-2014.pdf.

Referral involves a midwife sending the woman to obtain an opinion or treatment from another health professional or entity. Referral usually involves the transfer (all or in part) of responsibility for the care of the woman, usually for a defined time and for a particular purpose, such as care that is outside the referring practitioner's expertise or scope of practice.

Social media describes the online and mobile tools that people use to share opinions, information, experiences, images, and video or audio clips. It includes websites and applications used for social networking. Common sources of social media include, but are not limited to, social networking sites such as Facebook and LinkedIn, blogs (personal, professional and those published anonymously), WOMO, True Local, microblogs such as Twitter, content-sharing websites such as YouTube and Instagram, and discussion forums and message boards.

Substitute decision-maker is a general term for a person who is either a legally appointed decision-maker for the woman, or has been nominated to make healthcare decisions on behalf of a woman whose decision-making capacity is impaired.

Supervision includes managerial supervision, professional supervision and clinically focused supervision as part of delegation. For details see the NMBA Supervision guidelines for nursing and midwifery.

Therapeutic relationships are different to personal relationships. In a therapeutic relationship the midwife is sensitive to a woman's situation and purposefully engages with her using knowledge and skills in respect, compassion and kindness. In the relationship the woman's rights and dignity are recognised and respected. The professional nature of the relationship involves recognition of professional boundaries and issues of unequal power.

Unprofessional conduct includes conduct of a lesser standard that might reasonably be expected by the public or professional peers.

Woman or **women** is used to refer to those individuals who have entered into a therapeutic and/or professional relationship with a midwife. The word woman in midwifery is generally understood to be inclusive of the woman's baby, partner and family. Therefore, the words woman or women include all the women, babies, newborn, infants, children, families, carers, groups and/or communities, however named, that are within the midwife's scope and context of practice. Baby in this document refers to the newborn/s, infant/s and child/children as relevant to the midwife's scope of practice.

Woman-centred practice is a collaborative and respectful partnership built on mutual trust and understanding through good communication. Each woman is treated as an individual with the aim of respecting women's ownership of their health information, rights and preferences while protecting their dignity and empowering choice. Woman-centred practice recognises the role of family and community with respect to cultural and religious diversity.

Bibliography

The Australian Commission on Safety and Quality in Health Care website www.safetyandquality.gov.au provides relevant guidance on a range of safety and quality issues. Information of particular relevance to midwives includes:

- end-of-life care
- hand hygiene
- healthcare rights
- health literacy
- medication administration, and
- open disclosure and incident management

The Australian Human Rights Commission also provides resources that promote and protect human rights. Resources on workplace bullying include a fact sheet and a 'get help' section at https://www.humanrights.gov.au.

The Australian Health Practitioner Regulation Agency (AHPRA) works in partnership with the NMBA to regulate nurses and midwives in Australia.

The Congress of Aboriginal and Torres Strait Islander Nurses and Midwives (CATSINaM) website (http://catsinam.org.au/) 'promotes, supports and advocates for Aboriginal and Torres Strait Islander nurses and midwives and to close the gap in health for Aboriginal and Torres Strait Islander peoples'.

The National Aboriginal and Torres Strait Islander Health Plan 2013–2023 provides an evidence-based framework for a coordinated approach to improving Aboriginal and/or Torres Strait Islander people's health. For additional information go to www.health.gov.au/NATSIHP.

The National Health and Medical Research Council website www.nhmrc.gov.au provides relevant information on informed consent and research issues.

The national Nurse & Midwife Support service provides 24 hour access to health support anywhere in Australia.

The Therapeutic Goods Administration website www.tga.gov.au provides relevant information on therapeutic goods.

The Nursing and Midwifery Board of Australia website is the best place to find up to date information, standards and guidelines for nurses and midwives (www.nursingmidwiferyboard.gov.au).

Where to find the International Council of Nurses Code of Ethics and the International Confederation of Midwives Code of Ethics

For the International Council of Nurses Code of ethics for nurses, please visit: www.icn.ch/nursing-policy/regulation-and-education

For the International Confederation of Midwives Code of ethics for midwives, please visit: www.internationalmidwives.org/assets/files/definitions-files/2018/06/eng-international-code-of-ethics-for-midwives.pdf

Glossary

Abortion the intentional termination of pregnancy by drugs or surgical procedure.

Accused the person charged with a criminal offence.

Act an Act of Parliament – a law passed by parliament. Also known as a statute or a piece of legislation.

Advance directive see the section 'How do decisions get made if an adult patient lacks the capacity to make a health care decision?' in Chapter 5.

Assault is the term that is commonly referred to (along with 'battery') when discussing the criminal offence of physically touching someone without consent; and the civil action of trespass against a person without consent. Traditionally, assault referred to an act that led a person to fear physical contact, rather than the contact itself (see battery and trespass).

Assisted Reproductive Technologies (ART) the application of laboratory or clinical techniques to gametes and/or embryos for the purposes of reproduction.

Assisted suicide is the intentional ending of a competent person's life, at their request, where assistance is provided by another person, but the patient does the final act that causes death.

Autonomy the ethical duty to support a person's right to make decisions about their life (also known as self-determination).

Battery is the term that is commonly referred to (along with 'assault') when discussing the criminal offence of physically touching someone without consent; and the civil action of trespass against a person without consent. Traditionally, battery referred to the actual infliction of unlawful contact with a person, rather than just fear of such contact (see assault and trespass).

Beneficence the ethical duty to benefit others.

Burden of proof where one party in a legal proceeding has the burden of demonstrating that all the legal elements are present for them to succeed in the action.

Capacity the mental ability of an individual to make decisions (otherwise known as competence). For a person to have capacity to make health decisions they must be able to comprehend and retain information that is important to the decision and be able to use the information and weigh it in the balance as part of the process of arriving at a decision.

Case a court decision.

Case law see common law.

Causation a determination of whether the damage to the person would have occurred but for the act or omission by the nurse or midwife in this context.

Chemical restraint the use of pharmaceuticals to restrict movement.

Common law law developed by judges through court decisions – also called case law.

Common law system the system of law which exists in Australia which was inherited from the British upon colonisation.

Community treatment order an order that requires a person to involuntarily receive care and treatment for a mental illness in the community.

Competence see capacity.

Confidentiality a principle that information disclosed to a health professional in the context of a professional relationship should not be disclosed to any other person, except as required by law.

Damage harm.

Defendant the person against whom a civil action is brought.

Doctrine of Precedent a lower court must follow a precedent established by a higher court within that legal system (e.g. the Supreme Court of Queensland must follow a precedent established by the Queensland Court of Appeal).

Duty of Care legal obligation imposed upon an individual to take reasonable care when undertaking actions that the person could foresee may cause harm to others.

Elder abuse an act that results in harm to an older person, including physical, sexual, financial, psychological and social abuse or neglect.

Enduring attorney and **enduring guardian** – see the section 'How do decisions get made if an adult patient lacks the capacity to make a health care decision?' in Chapter 5.

Ethical dilemma arising from a situation where there may be opposing, but equally morally legitimate approaches to resolve a dilemma.

Ethical distress moral distress (guilt, concern, distaste) arising from action or inaction – sometimes actions or inaction imposed upon a person by another health professional, organisation or government.

Ethical violation incompetence or deliberate wrong-doing in the context of professional practice.

Euthanasia the intentional ending of a competent person's life, at their request, where another person's actions cause the death of the patient.

***Gillick*-competent** A child who 'achieves a sufficient understanding and intelligence to enable him or her to understand fully what is proposed' (*Gillick and West Norfolk and Wisbech Area Health Authority and Department of Health and Social Security* [1986] AC 112) and therefore can consent to medical treatment.

Guardian in relation to adults lacking capacity, see the section 'How do decisions get made if an adult patient lacks the capacity to make a health care decision?' in Chapter 5.

Jurisdiction the geographic area a government controls which it is able to make laws in relation to.

Justice the ethical duty to ensure distributive justice (the fair distribution and allocation of health services); rights-based justice (to respect patient rights); and legal justice (respect morally just laws and be accountable for one's acts or failures to act).

Legislation law created by parliament or a legislature; also known as a statute. Referred to in Chapter 3 as 'parliament-made law'.

Mechanical restraint the application of devices (straps, manacles, harnesses, bed rails, chairs that are difficult to get out of, etc.) to a person's body to restrict movement.

Negligence conduct that is wrong because it falls short of what a reasonable person is expected to do to protect others from foreseeable risks of harm.

Non-maleficence the ethical duty to not harm others.

Physical restraint the application of physical force to a person's body to restrict movement.

Plaintiff the person bringing a civil action against someone (the defendant) whom it is alleged has caused them harm.

Precedent where a case establishes a principle or rule.

Prosecutor the government public prosecutor who makes a decision regarding whether to pursue a criminal matter against an accused and who brings such matters against the accused to the courts.

Seclusion the confinement of a person in a locked room.

Standard of care standard against which a nurse's or midwife's professional practice is measured to determine whether they have breached their duty of care.

Standard of proof the level of proof required for a party to be successful in a case before court; that is, beyond reasonable doubt (for criminal matters) or on the balance of probabilities (for civil matters).

Statute see Legislation.

Statutory power of Attorney where legislation grants power of attorney to a person to make health-related decisions for an individual who is not competent to make decisions for him- or herself.

Substitute decision-maker see the section 'How do decisions get made if an adult patient lacks the capacity to make a health care decision?' in Chapter 5.

Surrogacy the situation where a woman (the surrogate) agrees with another person or couple to become pregnant with the intention of giving the child born to that person or persons.

Tort law wrongful conduct involving a breach of a duty owed to society but which does not amount to a criminal act.

Trespass (to the person) includes:
1. assault, which is any act which makes a person fear physical contact;
2. battery, intentional contact with a person which that person has not permitted; and
3. false imprisonment, obstructing or limiting a person's freedom of movement.

Vicarious liability an organisation or individual becomes liable for the negligence of another person.

References

ABC News 2010, 'Liver Transplant Mum Dies in Singapore', 1 April, accessed 15 July 2018, <http://www.abc.net.au/news/2010-04-01/liver-transplant-mum-dies-in-singapore/389278>.

ABC News 2013, 'Nurse Roger Dean Admits Arson Murder of 11 Quakers Hill Nursing Home Residents', 27 May, accessed 15 July 2018, <http://www.abc.net.au/news/2013-05-27/nurse-admits-murder-of-11-nursing-home-patients/4715024>.

Aboriginal and Torres Strait Islander Social Justice Commissioner. 2005, *Social Justice Report 2005* Report 3, Human Rights and Equal Opportunity Commission, Canberra.

ABS (Australian Bureau of Statistics). 2008, *One in Five Australians Have a Mental Illness: ABS*, Media release, 23 October 2008.

ABS (Australian Bureau of Statistics). 2012, *Cat. 3302.0.55.003, Life Tables for Aboriginal and Torres Strait Islander Australians 2010–2012, table A2.2, appendix 2, 'Estimating Revised Life Expectancy Measures for 2005–2007'*, accessed 19 September 2018, <http://www.abs.gov.au/ausstats/abs@.nsf/Latestproducts/A308E69131071890CA257C230011C882?opendocument>.

ABS (Australian Bureau of Statistics). 2018, *Cat. 3238.0.55.001, Estimates of Aboriginal and Torres Strait Islander Australians, June 2016*, accessed 19 September 2018, <http://www.abs.gov.au/ausstats/abs@.nsf/mf/3238.0.55.001>.

AHPRA (Australian Health Practitioners Regulatory Agency). 2014a, *Social Media Policy*, <http://www.nursingmidwiferyboard.gov.au/Codes-Guidelines-Statements/Policies/Social-media-policy.aspx>.

AHPRA (Australian Health Practitioners Regulatory Agency). 2014b, *Guidelines for Mandatory Notifications*, <http://www.nursingmidwiferyboard.gov.au/Codes-Guidelines-Statements/Codes-Guidelines/Guidelines-for-mandatory-notifications.aspx>.

Attorney General's Department of New South Wales. 2008, *Capacity Toolkit*, accessed 26 July 2018, <https://www.justice.nsw.gov.au/diversityservices/Documents/capacity_toolkit0609.pdf>.

Australian Commission on Safety and Quality in Health Care 2008, *Australian Charter of Healthcare Rights*, accessed 15 July 2018, <https://www.safetyandquality.gov.au/national-priorities/charter-of-healthcare-rights/>.

Australian Commission on Safety and Quality in Health Care 2015, *National Consensus Statement: Essential Elements for Safe High Quality End of Life Care, Sydney*, accessed 10 August 2018, <https://www.safetyandquality.gov.au/wp-content/uploads/2015/05/

355

National-Consensus-Statement-Essential-Elements-forsafe-high-quality-end-of-life-care.pdf>.

Australian Commission on Safety and Quality in Health Care 2017, *Clinical Governance for Nurses and Midwives*, Australian Commission on Safety and Quality in Health Care, Sydney, <https://www.safetyandquality.gov.au/wp-content/uploads/2017/12/Clinical-governance-for-nurses-and-midwives.pdf>.

Australian Health Ministers' Advisory Council 2016, *Cultural Respect Framework 2016–2026 for Aboriginal and Torres Strait Islander Health*, accessed 15 September 2018, <https://www.coaghealthcouncil.gov.au/Portals/0/National%20Cultural%20Respect%20Framework%20for%20Aboriginal%20and%20Torres%20Strait%20Islander%20Health%202016_2026_2.pdf>.

Australian Health Ministers' Advisory Council 2017, *Discussion Paper Mandatory Reporting under the Health Practitioner Regulation National Law*, <https://www.coaghealthcouncil.gov.au/Portals/0/Mandatory%20reporting%20under%20the%20Health%20Practitioner%20Regulation%20National%20Law.pdf>.

Australian Human Rights Commission 2008, *Indigenous Health Equality Summit Statement of Intent*, accessed 20 September 2018, <http://www.hreoc.gov.au/Social_Justice/health/statement_intent.html>.

Australian Institute of Health and Welfare 2015, *Aboriginal and Torres Strait Islander Health Performance Framework 2014 Report: Detailed Analyses*, cat. no. IHW 167 AIHW: Canberra.

Australian Institute of Health and Welfare 2017, *Older Australia at a Glance*, <https://www.aihw.gov.au/reports/older-people/older-australia-at-a-glance/contents/demographics-of-older-australians/australia-s-changing-age-and-gender-profile>.

Australian Law Reform Commission 2017, *Elder Abuse: A National Legal Response*, <https://www.alrc.gov.au/publications/elder-abuse-report>.

Australian Nursing Federation 2011 *Member Advice: What You Need to Know about Social Networking*, Australian Nursing Federation, Canberra, <http://www.anfvic.asn.au/39548.html>.

Australian Patient Safety Foundation 2000, *Iatrogenic Injury in Australia*, Department of Health and Aged Care: Canberra.

Bauer, M. & Fetherstonhaugh, D. 2016, *Sexuality and People in Residential Aged Care Facilities: A Guide for Partners and Families*, La Trobe University: Melbourne, <http://dementiakt.com.au/wp-content/uploads/2016/08/SexualityConsumerGuide.pdf>.

Beauchamp, T. & Childress, J. 2009, *Principles of Biomedical Ethics*, 6th edn, Oxford University Press: Oxford.

Beauchamp, T. & Childress, J. 2013, *Principles of Biomedical Ethics*, 7th edn, Oxford University Press: Oxford.

Bennett, B. & Douglas, H. 2018, Abortion. In B. White, F. McDonald & L. Willmott (eds), *Health Law in Australia*, 3rd edn, Thomson Reuters: Sydney, 437–495.

Bennett, B. & Trowse, P. 2018, Surrogacy. In B. White, F. McDonald & L. Willmott (eds), *Health Law in Australia*, 3rd edn, Thomson Reuters: Sydney, 497–521.

Best, O. & Fredericks, B. eds. 2018, *Yatdjuligin: Aboriginal and Torres Strait Islander Nursing and Midwifery Care*. Cambridge: Cambridge University Press.

Bowman, K. & Hui, E. 2000, Bioethics for clinicians: 20. Chinese bioethics, *Canadian Medical Association Journal*, 163: 11, 1481–1485.

The Bristol Royal Infirmary Inquiry 2001, *The Report of the Public Inquiry into Children's Heart Surgery at the Bristol Royal Infirmary 1984–1995: Learning from Bristol*, The Stationery Office: Norwich.

Brock, D. 1989, Justice, health care and the elderly, *Philosophy and Public Affairs*, 18: 3, 297–312.

Butler, R.N. 1975, Psychiatry and the elderly: An overview, *American Journal of Psychiatry*, 132: 9, 893–900.

Callahan, D. 1995, *Setting Limits: Medical Goals in an Aging Society*, Georgetown University Press: Washington, DC.

Callahan, D. 1996, Aging and the ends of medicine. In T. Mappes & D. DeGrazia (eds), *Biomedical Ethics*, 4th edn, McGraw Hill: New York, 577–583.

Commonwealth of Australia 1997, *Bringing them Home: National Inquiry into the Separation of Aboriginal and Torres Strait Islander Children from their Families*, accessed 17 September 2018, <https://www.humanrights.gov.au/sites/default/files/content/pdf/social_justice/bringing_them_home_report.pdf>.

Commonwealth of Australia 2017a, *Aboriginal and Torres Strait Islander Health Performance Framework 2017 Report*, accessed 19 September 2018, <https://www.pmc.gov.au/sites/default/files/publications/indigenous/hpf-2017/tier3/314.html>.

Commonwealth of Australia 2017b, *Future of Australia's Aged Care Sector Workforce*, Canberra.

Commonwealth of Australia, Department of Health and Ageing, Office for Aboriginal and Torres Strait Islander Health 2008, *The Link between Primary Health Care and Health Outcomes for Aboriginal and Torres Strait Islander Australians*, accessed 19 September 2018, <https://www.health.gov.au/internet/main/publishing.nsf/Content/EF81F462A8E8482BCA257BF0001ED78 8/$File/2008%20OATSIH%20Primary%20Health%20Care%20lit%20 review%20FINAL%20ll.pdf>.

Council of Australian Governments 2008, *Intergovernmental Agreement for a National Registration and Accreditation Scheme for the Health Professions*.

Council of Australian Governments 2012, *National Indigenous Reform Agreement 2012*, accessed 16 September 2018, <http://www.federalfinancialrelations. gov.au/content/npa/health_indigenous/indigenous-reform/national-agreement_sept_12.pdf>.

Crossthwaite, J. 1994, Feminism and medical ethics, *Monash Bioethical Review*, 13: 3, 13–19.

Daar, A.S. & Khitamy, A. 2001, Bioethics for clinicians: 21. Islamic bioethics, *Canadian Medical Association Journal*, 164: 1, 60–63.

Daniels, N. 1988, *Am I My Parents' Keeper? An Essay on Justice between the Young and the Old*, Oxford University Press: New York.

Donnelly, M. & Kilkelly, U. 2011, Child-friendly healthcare: Delivering on the right to be heard, *Medical Law Review*, 19: 1, 27.

Dworkin, R. 1977, *Taking Rights Seriously*, Harvard University Press: Cambridge, MA.

Ells, C. & Caniano, D. 2002, The impact of culture on the patient-surgeon relationship, *Journal of the American College of Surgeons*, 195: 4, 520–530.

Forrester, K. & Griffiths, D. 2014, *Essentials of Law for Health Professionals*, 4th edn, Elsevier: Sydney, chaps 1–2.

Freegard, H. 2012, End of life. In H. Freegard & L. Isted (eds), *Ethical Practice for Health Professionals*, 2nd edn, Cengage Learning: Sydney, chap. 18.

Garvey, G., Towney, P., McPhee, V., Little, M. & Kerridge, I. 2004, Is there an Aboriginal bioethic?, *Journal of Medical Ethics*, 30, 570–575.

Gillam, L. & Sullivan, J. 2011, Ethics at the end of life: Who should make decisions about treatment limitation for young children with life-threatening or life-limiting conditions? *Journal of Paediatrics and Child Health*, 47, 594–598.

Gilligan, C. 1982, *In A Different Voice*, Harvard University Press: Cambridge, MA.

Gillon, R. 2001, Is there a 'new ethics of abortion'? *Journal of Medical Ethics*, 27: 2, ii5–ii9.

Gregory, J. 2008, Manslaughter charges against nurses dropped, *Courier Mail*, 21 April.

Griffiths, K., Coleman, C., Lee, V. & Madden, R. 2016, 'How colonisation determines social justice and Indigenous health: A review of the literature', *Journal of Population Research*, 33: 1, 9–30.

The Guardian. 2009, 'Death tourism' leads Swiss to consider ban on assisted suicide, *The Guardian*, 29 October, accessed 15 December 2018, <http://www.guardian.co.uk/society/2009/oct/28/swiss-consider-ban-assisted-suicide>.

Hanson, R.M., Phythian, M.A., Jarvis, J.B. & Stewart, C. 1998, The true cost of treating children, *Medical Journal of Australia*, 169: 8, 39–41.

Harris, J. 1998, Rights and reproductive choice. In J. Harris & S. Holm (eds), *The Future of Human Reproduction: Choice and Regulation*, Oxford University Press: Oxford, 5–37.

Health Policy Analysis 2013, *Analysis of Hospital-Acquired Diagnoses and Their Effect on Case Complexity and Resource Use – Final Report*, Australian Commission on Safety and Quality in Health Care: Sydney.

Henry, B., Houston, S. & Mooney, G. 2004. Institutional racism in Australian healthcare: A plea for decency, *Medical Journal of Australia* 180: 10: 517–520.

Hesketh, T. & Xing, Z.W. 2006, Abnormal sex ratios in human populations: Causes and consequences, *Proceedings of the National Academy of Sciences of the United States of America*, 103: 36, 13271–13275.

Higgins, I., Van Der Reit, P., Slater, L. & Peek, C. 2007, The negative attitides of nurses towards elder patients in the acute hospital setting: A qualiatative descriptive study, *Contemporary Nurse*, 26, 225–237.

Ibrahim, J. & Davis, M. 2013, Impediments to applying the 'dignity of risk' principle in residential aged care services, *Australasian Journal on Aging*, 32: 3, 188–193.

ICM (International Confederation of Midwives). 2014, International Code of Ethics for Midwives, The Netherlands, accessed 19 July 2018, <http://internationalmidwives.org/assets/uploads/documents/CoreDocuments/>

CD2008_001%20V2014%20ENG%20International%20Code%20of%20 Ethics%20for%20Midwives.pdf>.

ICN (International Council of Nurses). 2012, ICN Code of Ethics, Switzerland, accessed 19 July 2018, <http://www.icn.ch/images/stories/documents/about/ icncode_english.pdf>.

Illingworth, P. & Parmet, W. 2006, Bioethics: Expanding our horizons. In P. Illingworth & W. Parmet (eds), *Ethical Health Care*, Pearson: New Jersey, 1–15.

Jackson, K. & Parker, M. 2009, Full-steam ahead on the SS 'external regulator'? Mandatory reporting, professional independence and patient harm, *Journal of Law and Medicine*, 17: 1, 29–45.

Jiwani, B. 2001, *An Introduction to Health Ethics Committees: A Professional Guide for the Development of Ethics Resources*, Provincial Health Ethics Network: Alberta, Canada.

Jones, C. 2012, Life in a public mental ward: Enough to drive you insane, *Sydney Morning Herald*, 15 March.

Kable, A., Kelly, B. & Adams, J. 2018, Effects of adverse events on acute care nurses in an Australia context: A qualitative study, *Nursing & Health Sciences*, 20: 2, 238–246.

Kaspiew, R., Carson, R. & Rhoades, H. 2016, *Elder Abuse: Understanding Issues, Frameworks and Responses*. Research Report 35, Australian Institute of Family Studies 5.

Kearney, N., Miller, M., Pail, J. & Smith, K. 2000, Oncology health professionals' attitudes towards elderly people, *Annals of Oncology*, 11: 5, 599–601.

Kelaher, M., Ferdinand, A. & Paradies, Y. 2014, Experiencing racism in health care: The mental health impacts for Victorian Aboriginal communities, *Medical Journal of Australia*, 201: 1, 44–47.

Kenny, N. & Giacomini, M. 2005, Wanted: A new ethical field for health policy analysis, *Health Care Analysis*, 13: 4, 247–260.

Kerridge, I., Lowe, M. & Stewart, C. 2013, *Ethics and Law for the Health Professions*, 4th edn, Federation Press: Sydney.

Khanal, N., Lawton, P., Cass, A. & McDonald, S. 2018, Disparity of access to kidney transplantation by Indigenous and non-Indigenous Australians, *Medical Journal of Australia*, 209: 6, 261–266.

King, L. (trans.) 2008, *The Code of Hammurabi*, The Avalon Project – Documents in Law, History and Diplomacy, http://avalon.aw.yale.edu/ancient/hamframe. asp)

Kingston, M., Evans, S., Smith, B. & Berry J. 2004, Attitudes of doctors and nurses towards incident reporting: A qualiatative analysis, *Medical Journal of Australia*, 181: 1, 36–39.

Kochardy, M. 2010, Impairing the practice of nursing: Implications of mandatory notification on overseas trained nurses in Australia, *Journal of Law and Medicine*, 17: 5, 708–718.

Levinson, W., Gorawara-Bhat, R. & Lamb, J. 2000, A study of patient clues and physician responses in primary care and surgical settings, *Journal of the American Medical Association*, 284: 8, 1021–1027.

Little, M. 1996, Why a feminist approach to bioethics? *Kennedy Institute of Ethics Journal*, 6: 1, 1–18.

Macaldowie, A., Wang, Y.A., Chambers, G.M. & Sullivan, E.A. 2010, Assisted reproductive technology in Australia and New Zealand 2010, *Assisted reproduction technology series no. 16. Cat. no. PER 55*, Canberra: AIHW, accessed 7 August 2018, <https://www.aihw.gov.au/getmedia/6feb5bf2-43df-401f-bbf f-4f2c764a773f/14533.pdf>.

McCallum, J. 1997, Health and aging: The last phase of the epidemiological transition. In A. Borowski, S. Encel & E. Ozanne (eds), *Aging and Social Policy in Australia*, Cambridge University Press: Melbourne, 54–73.

McDonald, F. 2003, 'To become old is to become institutionalised and imprisoned': Comparing regulatory frameworks for the use of restraints in long-term care facilities, *Health Law Review*, 12: 1, 22–28.

McGrath, P. & Phillips, E. 2008, Western notions of informed consent and indigenous cultures: Australian findings at the interface, *Journal of Bioethical Inquiry*, 5, 21–31.

McGuinness, S. 2013, Law, reproduction and disability: Fatally 'handicapped?', *Medical Law Review*, 21: 2, 213–242.

Marmot, M., Allen, J., Goldblatt, P., Boyce, T., McNeish, D., Grady, M. & Geddes, I. 2010, *The Marmot Review: Fair Society, Healthy Lives*, The Marmot Review: London.

Massó Guijarro, P., Aranaz Andrés, J., Mira, J., Perdiguero, E. & Aibar, C. 2010, Adverse events in hospitals: The patient's point of view, *Quality and Safety in Health Care*, 19, 144–147.

Mathews, B. 2011, Female genital mutilation: Australian law, policy and practical challenges for doctors, *Medical Journal of Australia*, 194, 139–141.

Mathews, B. & Smith, M. 2018, Children and consent to medical treatment. In B. White, F. McDonald & L. Willmott (eds), *Health Law in Australia*, 3rd edn, Thomson Reuters: Sydney, 159–206.

Mill, J. S. 1985, *On Liberty*, Penguin: Harmondsworth.

Morgan, V., Morgan, F., Valuri, G., Ferrante, A., Castle, D. & Jablensky, A. 2012, A whole of population study of the prevalence and patterns of criminal offending in people with schizoprehnia and other mental illnesses, *Psychological Medicine*, 13, 1–12.

Nelson, H. 1992, Against caring, *Journal of Clinical Ethics*, 3: 1, 8–15.

NHMRC (National Health and Medical Research Council). 2017, *Ethical Guidelines on the Use of Assisted Reproductive Technology in Clinical Practice and Research*, National Health and Medical Research Council, Melbourne, accessed 7 August 2018, <https://www.nhmrc.gov.au/_files_nhmrc/file/ guidelines/ethics/16506_nhmrc_-_ethical_guidelines_on_the_use_of_ assisted_reproductive_technology-web.pdf>.

NMBA (Nursing and Midwifery Board of Australia). 2007, *A National Framework for the Development of Decision-making Tools for Nursing and Midwifery Practice*, Nursing and Midwifery Board of Australia, Melbourne, accessed 26 July 2018, <http://www.nursingmidwiferyboard.gov.au/Codes-Guidelines-Statements/Frameworks.aspx>.

NMBA (Nursing and Midwifery Board of Australia). 2016, *Position Statement on Nurses, Midwives and Vaccination*, Nursing and Midwifery Board of Australia,

Melbourne, accessed 4 August 2018, <http://www.nursingmidwiferyboard.
gov.au/Codes-Guidelines-Statements/Position-Statements/vaccination.aspx>.

NMBA (Nursing and Midwifery Board of Australia). 2018a, *Code of Conduct
for Nurses*, Nursing and Midwifery Board of Australia, Melbourne, accessed
19 July 2018, <http://www.nursingmidwiferyboard.gov.au/Codes-Guidelines-
Statements/Professional-standards.aspx>.

NMBA (Nursing and Midwifery Board of Australia). 2018b, *Code of Conduct for
Midwives*, Nursing and Midwifery Board of Australia, Melbourne, accessed
19 July 2018, <http://www.nursingmidwiferyboard.gov.au/Codes-Guidelines-
Statements/Professional-standards.aspx>.

O'Neill, D. 2011, Reflections on aging, *British Medical Journal*, 342, 3395.

Productivity Commission 2005, *Australia's Health Workforce: A Report*, Commonwealth of Australia: Canberra.

Purtilo, R. 1999, *Ethical Dimensions in the Health Professions*, 3rd edn, W.B. Saun-
ders: Philadelphia.

Queensland Law Reform Commission 2018, *Review of Termination of Pregnancy
Laws Report No 76*, QLRC, Brisbane.

Queensland Public Hospitals Commission of Inquiry 2005, *Final Report 2005*,
Queensland Parliament.

Queensland University of Technology 2018, *End of Life Law in Australia*,
accessed 10 August 2018, <https://end-of-life.qut.edu.au>.

Quill, T., Dresser, R. & Brock, D. 1997, The rule of double effect: A critique of
its role in end-of-life decision making, *New England Journal of Medicine*, 337,
1768.

Reason, J. 1990, *Human Error*, Cambridge University Press: Cambridge.

Reconciliation Australia n.d., *The United Nations Declaration on the Rights of
Indigenous Peoples (UNDRIP)*, accessed 18 September 2018, <https://www.
reconciliation.org.au/wp-content/uploads/2017/11/Reconciliation-Australia-
United-Nations-Declaration-on-the-Rights-of-Indigenous-Peoples-UNDRIP.pdf>.

Robinson, C. 1999, Sexual misconduct: The Canadian experience. In J. Bloom,
C. Nadelson & M. Nottman (eds), *Physician Sexual Misconduct*, American
Psychiatric Publications: London and Washington, DC, 127.

Ross, C. & Goldner, E. 2009, Stigma, negative attitudes and discrimination
towards mental illness within the nursing profession: A review of the literature, *Journal of Psychiatric and Mental Health Nursing*, 16: 6, 558–567.

Royal Commission into Aboriginal Deaths in Custody 1991, *Royal Commission
into Aboriginal Deaths in Custody: National Report*, Australian Government
Printing Service: Canberra.

Royal Commission into Deep Sleep Therapy 1990, *Report of the Royal Commission
into Deep Sleep Therapy*, NSW Government Premier's Department: Sydney.

Royal Commission on New Reproductive Technologies 1993, 'Judicial Interven-
tion in Pregnancy and Birth' in Royal Commission on New Reproductive
Technologies, *Proceed with Care: Final Report of the Royal Commission on New
Reproductive Technologies*, The Commission: Ottawa, 2, 949–965.

Sharpe, V. 2004, Introduction: Accountability and justice in patient safety
reform. In V. Sharpe (ed.), *Accountability: Patient Safety and Policy Reform*,
Georgetown University Press: Washington, DC, 1.

Sherwin, S. 1992, *No Longer Patient: Feminist Ethics and Health Care*, Temple University Press: Philadelphia.

Shetty, P. 2012, India's unregulated surrogacy industry, *The Lancet*, 380: 9854, 1633–1634.

Smith, M. & Bennett, B. 2018, Assisted reproductive technology. In B. White, F. McDonald & L. Willmott (eds), *Health Law in Australia*, 3rd edn, Thomson Reuters: Sydney, 437–472.

Standing Committee on Law and Justice 2016, *Remedies for Serious Invasions of Privacy in New South Wales*, NSW Parliament: Sydney.

Staunton, P. & Chiarella, M. 2012, *Law for Nurses and Midwives*, Chatswood NSW 7th edn, Elsevier.

Steinbock, B., Arras, J. & London, J. 2003, Introduction: Moral reasoning in the medical context. In B. Steinbock, J. Arras & J. London (eds), *Ethical Issues in Modern Medicine*, 5th edn, Mayfield Publishing Company: Mountain View, CA.

Stewart, C. 2018, Euthanasia, suicide and assisted dying. In B. White, F. McDonald & L. Willmott (eds), *Health Law in Australia*, 3rd edn, Thomson Reuters: Sydney, 525–570.

Stewart, C. & Biegler, P. 2004, A primer on the law of competence to refuse medical treatment, *Australian Law Journal*, 78, 325.

Swisher, L. & Krueger-Brophy, C. 1998, *Legal and Ethical Issues in Physical Therapy*, Butterworths: Boston, MA.

Sydney Morning Herald. 2018, Japan Nurse Arrested Over Hospital Deaths 'Put Cleanser in Drips' of Patients, *Sydney Morning Herald*, 13 July, accessed 15 July 2018, <https://www.smh.com.au/world/asia/japan-nurse-arrested-over-hospital-deaths-put-cleanser-in-drips-of-patients-20180712-p4zr7f.html>.

Szoke, H. 2002, The nanny state or responsible government? *Journal of Law and Medicine*, 9, 470.

Szoke, H., Neame, L. & Johnson, L. 2006, Old technologies and new challenges: Assisted reproduction and its regulation. In I. Freckelton & K. Petersen (eds), *Disputes and Dilemmas in Health Law*, Federation Press: Sydney, 187–216.

Taplin, S. 2017, Prenatal reporting to child protection: Characteristics and service responses in one Australian jurisdiction, *Child Abuse & Neglect*, 65, 68–76.

Task Force on Quality in Australian Health Care. 1996, *Final Report of the Task Force in Australian Health Care*, Department of Health and Aging: Canberra.

Tavella, R., McBride, K., Keech, W., Kelly, J., Rischbieth, A., Zeitz, C., Beltrame, J., Tideman, P. & Brown, A. 2016, Disparities in acute in-hospital cardiovascular care for Aboriginal and non-Aboriginal South Australians, *Medical Journal of Australia*, 205: 5, 222–227.

Tschudin, V. & Farr, B. 1994, Nursing ethics VI: Particular features, *Nursing Standard*, 9: 4, 51–57.

The Uluru Statement from the Heart. 2017, accessed 19 September 2018, <https://www.referendumcouncil.org.au/sites/default/files/2017-05/Uluru_Statement_From_The_Heart_0.PDF>.

United Kingdom Department of Health. 1994, *The Allitt Inquiry: Independent Inquiry Relating to Deaths and Injuries on the Children's Ward at Grantham and Kesteven General Hospital*, HMSO: London.

United Nations. 2018, *Aging and Health*, <http://www.who.int/news-room/ fact-sheets/detail/ageing-and-health>.

United Nations. n.d., *Aging*, <http://www.un.org/en/sections/issues-depth/ageing/>.

Veatch, R. 1988, Justice and the economics of terminal illness, *The Hastings Center Report*, 18: 4, 34–40.

Veatch, R. 1995, Resolving conflicts among principles: Ranking, balancing, and specifying, *Kennedy Institute of Ethics Journal*, 5: 3, 199–218.

Victorian Mental Illness Awareness Council. 2013, *Zero Tolerance for Sexual Assault: A Safe Admission for Women*, Victorian Mental Health Awareness Council: Melbourne.

Viens, A. & Singer, P. 2008, Introduction. In P. Singer & A. Viens (eds), *The Cambridge Textbook of Bioethics*, Cambridge University Press: Cambridge, 1–8.

Vigod, S., Bell, C. & Bohnen, J. 2003, Privacy of patients' information in hospital lifts: Observational study, *British Medical Journal*, 327, 1024.

Wahlquist, C., Allam, L. & Evershed, N. 2018, Police said HN was 'good as gold' to be in custody, three days later he was dead, *Guardian Australia*, 1 September, accessed 16 September 2018, <https://www.theguardian.com/ australia-news/2018/sep/01/police-said-hn-was-good-as-gold-to-be-in- custody-three-days-later-he-was-dead>.

Weithorn, L. & Campbell, S.B. 1982, The competency of children and adolescents to make informed treatment decisions, *Child Development*, 53, 1589–1598.

White, B., Willmott, L. & Then, S.N. 2018, Adults who lack capacity: Substitute decision-making. In B. White, F. McDonald & L. Willmott (eds), *Health Law in Australia*, 3rd edn, Thomson Reuters: Sydney, 571–623.

WHO (World Health Organization). *Palliative Care*, <https://www.who.int/en/ news-room/fact-sheets/detail/palliative-care, accessed 15 December 2018>.

WHO (World Health Organization). 2002, *The Toronto Declaration on the Global Prevention of Elder Abuse*, <http://www.who.int/ageing/projects/elder_abuse/ alc_toronto_declaration_en.pdf>.

Willmott, L., White, B. & Then, S.N. 2018, Withholding and withdrawing life-sustaining medical treatment. In B. White, F. McDonald & L. Willmott (eds), *Health Law in Australia*, 3rd edn, Thomson Reuters: Sydney, 571–627.

Wilson, R., Runciman, W., Gibberd, R., Harrison, B., Newby, L. & Hamilton, J. 1995, The quality in Australian health care study, *Medical Journal of Australia*, 163: 9, 458–471.

Wolf, Z. 2007, Health care providers' experiences with making fatal medication errors. In M. Cohen (ed.), *Medication Errors*, 2nd edn, American Pharmacists Association: Washington, DC, 43–51.

Wu, A. 2004, Is there an obligation to disclose near misses? In V. Sharpe (ed.), *Accountability: Patient Safety and Policy Reform*, Georgetown University Press: Washington, DC, 135–142.

Wyman, M., Shiovitz-Ezra, S. & Bengel, J. 2018, Ageism in the health care system: Providers, patients, and systems. In L. Ayalon & C. Tesch-Römer (eds), *Contemporary Perspectives on Ageism, International Perspectives on Aging*, Springer International: Basel, 193–212.

Index